WHIPLASH INJURIES

THE CERVICAL ACCELERATION/ DECELERATION SYNDROME

WHIPLASH INJURIES

THE CERVICAL ACCELERATION/ DECELERATION SYNDROME

STEPHEN M. FOREMAN, DC, DABCO

*Assistant Professor, Department of Diagnosis and
Postgraduate Faculty, Los Angeles College of
Chiropractic, Whittier, California
Co-founder, American College of Forensic Sciences*

ARTHUR C. CROFT, DC, MS, DABCO

*Postgraduate Faculty, Los Angeles College of
Chiropractic, Whittier, California
Co-founder, American College of Forensic Sciences
Clinic Director, Alvarado Chiropractic Group
San Diego, California*

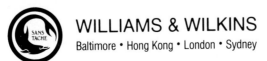

WILLIAMS & WILKINS
Baltimore • Hong Kong • London • Sydney

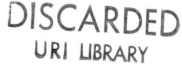

Editor: Jonathan W. Pine, Jr.
Associate Editor: Victoria M. Vaughn
Copy Editor: Bill Cady
Design: JoAnne Janowiak
Illustration Planning: Wayne Hubbel
Production: Theda Harris

Copyright © 1988
Williams & Wilkins
428 East Preston Street
Baltimore, MD 21202, U.S.A.

Japanese Edition. 1988

Accurate indications, adverse reactions, and dosage schedules for drugs are provided in this book, but it is possible that they may change. The reader is urged to review the package information data of the manufacturers of the medications mentioned.

Printed in the United States of America

Library of Congress Cataloging-in-Publication Data

Foreman, Stephen M.
  Whiplash injuries.

  Includes index.
  1. Whiplash injuries—Chiropractic treatment.
I. Croft, Arthur C. II. Title. [DNLM: 1. Cervical
Vertebrae—injuries. WE 725 F715w]
RZ275.W48F67   1988   617'.371   87-10624
ISBN 0-683-03314-X

88 89 90 91 92
10 9 8 7 6 5 4 3

To my parents, who shaped my past; to my wife, Geri, whose love and support is ever present; and to my sons Joseph, Benjamin, Michael, Timothy and Neil, who represent the future.

SMF

To the memory of my parents.

ACC

Foreword

Whiplash Injuries: The Cervical Accelera-
tion/Deceleration Syndrome, by Drs. Stephen
M. Foreman and Arthur C. Croft, is a comprehensive study of the biomechanical
behavior of the cervical spine in health,
trauma, and disease. This book contains a
wealth of information gleaned from extensive review of the literature in addition to
the authors' extensive personal, clinical,
and research experience.

The thorough manner in which this book
covers the entire spectrum of whiplash
injuries is indeed commendable. It amply
covers the basic principles and fundamentals of embryology, normal anatomy, and
the biomechanics of the spine in general
and of the cervical region in particular. The
authors continue with an in-depth study of
the physical examination and state-of-the-
art diagnostic imaging and then proceed in
logical sequence into a comprehensive
study of the manifestations of traumatic
insult to the osseous and soft tissue components of the cervical spine.

This succinct, narrative text is further
augmented by a plethora of superb illustrations that are of help in clarifying many
important points and add immensely to the
value of this volume. In addition, an extensive glossary of pertinent terms is available
at the end of the book for ready reference.

In summary, Drs. Foreman and Croft
have succeeded in creating a book of fundamental importance that is written in a
language readily understandable to every
student, professor, and practicing physician. A text of this significance that covers
all the important features of whiplash
injury so thoroughly and elegantly has long
been needed and represents an important
contribution to the healing arts.

Russell Erhardt, DC, DABCR
Diplomate of the American Chiropractic
Board of Roentgenologists Board,
Qualified Chiropactic Orthopedist

Foreword

My interest in injuries and disorders of the cervical spine began in 1936. There was very little written about injuries of the cervical spine at that time, and I was unable to explain the majority of my patients symptoms. I later began my research and found that irritation of the cervical nerve roots was responsible for many of their complaints. This, of course, was only the beginning of my involvement with cervical spine injuries.

Now that I have reviewed this phenomenal dissertation, I am convinced that this book is the most remarkable compilation of scientific and factual data thus far published concerning the many facets of the cervical spine. This text should be of great value to all doctors, physicians, and other health care providers whose primary concern is a conceptual knowledge of the injuries that occur to the most susceptible portions of the human body in acceleration/deceleration accidents.

Ruth Jackson, MD, FACS

Preface

A wealth of information on whiplash injuries has accumulated in the literature over the past few decades, but to date, there are no currently available reference books devoted extensively to this subject. This textbook was created to fill that void. It is designed as a compendium of information on the subject of acceleration/deceleration trauma to the cervical spine. It has been our desire to provide those that deal with this type of injury on a daily basis with the history, research, current thinking, diagnosis, physiology, and prognosis for all facets of the whiplash injury. We have borrowed from other disciplines, such as neurology and radiology, only that material relevant to our discussion, so that the material presented is both complete and to the point.

This book is intended for those individuals who deal routinely with cervical spine trauma, including emergency room physicians, chiropractors, osteopaths, general practitioners, neurologists, psychiatrists, orthopaedic surgeons, radiologists, neurosurgeons, nurse practitioners, and physical therapists. All will find the information in this book useful and clinically relevant—information that can definitely affect the way they examine and treat their patients.

This book is also intended for those outside of the health care profession whose job it is to mediate disputes arising from this type of injury. These include attorneys, both for the plaintiff and for the defense,

claims adjusters, and accident reconstructionists. We realize that there is a real need in these areas for a definitive textbook on the subject of whiplash injuries that can be used as a reference to better understand the soft tissue injury, why it happens, how it happens, the usual and customary diagnostic workup, and the appropriate management of the typical case, as well as providing a method for prognosticating future disability based on actual research studies. With the glossary provided and the straightforward explanative text, we believe that we have provided such a tool.

We have constantly strived to present the best information available, and we have attempted always to present all contemporary schools of thought on a subject. To this end, the reader will find no philosophical digression that might be expected of a book intended for one particular subspecialty or group. This book was written primarily as a reference textbook and not as a guide to treatment, and although some areas of treatment are discussed briefly, we have omitted most of this aspect of the subject. We do, however, expect to cover this area more thoroughly in subsequent editions, and certainly this is an area where much research is needed. The authors are currently engaged in compiling research data on the subject of treatment protocol, and it is hoped that eventually some standard of care will emerge.

As the intended readership includes students and professionals from outside the health care professions, we have attempted to explain concepts adequately. The Glossary will be helpful in this regard, especially for Chapter 1 which covers some basic physics.

This textbook is arranged in a logical sequence, beginning with the mechanics of the whiplash phenomenon and how it interfaces with the biomechanics of the cervical spine (Chapter 1). It then proceeds to cover the the physical examination of the patient who has suffered this type of trauma (Chapters 2 and 3). In Chapter 2, we discuss in-office orthopaedic and neurological tests germane to cervical spine injury. In Chapter 3, we cover testing procedures that would usually be ordered after the initial examination. These include electrodiagnostic procedures such a electroencephalography and electromyography, bone scans, magnetic resonance imaging (MRI) studies, computed tomography (CT) scans, thermography, and fluorovideo motion studies.

In Chapter 4 are covered routine radiographic procedures that can be performed in the office. Chapter 5, written by William V. Glenn, Jr., MD, is a general overview of CT, MRI, and three-dimensional CT imaging of the cervical spine. This is an area in which our technology is constantly changing. For those health care providers whose training was completed prior to the early 1980's, this chapter will be extremely informative.

The general subject of fracture and dis-

location is covered in Chapter 6. In Chapter 7, the developmental anatomy and normal anatomy of the cervical spine are described. The subject of soft tissue injury is covered in some detail in Chapter 8. We believe that logical approaches to treatment can only result from a thorough understanding of the physiology of the healing process.

Nervous system trauma is the subject of Chapter 9. In this chapter, both the common and the unusual forms of injury seen in cervical spine trauma are outlined. Chapter 10 is a general overview of the temporomandibular joint and how it is adversely affected by the dynamics of acceleration/deceleration trauma. Contributed by our widely published dental colleague Lawrence A. Weinberg, DDS, it is (at our request) written in essentially nondental language.

Finally, the subject of prognosis is covered in detail in Chapter 11. We have provided a method of scaling cervical acceleration/deceleration injuries so that they can be better quantified initially, thereby providing all parties concerned with a reasonable estimate of any future disability that may result. This prognosis index is based strictly upon published research.

We sincerely hope that you find this textbook useful and its presentation enjoyable.

Stephen M. Foreman
Arthur C. Croft

Acknowledgments

The preparation of this book has, in many ways, been a group effort. A wide variety of people have contributed to this work, and their contributions deserve special recognition at this time.

We are especially thankful to those physicians who wrote the Forewords for this text: Ruth Jackson, MD, FACS, and Russell Erhardt, DC, DABCR. Their opinions are a welcome addition.

We are grateful for the work of our contributing authors: William V. Glenn, Jr., MD, and Lawrence Weinberg, DDS, MS, FACD, FICD. Each has contributed his own expertise to these chapters. Their time and efforts have been given unselfishly, often at the expense of other projects.

Others have graciously opened their personal files for our use and have provided the vast majority of the radiographs in this text. Without their generosity this book would have been barren of many of the excellent radiographic cases. These special contributors are: Cynthia Baum, DC; Debbie Forrester, MD; William V. Glenn, Jr., MD; Joseph Howe, DC; Mark Jenkins, MD; G. Sherman Johnson, DC; Charles W. Kerber, MD; Joyce Pais, MD; Stephen Rothman, MD; J. Rodney Shelley, DC; and Stephen Wendling, MD.

We wish to recognize the typing skills and efforts of Christine Prario and Lisa L. Wyatt. Their dedication and enthusiasm often went above and beyond the call of duty. Our thanks are also extended to Glynna Rangel, DC, who typed the Glossary, Preface, and Acknowledgments.

Special thanks are also due Charles W. Kerber, MD, who provided an experienced editorial perspicuity that can only be developed from years of writing, and Gary D. Schultz, DC, and Marie Bochniak, DC, who provided editorial assistance. Their encouragement and criticisms are greatly appreciated.

Thanks are due the following people: Brian O'Neill, president of the Insurance Institute for Highway Safety; David Hubbard, Jr., MD, for his neurological expertise; Joan Schaefer, of the Nicolet Biomedical Instrument Company; Irene Dickery, of Qmax Medical; William Klink, of Hughes Aircraft Company; A. B. Shuman, of Mercedes-Benz of North America, Inc.; Deborah Durban, x-ray technician and model; Bruce Prario, for modeling; and to our staffs, for all their understanding and help.

Art would like to extend thanks to his partners, William Remsen, DC, MS, and John Krage, DC, for their help and understanding during the writing of this book.

To our editor Jonathan W. Pine, Jr., and our associate editor Victoria M. Vaughn, your expertise is appreciated. Thank you for bringing this book to publication.

Lastly, I would like to extend a very personal thank-you to my co-author Art Croft.

His abilities as an author and as a medical illustrator are only surpassed by his infinite patience in the face of a never-ending series of phone calls and letters from me. I have driven this fine friend truly mad, but with time and therapy, I am told, he is expected to recover.

Stephen M. Foreman
Arthur C. Croft

Contributors

Arthur C. Croft, DC, MS, DABCO
Postgraduate Faculty, Los Angeles College of
  Chiropractic
Whittier, California
Clinic Director, Alvarado Chiropractic Group
San Diego, California

Stephen M. Foreman, DC, DABCO
Assistant Professor, Department of Diagnosis
  and Postgraduate Faculty
Los Angeles College of Chiropractic
Whittier, California

William V. Glenn, Jr., MD
Private Practice of Radiology
Manhattan Beach, California

Lawrence A. Weinberg, DDS, MS, FACD,
  FICD
Former Associate Professor of Prostodontics
New York University College of Dentistry
New York, New York
Past President, American Academy of
  Craniomandibular Disorders
Private Practice of Dentistry
New York, New York

Contents

1

Biomechanics

ARTHUR C. CROFT, DC, MS, DABCO

"[The science of life] is a superb and dazzling lighted hall which may be reached only by passing through a long and ghastly kitchen."
Claude Bernard (1813–1878)

The clinical syndrome of whiplash, first described by Crowe in 1928 (1), has proved to be one of the more enigmatic conditions seen in everyday clinical practice. Its rather unsavory reputation, owing to its common association with litigation, discouraged most researchers from delving into this "Pandora's box." It later became clear that the chief complaints described by those unfortunate enough to sustain this type of injury were, in fact, fairly consistent. By common sense, the most common and consistent complaint, neck pain, would be explainable, but other symptoms, such as headache, blurred vision, Horner's syndrome, tinnitus, dizziness, nausea, paresthesias, numbness, and back pain, defied casual clinical explanation. To add insult to injury, these patients often were thought of as malingerers who fabricated their claims of pain and suffering in hopes of securing a large settlement from a third party, or they were labeled as hypochon-

driacs who perhaps used their injury for some sort of secondary gain.

With the passing of time, however, data began to accumulate, and it became more and more obvious that litigation was neither the cause of nor the cure for this type of injury. Early retrospective studies by Macnab (2) shed new light on the "suspicious" association between whiplash and monetary settlement. In a review of 266 medicolegal cases, he found that 45% continued to have symptoms 2 years after settlement of court actions. In reality, the percentage was probably higher than this, but in order to avoid any type of bias, those who did not respond to his questionnaire were automatically considered "cured," when many nonresponders were, in fact, probably not "cured." Ebbs et al. (3), in a similar type of study, found that 36 of 137 patients who were followed for more than a year continued to have neck pain. Norris and Watt (4) found that 44–90% of patients

1

in their series remained symptomatic at 6 months (the variance in percentages is associated with grouping as to the severity of the injury—see Chapter 8).

Other researchers (5, 6) have demonstrated that whiplash alone (in the absence of blunt head trauma) may result in surface hemorrhages on the brain, cerebral concussion, and subdural hematoma. Cerebral concussion, which can sometimes be demonstrated by electroencephalography, very often results in postconcussion headaches or the so-called posttraumatic headache syndrome. Russell (7) found that even after 6 months, 60% of the group that he studied continued to have headaches. Denker and Perry (8) reported similar findings, with 33% symptomatic at 1 year and 15–20% symptomatic at more than 3 years. In one study, 31% were said to have headaches after 5 years (9). Many of these cases resulted from direct head trauma.

Many studies have been conducted to study the effects of whiplash on the spine and supporting soft tissues. By using anthropomorphic dummies, laboratory animals, cadavers and, in limited studies, human volunteers, researchers have formulated mathematical models that help to quantify the forces of linear and angular acceleration that the spine and skull are subjected to at various collision speeds. These experiments have also allowed certain statements to be made about other variables, such as closing speeds of vehicles, relative sizes of vehicles, road conditions, vectors of impact, seatback height and stiffness, and the use of seat belts and shoulder harnesses, head restraints, and air bags. These variables necessarily must be included in the equation.

These facts or hypotheses coupled with laboratory data obtained by Unterharnscheidt (10), Wickstrom et al. (11), Macnab (12), and others who have produced experimental lesions in laboratory animals, as well as clinical information available from surgery reports and autopsy reports, have provided a tremendous understanding of both the pathophysiological and the biomechanical processes involved in acceleration/deceleration trauma.

A few words about the term "whiplash" are appropriate here. Many have suggested

this term be abandoned forever and be replaced with more up-to-date and descriptive phraseology such as "acceleration/deceleration trauma" or "hyperextension/hyperflexion trauma." The latter phrase would technically imply first a hyperextension injury and second the hyperflexion injury. If the injuries occurred in the reverse order; i.e., the first phase of injury was the hyperflexion phase, it would then be more appropriate to use the phrase "hyperflexion/hyperextension injury." This point is perhaps a moot one, in that there is controversy over whether a brief hyperflexion movement precedes a typical hyperextension movement. In the long run, the term "whiplash" is firmly entrenched in our language and is, in fact, perhaps more fundamentally descriptive than any of these other phrases. Anyone of these terms can be and probably is commonly misused, and the world will be no less confused by abandoning the term "whiplash." Throughout this text, therefore, all three terms are used synonymously, although I prefer the phrase "cervical acceleration/deceleration syndrome" (CADS).

Physical Properties of Vertebrae and Soft Tissues

BONE

In this chapter, I discuss the physical properties of bone and the soft tissues; the relevant developmental anatomy of the vertebrae is discussed in some detail in Chapter 7. Unfortunately, the vast majority of data concerning the relevant biomechanical properties of bone is based upon studies of the bone of the lumbar spine. In some instances, these data are applicable to other bone, whereas in other cases, this is probably not wise. I do, however, mention salient studies and include the reference as well as the spinal level under discussion.

Because the vertebrae bear increasingly heavier loads and forces as they course caudally in the body, they gradually become heavier and sturdier. The compression strength of lumbar and thoracic vertebrae have been studied by numerous researchers over the years. In their excellent work on clinical biomechanics, White and Panjabi (13) describe only one study in which this property of cervical vertebrae was examined, and it is more than 100 years old (14)! In this study, Messerer found the compression strengths of cadaver vertebrae in the cervical spine to be slightly under 2 kilonewtons (kN) (0.45 lbf). Since White and Panjabi's work, Pintar et al. (15) have also tested the compression strength of cervical vertebrae (C2–C7). They found a mean compression strength of 2.6 kN for C2–C7, whereas Bell et al. (16) found a mean compression strength of 8 kN (1.8 lbf) for L4. The greater strength of the lumbar vertebrae is thought to be a function of their larger size only. With advancing age, however, the mass of bone decreases dramatically. This occurs sooner in the axial skeleton than in the peripheral skeleton. It has been demonstrated by Bell et al. (16) that a 25% decrease in osseous tissue results in a 50% decrease in strength. The relative compressive load-carrying capacity of cortical versus cancellous bone has been found to vary with advancing age. In subjects under 40 years of age, cancellous bone has the major load-carrying capacity, whereas in those over 40 years of age, cortical bone bears most of the load (17) (Fig. 1.1). This is due to the loss of trabeculation which acts to absorb and distribute forces of vertical loading.

In much of the early research on the compressive strength of bone, cadaver bone that had been frozen or stored for long periods of time was utilized. In more recent studies, however, bone from fresh(er) specimens has been utilized and has revealed the importance of marrow as an energy-absorbing and load-distributing structure. After applying axial compressive loading to fresh lumbar specimens with discs intact, Farfan (18) observed that blood-tinged fluid and then marrow were expelled from the vertebral body. The disc surface remained dry. According to Farfan (19), this has also been reported by Roaf. The first structure to fail was the endplate, and this occurred with a loud snap. The result resembled a Schmorl's node.

Hayes and Carter (20), using bovine specimens, found that compressive strength as well as energy-absorbing capacity was

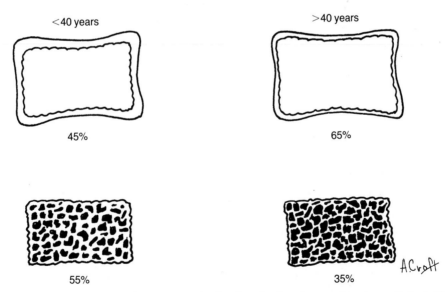

Figure 1.1.   Relative compressive loading capacity of cortical and cancellous bone. Before 40 years of age, a person's cortical bone bears about 45% of the compressive load, whereas the cancellous bone carries about 55% of the load. After 40 years of age, however, this ratio inverts; cortical bone bears up to 65% of the compressive load, while the cancellous bone supports only 35% of the load. (After Rockoff et al. (17); adapted from Panjabi MM, White AA: Physical properties and functional biomechanics of the spine. In White AA, Panjabi MM (eds): *Clinical Biomechanics of the Spine.* Philadelphia, JB Lippincott, 1978, p 26.)

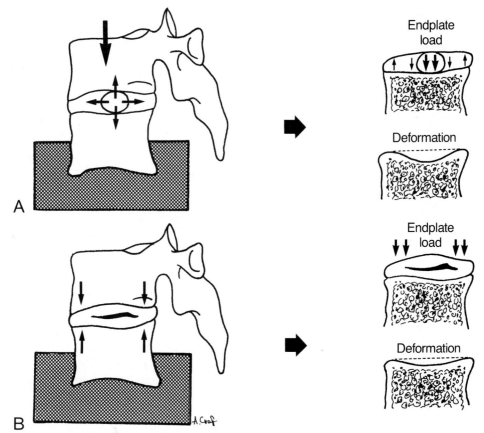

Figure 1.2.   Mechanism of endplate failure. **A.** Vertical compression of the normal healthy disc with the nucleus intact results in a relatively even distribution of forces which are most concentrated at the center of the endplate. This is facilitated by the hydrodynamics of the nucleus pulposus. High bending stress results in central endplate fractures and Schmorl's node formation. This occurs before annular injury. **B.** Direct vertical loading of a degenerated disc results in loads that, without the effect of the nucleus, are transferred via the anulus to the periphery of the endplate. High bending stress results in fracture of the peripheral endplate. This occurs before annular injury. (Adapted from Panjabi MM, White AA: Physical properties and functional biomechanics of the spine. In White AA, Panjabi MM (eds): *Clinical Biomechanics of the Spine.* Philadelphia, JB Lippincott, 1978, p 29.)

enhanced by bone marrow, and this phenomenon was most pronounced at higher rates of loading.

Perry (21) studied this phenomenon of endplate fracture upon vertical loading in great depth and made several interesting and noteworthy observations regarding the condition of the intervertebral disc. He found, as have others, that variation in endplate strength is largely a function of age. He noted, however, that there were two basic patterns of endplate failure—central and peripheral. Generally, the former was seen in specimens with normal discs,

whereas the latter was seen in specimens with degenerated discs.

With an intact disc and nucleus pulposus, a vertical compressive force produces an increased intranuclear pressure that results in a bulging of the nucleus into the adjacent endplates while tensile forces are produced at the outer annular fibers. It is noteworthy that herniations as a result of pure axial load are always into the cancellous bone and not peripherally through the anulus (Fig. 1.2).

White and Panjabi (22) use the example of a sealed tin can filled with water to explain the phenomenon of endplate fracture. According to basic principles of physics, when this tin can is heated, stresses will be greater at the ends than at the walls, resulting in outward bulging only at the ends. This same principle is applicable to the endplates under increasing nuclear pressure.

The notion that osteoporosis decreases the vertebra's ability to resist axial loading is universally accepted. Another well-known principle of engineering is Euler's formula. According to this formula, the strength of a column of given material is directly proportional to the square of its cross-sectional area and inversely proportional to the square of its unsupported length. This principle can be applied to our biological system in the following way: To understand the inherent strength of vertebra under compressive load is easy if the interconnected meshwork in the trabeculae

of the spongiosa of normal healthy bone is taken into consideration. In osteoporosis, however, much of this reinforcement (i.e., trabeculation) is lost (both horizontal ties and vertical ties). This means, then, that a reduction of 50% of the trabeculae (area) will result in a corresponding lack of strength such that the vertebra is now only 25% of its original strength. If the loss of horizontal supports is taken into consideration, another part of the equation essentially must be increased (i.e., unsupported length becomes greater). This results in a further loss of strength (23).

DISC

Most of the research on the biomechanical properties of discs has been carried out on lumbar discs. Many of the physical properties of discs are consistent through-

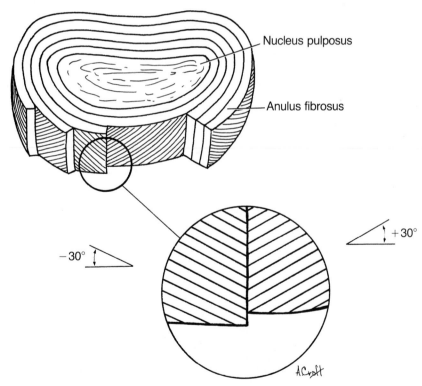

Figure 1.3. The intervertebral disc is composed of the nucleus pulposus surrounded by the anulus fibrosus. This latter structure consists of concentric laminated bands of fibers that are oriented in staggered opposing directions. These fibers run at angles of roughly 30° to the horizontal. (Adapted from Panjabi MM, White AA: Physical properties and functional biomechanics of the spine. In White AA, Panjabi MM (eds): *Clinical Biomechanics of the Spine.* Philadelphia, JB Lippincott, 1978, p 3.)

out the spine, however, and only those properties that can reasonably be expected to remain relatively constant, whether in the cervical, thoracic, or lumbar spine, are considered here.

The intervertebral disc is composed of a tough outer component, the anulus fibrosus, and a mucoid center, the nucleus pulposus. The anulus is composed of laminated fibrocartilage with its concentric layers arranged in a staggered pattern at about 30° to the horizontal (Fig. 1.3).

Cervical discs probably play a larger part in the overall biomechanics of spinal movement, in that they possess greater proportional height and their nuclei have a greater capacity to swell (Fig. 1.4). The increased disc height allows for a greater range of motion, and the greater nuclear capacity allows for an enhanced shock absorption and load distribution.

The nucleus pulposus, located roughly at the center of the disc, is composed chiefly of mucopolysaccharides (most notably chondroitin sulfate) supported by a retinacular fiber mesh. In the mature nucleus, some collagen fiber is also present (24).

The outer portion of the anulus remains firmly attached to the vertebra by Sharpey's fibers. This peripheral attachment is said to be stronger than the more central attachment to cartilaginous endplates (25). This fact becomes important in the evaluation of clinical stability because, as is described later, significant acceleration/deceleration forces can produce hyperextension and hyperflexion injuries whereby the anulus is avulsed from the vertebra.

The inner portion of anulus that surrounds the nucleus is softer and, as pointed out by Farfan, is subjected to less torsional force than the more peripheral fibers.

Both anulus and nucleus are devoid of blood vessels in the human after the age of 8 (26, 27), and the topic of innervation remains controversial. There is some evidence that unmyelinated pain fibers are to be found in the posterior anulus and perhaps even the nucleus (28). It is also conceivable that innervation is a result of injury to the disc, in that branches of the recurrent meningeal nerve (sinuvertebral nerve) may grow into the disc only after it is damaged.

The load displacement curve of the intervertebral disc is sigmoid. At low loads, the disc remains relatively flexible, while at higher loads, the disc becomes stiffer and more resistant, providing greater stability (25). More interesting, however, is the fact that the disc possesses great *anisotropy*. In other words, its strength and stiffness vary depending on the type and direction of force applied. This is the result of the complex lamellar arrangement of fibers oriented at alternating angles. Markolf (29), studying lumbar and thoracic specimens, found that the discs became stiffer under compressive loads than under tensile loads because of the increased nuclear pressure seen with compression of the disc. It can be surmised from this that a disc under tension is more easily injured. This again will be significant in the clinical setting as the various vectors and forces of injury that occur during the acceleration/deceleration trauma are examined.

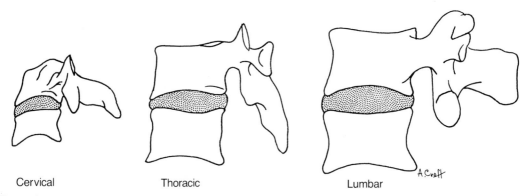

Cervical   Thoracic   Lumbar

Figure 1.4. Relative proportions of the disc and vertebral body in cervical, thoracic, and lumbar spines.

The disc, as a viscoelastic structure, also displays the properties of *creep* and *hysteresis*. As discs degenerate, however, they become less viscoelastic.

When a viscoelastic material is subjected to a suddenly applied constant load, it deforms gradually and the deformation-time curve approaches a steady state value asymptotically. This is known as creep. White and Panjabi (30) have reported that degenerative discs, compared with healthy discs, display less of this phenomenon, which implies a diminished capacity for shock attenuation and load distribution.

Hysteresis is a phenomenon exhibited by all viscoelastic materials and, after repetitive loading and unloading cycles, results in an overall loss of energy. Virgin (31) is credited with the first observation of this property in discs and noted that hysteresis decreased after a second load. Virgin also noted that the larger the load, the larger the hysteresis and that it was most marked in the very young and was diminished in degenerative discs.

Some have suggested that a disc may be capable of repair by a self-sealing mechanism (32). Virgin (31), like Perry, observed that after compressing discs under loads severe enough to permanently deform the anulus, there was no evidence of herniation of nuclear material. He found that discs could support more than 1000 lb (4.4 kN). When a stab wound was made in the posterolateral part of the disc, extending all the way into the nucleus, and the disc was compressed, there was still no herniation. This has been demonstrated by others also (32, 33). As mentioned earlier, these experiments have been carried out on lumbar segments.

These experiments would indicate that some other factor must be involved in the production of disc herniation. It would seem that a combination of bending and torsional loads are necessary to produce this type of injury (34). Roaf (35) considered the combination of rotation and compression capable of producing all known disc injuries. Farfan (36) noted that degenerated discs were found to exhibit appreciable lateral motion (lateral shear) when subjected to torsion, whereas normal discs seemed to have sufficient reserve tissue to prevent the rotating joint from developing a side-to-side shearing motion. Liu et al. (37) found that lateral shear stress was generally greater than that of anterior-posterior sheer stress. This was also observed by Liu et al. (38). I believe that this type of degeneration is usually the result of trauma or, more often, numerous microtraumas and that the instability it produces in the disc results in the subsequent development of degenerative and proliferative changes in the uncovertebral and facet joints as well as in the amphiarthrodial joints. The only disc protrusions produced in Farfan's study (36) occurred in the degenerated disc group subjected to torsion.

Roaf (35) states that when bending occurs, the normal disc bulges into the concavity and this suggests that denucleation actually increases the bulging. This bulging occurs in the lateral flexion or flexion and extension in the sagittal plane (Fig. 1.5)

Farfan and his colleagues (39–41) have also tested the torque strength of the intervertebral joint. A rate of loading of 3.6°/min

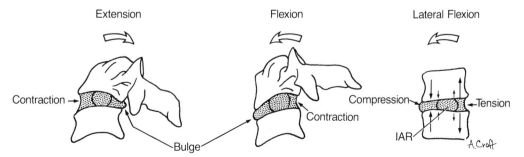

Figure 1.5.   In the normal disc, lateral bending and flexion and extension produce disc bulging. This occurs in the concavity with lateral flexion, anteriorly with flexion, and posteriorly with extension. The instantaneous axis of rotation (IAR) separates the zones of compression and tension.

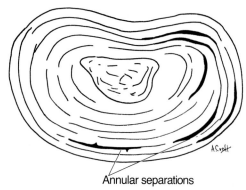

Annular separations

Figure 1.6. The natural cause for radial tears in the anulus is unknown. Peripheral separations have been produced by Farfan (18) with the application of torque.

(0.00108 radians/sec) was used, and the typical S-curve seen in the load/deflection curves for bone, mesentery, or fascia were also seen in the torque/rotation curve of discs. Farfan and his colleagues were unable to reproduce any radial tears in the disc with the application of torque. They were able to produce, however, peripheral separations in the anulus that were accompanied by a loud snapping noise. This may be the source of the loud snap or pop that many patients claim to hear just prior to the onset of back pain (Fig. 1.6).

Compression of a healthy disc produces complex stresses and a distribution of forces within (Fig. 1.7). In the degenerated disc, however, the hydraulics of the disc mechanism are altered due to the lack of nuclear buildup (pressure) and consequent inability to distribute the load at the endplates. Greater load is now placed on the periphery, and there is less peripheral tension, more axial stress, and much greater stress on the fibers (42) (Fig. 1.8).

The last force that acts upon the disc is shear stress or shear loading. With this force, the load is conceived to be applied at right angles to an axis in such a way that no bending moment is applied (in other words, there is pure rotation) (Fig. 1.9). Shear stress occurs in the disc in both axial and horizontal planes in such a way that the periphery always receives the greatest stress.

An excellent study of the viscoelastic properties of discs was undertaken by Lafferty and Kahler (43) utilizing rhesus monkey lumbar spines. In their study, kelvin

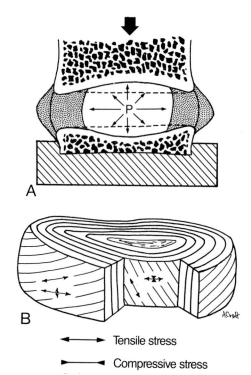

A

B

→ Tensile stress

► Compressive stress

Figure 1.7. Vertical compression of a normal disc produces a complex distribution of stresses throughout the disc, largely as a result of the fluid dynamics of the nucleus pulposus. **A.** Bulging occurs around the periphery and into the endplates. **B.** Distribution of stresses: In the inner layers of the anulus, the axial stress is compressive, whereas in the outer layers, the axial stress is tensile. Tangential tensile stresses are greater in the outer layers than in the inner layers. (Adapted from Panjabi MM, White AA: Physical and functional biomechanics of the spine. In White AA, Panjabi MM (eds): *Clinical Biomechanics of the Spine.* Philadelphia, JB Lippincott, 1978, p 13.)

units were used to represent the stress and the strain of the viscoelastic properties of the disc, with the phenomenon of creep taken into account. The viscoelastic properties are best described by the series spring and dashpot. These linear elements must then be represented by kelvin units (parallel spring and dashpot). Analysis of these data provides the following creep function response:

$$\frac{\epsilon}{\sigma} = \frac{1}{k_3} + \frac{t}{C_3} + \frac{1}{k_1}\left[1 - \exp\left(\frac{-k_1 t}{C_1}\right)\right]$$
$$+ \frac{1}{k_2}\left[1 - \exp\left(\frac{-k_2 t}{C_2}\right)\right]$$
(Eq. 1.1)

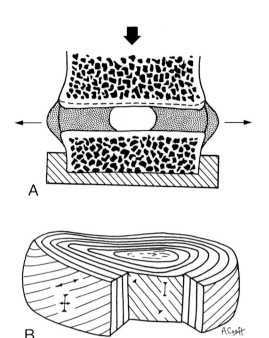

$$\frac{1}{G} = \frac{1}{k} + \frac{t^{(1-\beta)}}{A(1-\beta)} \qquad \text{(Eq. 1.2)}$$

where G is defined as the ratio of stress to strain for shear, tensile, and compressive loading and is the deflection torque ratio for torsional stress. Values for the three constants—k, β, and A—could be selected such that this nonlinear, two-element equation (1.2) represents data to within 1% of the experimental mean for compression, tension, shear, and torsion (Table 1.1).

In summary, the disc may be subjected to compression, tension, and torsion (resulting in shear) forces. White and Panjabi (42) state that the risk of disc failure is greater with tensile loading than with compressive loading. Others (34, 35) have found compression coupled with torsion to be most responsible for disc injury.

LIGAMENT

There are several important ligaments in the spine. A very brief description of each follows. Chapter 7 contains a more in-depth discussion of these important structures.

The *anterior longitudinal ligament* runs from the basiocciput to the sacrum attaching firmly to the anterior parts of all vertebrae and discs. The *anterior atlantooccipital membrane* spans between the basiocciput and the anterior arch of the atlas. The *atlantoepistrophic ligament* is found deep to the anterior longitudinal ligament and connects the anterior portion of the axis to the inferior anterior arch of the atlas (see Fig. 7.40).

The *posterior longitudinal ligament*, like its anterior counterpart, runs the entire length of the spine. Both the anterior and posterior longitudinal ligaments are thicker in the thoracic region. The cephalad portion of the posterior longitudinal ligament is named the *tectorial membrane*. Adjacent to it can be found the *accessory (deep) portion of the tectorial membrane* that spans the posterolateral portions of the body of the axis and the anterior foramen magnum (see Fig. 7.39).

Deep to the tectorial membrane lies the *cruciform ligament*, so named because it is shaped like a cross. It has an upper vertical component and a lower vertical component. These run between the anterior aspect of the foramen magnum and the posterior

Figure 1.8. Vertical compression in a degenerated disc. **A.** The endplates are loaded at the periphery only. This results in tensile and compressive forces that are markedly different from those seen in a healthy disc (Fig. 1.7). **B.** Distribution of stresses: In the inner layers of the anulus, the axial stress produces relatively high compressive forces, whereas in the outer layers, the tangential stress is much lower, while the anulus fibers are subjected to nearly twice the stress. (Adapted from Panjabi MM, White AA: Physical properties and functional biomechanics of the spine. In White AA, Panjabi MM (eds): *Clinical Biomechanics of the Spine.* Philadelphia, JB Lippincott, 1978, p 14.)

where ϵ equals strain which is the deformation/disc height, σ equals stress which is the force/disc area, t equals time, k equals elastic modulus, and C equals the viscous coefficient.

The mathematical model devised by Lafferty and Kahler represents their experimental data to within 1% of the mean. Although additional kelvin units were needed, because of the time dependency of the viscous coefficient (in other words, the creep phenomenon), in order to accurately represent the data, the final analysis of this model gives the creep response as:

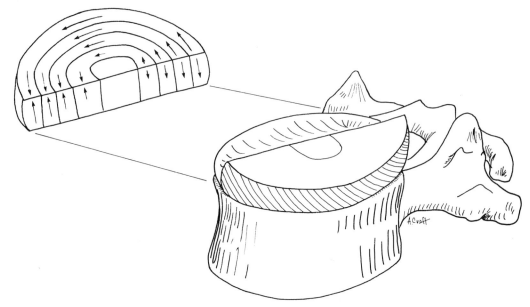

Figure 1.9. Shear forces occurring within the disc, exerting pressure in horizontal and axial directions. The outer portions of the disc reach physiological limits before the inner portions, which receive less shear, do. (Adapted from Panjabi MM, White AA: Physical properties and functional biomechanics of the spine. In White AA, Panjabi MM (eds): *Clinical Biomechanics of the Spine*. Philadelphia, JB Lippincott, 1978, p 16.)

body of the axis. The *transverse ligament of the atlas*, which acts as a sling holding the dens against the anterior arch of the atlas, comprises the horizontal component of the cruciform ligament.

Deep to the upper vertical limb of the cruciform ligament is the *apical suspensory ligament of the dens*. This structure suspends, as its name implies, the dens from the foramen magnum. The *alar ligaments* are strong fibrous bands that extend from the medial sides of the condyles of the occiput around the posterior surface of the dens. These ligaments have been referred to as

check *ligaments* because they limit the amount of rotation that can occur upon the dens (see Figs. 7.43 and 7.44).

Somewhat thinner than its anterior counterpart, the *posterior atlantooccipital membrane* extends from the superior aspect of the posterior arch of the atlas to the base of the occiput. The paired *ligamenta flava* run between the inferior aspect of the posterior arch of the atlas to the lamina of the axis below and are found at each interlaminar space down to the level of the first sacral segment (see Fig. 7.41).

The *capsular ligaments* are found throughout the spine. Their fibers run at angles perpendicular to the plane of the facet joint they span. They generally offer the least resistance to movement in the cervical spine (see Fig. 7.40).

The *intertransverse ligaments* unite transverse processes. They are not well developed in the cervical spine and probably contribute little to its integrity. The *interspinous ligaments* are also poorly developed in the cervical spine where they are largely replaced by the *ligamentum nuchae*. This fibroelastic septum extends from the external occipital protuberance to the spine of the

Table 1.1.
Model Parameters[a]

	k[b]	A	β
Compression	22.78	81.0	0.906
Tension	5.08	198.4	0.86
Shear	2.68	42.7	0.87
Torsion	7.10	68.3	0.82

[a]From Lafferty JF, Kahler RL: Viscoelastic properties of intervertebral discs. In Sances A, Thomas DJ, Ewing CL, Larson SJ, Unterharnscheidt F (eds): *Mechanisms of Head and Spine Trauma*. Goshen, NY, Aloray, 1986, p 487.

[b]Values are in newtons per millimeter squared.

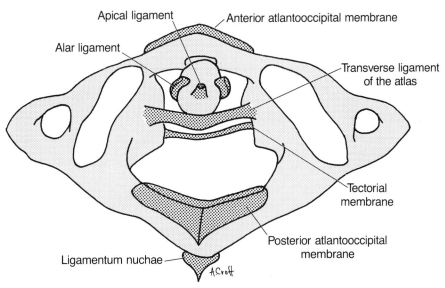

Figure 1.10. Ligaments of the upper cervical spine. (Adapted from Panjabi MM, White AA: Physical properties and functional biomechanics of the spine. In White AA, Panjabi MM (eds): *Clinical Biomechanics of the Spine.* Philadelphia, JB Lippincott, 1978, p 200.)

seventh cervical vertebra. Its strength in humans is limited. The *supraspinous ligament* attaches subsequent spinous processes together. It originates at the ligamentum nuchae (therefore, it is not found in the neck) and extends as far as the sacrum (see Fig. 7.42). Also worthy of mention is the *joint capsule of the uncovertebral joint*. Its contribution to spinal biomechanics has not been described. Figures 1.10 and 1.11 summarize this section.

Spinal Ligaments

Ligaments are uniaxial in nature, meaning that they are designed to carry loads primarily in one direction only—the direction in which their fibers run. White and Panjabi (44) compare them to rubber bands. They resist tensile forces but, when subjected to compression, buckle easily. In fact, their fiber orientation is always in line with the tensile forces they are designed to resist.

The spinal ligaments have two important functions: First, they act to give strength and stability to the complex articulations of the spine. This is most complex in the cervical spine because of the need for so much range of motion. Normal biomechanics depends on the smooth transition of movement from one articulation to the next, with

each allowed a finite amount of displacement and contributing to the overall harmonious movement of the body. Second, they act to protect the spine and its contents against excessive forces. Because of their strength and their viscoelastic properties, they are able to absorb large amounts of energy. The spine is a remarkable structure acting as a solid bony encasement for the protection of the spinal cord while allowing a large freedom of motion. This combination of safety and free range of motion is largely dependent upon ligamentous integrity.

It has been suggested that separations that occur between the anterior longitudinal ligament and the vertebrae result in the formation of the so-called "traction spur" or anterior lipping seen commonly on lateral spinal x-rays and generally considered pathognomonic of degenerative disc disease. Longitudinal ligaments, like discs, degenerate with age (26, 45). This is generally true of all spinal structures.

Pintar et al. (46) studied the isolated spines of 27 fresh male cadavers by using in situ technique. They measured the biomechanical characteristics of the spinal ligaments, reporting tensile breaking force and deflection to failure at all spinal levels. They

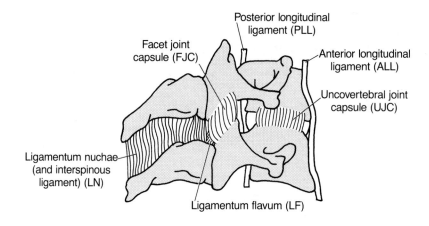

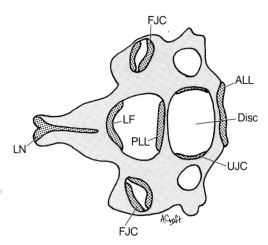

Figure 1.11. Ligaments of the lower cervical spine. (Adapted from Panjabi MM, White AA: Physical properties and functional biomechanics of the spine. In White AA, Panjabi MM (eds): *Clinical Biomechanics of the Spine.* Philadelphia, JB Lippincott, 1978, p 211.)

Table 1.2.
Failure Load and Deflection at Failure for Ligaments in the Upper Cervical Region[a]

Ligament	Level(s)[b]	Failure Load[c]	Deflection[d]
Anterior longitudinal	OC–C2	264 ± 132	12.8 ± 6.6
Alar	OC–C2	433 ± 196	11.3 ± 5.6
Apical	OC–C2	257 ± 152	11.8 ± 3.2
Joint capsule	OC–C2	280 ± 103	10.5 ± 5.2
Tectorial membrane	OC–C2	56 ± 72	11.9 ± 2.5
Ligamentum flavum	C1–C2	108 ± 97	10.3 ± 4.5

[a]Adapted from Pintar FA, Mykebust JB, Yoganandan N, Maiman DJ, Sances A: Biomechanics of human spiral ligaments. In Sances A, Thomas DJ, Ewing CL, Larson SJ, Unterharnscheidt F (eds): *Mechanisms of Head and Spine Trauma.* Goshen, NY Aloray, 1986, p 518.
[b]OC, occiput.
[c]Values are mean ± SD in newtons.
[d]Values are mean ± SD in millimeters.

Table 1.3.
Tensile Failure Load[a, b]

Levels	Anterior Longitudinal Ligament	Posterior Longitudinal Ligament	Ligamentum Flavum	Joint Capsules	Interspinous Ligament	Supraspinous Ligament
C2–C7	116 ± 91	82 ± 50	81 ± 45	224 ± 121	32 ± 12	
C7–T6	153 ± 72	90 ± 46	159 ± 55	204 ± 117	52 ± 38	110 ± 101
T6–T12	325 ± 164	112 ± 93	246 ± 82	202 ± 109	75 ± 66	292 ± 177
T12–S1	391 ± 214	95 ± 96	229 ± 129	284 ± 78	122 ± 41	546 ± 221

[a]Adapted from Pintar FA, Mykebust JB, Yoganandan N, Maiman DJ, Sances A: Biomechanics of human spiral ligaments. In Sances A, Thomas DJ, Ewing CL, Larson SJ, Unterharnscheidt F (eds): *Mechanisms of Head and Spine Trauma.* Goshen, NY, Aloray, 1986, p 515.
[b]Values are mean ± SD in newtons.

found that the anterior longitudinal ligament was strongest at the high cervical and lower thoracic and lumbar regions and that the posterior longitudinal ligament was strongest in the lower thoracic region. The anterior longitudinal ligament was found to be significantly stronger than the posterior longitudinal ligament, thereby confirming earlier studies by Nachemson and Morris (47). When force per unit area was measured, however, the posterior longitudinal ligament demonstrated greater strength (14.4 versus 9.8 N/mm^2).

The interspinous ligaments were found to be the weakest of those tested in the cervical spine. Table 1.2 provides a summary of the findings by Pintar et al. concerning the upper cervical spine, and Table 1.3 provides a summary of their findings relative to the remainder of the spine.

Pintar et al. also noted that ligaments in the cervical and lumbar spines displayed the greatest distensibility. These findings are summarized in Tables 1.2 and 1.4.

Their study indicates that ligaments farthest from the center of rotation demonstrate the greatest distensibility. The supraspinous ligament showed the greatest deflection at failure, whereas the posterior longitudinal ligament demonstrated the least.

The ligamentum flavum contains the highest amount of elastic fibers in the entire body, giving it its deep yellow color. This

Table 1.4.
Deflection at Failure[a, b]

Levels	Anterior Longitudinal Ligament	Posterior Longitudinal Ligament	Ligamentum Flavum	Joint Capsules	Interspinous Ligament	Supraspinous Ligament
C2–C7	6.4 ± 5.0	6.3 ± 6.5	8.9 ± 8.7	10.8 ± 7.7	7.3 ± 4.0	
C7–T6	7.7 ± 5.6	4.6 ± 3.2	8.2 ± 4.0	6.1 ± 2.7	8.0 ± 5.3	12.0 ± 4.6
T6–T12	14.0 ± 7.7	4.2 ± 2.3	9.6 ± 3.0	7.0 ± 3.7	7.5 ± 6.8	12.5 ± 5.4
T12–S1	16.0 ± 10.3	7.2 ± 6.7	10.3 ± 4.0	12.1 ± 3.5	12.8 ± 9.5	26.0 ± 6.4

[a]Adapted from Pintar FA, Mykebust JB, Yoganandan N, Maiman DJ, Sances A: Biomechanics of human spinal ligaments. In Sances A, Thomas DJ, Ewing CL, Larson SJ, Unterharnscheidt F (eds): *Mechanisms of Head and Spine Trauma.* Goshen, NY, Aloray, 1986, p 519.
[b]Values are mean ± SD in millimeters.

serves several purposes. First, it has been shown that a normal state of pre-tension exists in this ligament in the resting state, which produces a preloading of the disc (48). This may serve as a protective mechanism. Second, during extension of the neck the elasticity of the ligament helps to prevent it from buckling into the spinal cord. This most likely would be a problem, especially if the ligament were first stretched by extreme flexion (49). Third, the elastic nature of this structure may serve to act as a natural brake to forward flexion (especially in the cervical spine), thereby preventing any damage that might otherwise result from the abrupt stop that would occur as the limits of a nonelastic ligament were met at the end of range of motion.

From a functional standpoint, it is well accepted that ligament strengths increase with the rate of loading. This is also true of bone (50, 51). Very little resistance is offered to muscular movement of the spine in normal physiological ranges of motion. In the range of motion occurring during trauma, however, where great forces are applied to the spine, the stiffness offered by the ligaments may increase manyfold.

MUSCLE

The physical properties of a muscle vary depending upon whether it is in a passive or an active state. White and Panjabi use a three-element mathematical model to describe this phenomenon (Fig. 1.12). The parallel and series elements of a given muscle will have a constant stiffness value, whereas the contractile element is variable and dependent upon muscle activity.

Figure 1.12. Functional model of a skeletal muscle. The three-element mathematical model consists of a parallel element that represents the passive elastic nature of muscle, along with a series element and contractile element that represent the active elastic nature of muscle. (Adapted from Panjabi MM, White AA: Physical properties and functional biomechanics of the spine. In White AA, Panjabi MM (eds): *Clinical Biomechanics of the Spine.* Philadelphia, JB Lippincott, 1978, p 50.)

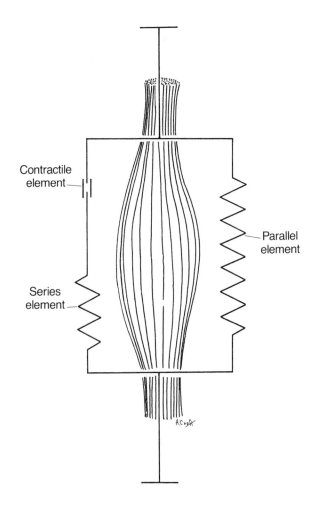

Contractile element

Series element

Parallel element

SPINAL CORD

The spinal cord, like other tissues, displays properties of viscoelasticity. Brieg (52) studied the biomechanics of the spinal cord and noted that when the cord is suspended by its own weight, it lengthens by more than 10%. When an attempt was made to increase this stretch, however, the stiffness of the cord increased in a behavior qualitatively similar to that of ligaments. Spinal cord without pia mater behaved like a cohesive semifluid mass.

It was also noted that when there was a change from full flexion to full extension, the cord's shape changed from round to oval. The spinal canals and the spinal cord are lengthened during flexion and shortened during extension. The dentate ligaments and perhaps also the nerve roots help to suspend the cord safely in the center of the spinal canal.

Normal Functional Biomechanics and Kinetics of the Cervical Spine

COORDINATE SYSTEM

In order to facilitate easy understanding of the descriptive terminology in this textbook the right-handed orthogonal coordinate system is utilized. Generally, the entire body is described in terms of the x, y, and z axes. Because the focus here is on the cervical spine, however, only this part is illustrated (53–57) (Fig. 1.13). There are different coordinate systems in common usage, and Chapter 8 includes a description of one of these variations.

TERMINOLOGY

Although a glossary of terms is included at the end of this textbook, several terms are defined here for ease of reading.

Degrees of Motion

"Degrees of motion" refers to the motion or freedom of a joint or set of joints taken as a group (such as the cervical spine). In the case of the spine, there is motion about all three orthogonal axes or planes (x, y, z), i.e., the horizontal plane (x, z), the sagittal plane (y, z), and the frontal or coronal plane (x, y). Normal movement is possible to either side of these planes (lateral flexion to the left and to the right; rotation to the left and to the right; and forward flexion and rearward extension), so the spine is said to possess six planes of motion or freedom.

Rotation

Very often the word "rotation" is used somewhat synonymously with rotation about the y axis. In a truer sense, however, the term merely implies a spinning or angular displacement of a body about some axis. Some authors use the term to imply rotation about the x axis (with $+\theta x$ being flexion and $-\theta x$ being extension). Unless otherwise specified in this text, rotation refers to rotary movement about the y axis; lateral flexion refers to side bending in the coronal plane or rotation about the z axis; flexion referes to forward rotation about the x axis ($+\theta x$); and extension refers to the opposite of flexion ($+\theta x$), with these latter two occuring in the sagittal plane.

Translation

"Translation" refers to a movement of a body part in relation to a fixed point. For example, when one vertebra is moving over its inferior contiguous neighbor, it is said to be in forward translation ($+\theta z$). Or, in the initial stage of a whiplash injury, the torso translates forward in relation to the head and neck which then accelerate secondarily.

Range of Motion

All motion or freedom of movement can be expressed in terms of range of motion. This includes the entire spectrum of pure movement through that plane or around the designated axis. Range of motion is generally expressed in degrees, whereas translation is expressed in centimeters or inches.

What is considered normal range of motion in the cervical spine has long been the subject of debate, especially since a patient's age, build, and any preexisting condition may affect this measurement. This controversy has often been solved by the

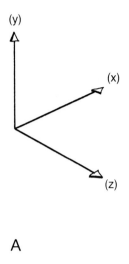

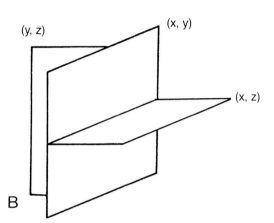

A

B

Figure 1.13. **A.** Right-handed orthogonal coordinate system. **B.** x, y indicates the frontal (coronal) plane; y, z indicates the sagittal plane; and x, z indicates the horizontal or axial plane. **C.** +z indicates forward translation; −z indicates rearward translation; +x indicates left lateral flexion; −x indicates right lateral flexion; +y indicates cephalad motion; and −y indicates caudad motion. **D.** Movements are typically described as rotations about these x, y, and z axes. Thus, rotation around the x axis would be synonymous with flexion and extension; rotation around the y axis would be synonymous with rotation to the left and right in the horizontal plane; and rotation around the z axis would be synonymous with left and right lateral flexion. Therefore, +θx is analogous to flexion, and −θx is analogous to extension; +θy is equivalent to axial rotation to the left, and −θy is equivalent to axial rotation to the right; +θz is equivalent to right lateral flexion, and −θz is equivalent to left lateral flexion.

individual clinician by expressing the range of motion as a percentage of normal or a percentage of limitation. This method then assumes that variables such as age, build, and preexisting disease have been factored into the equation. In other words, the normal range of motion for a 71-year-old man is certainly less than the normal range of motion for a 19-year-old woman. Although this method is generally considered acceptable, I prefer to express this measurement in absolute degrees. (The exception to this rule is flexion of the neck (+θx) which should be described as the distance by which the patient's chin, with closed mouth, misses the chest.)

The definitive study on normal range of motion in the cervical spine was conducted by Ferlic (58) in 1962. He found that individuals with short, thick muscular necks had a smaller range of motion than those with long slender necks. After studying a broad range of age groups, he concluded that over a period of six decades (ages 15–74), the average decrease in range of motion was 21% in the flexion-extension, 35% in

lateral bending, and 20% in rotation. As to the exact nature of this decrease in movement with increasing age, one can only speculate. Is it, in fact, normal for tissues to degenerate, contract, and become less elastic as a result of aging and free radical damage? Hunt (59) believes that cervical degenerative disc disease may be considered a normal process of aging. Macnab (60) suggests that cervical spondylosis and all its manifestations are the product of cervical disc degeneration.

Ferlic's findings concerning the normal

Table 1.5.
Normal Cervical Spine Range of Motion for All Age Groups[a, b]

Direction	Range of Motion
Flexion/extension	127 ± 19.5
Lateral flexion (left and right)	73 ± 15.6
Rotation (left and right)	142 ± 17.1

[a]Adapted from Ferlic D: The range of motion of the "normal" cervical spine. *Johns Hopkins Hosp Bull* 110:59–65, 1962.

[b]Values are mean ± SD in degrees.

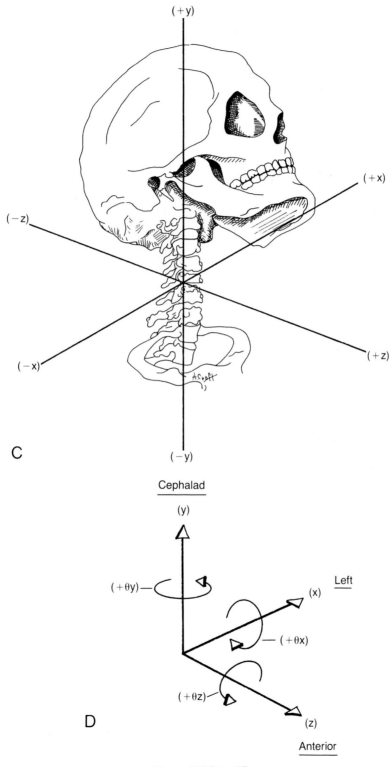

Figure 1.13 C and D.

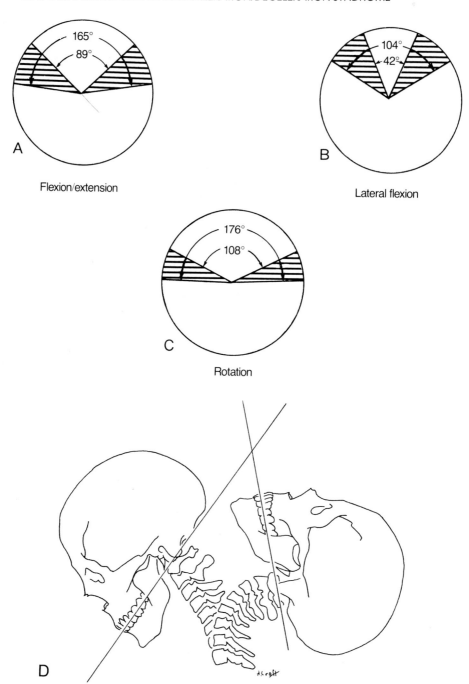

Figure 1.14.   A–C. Normal ranges of motion in the cervical spine after Ferlic (58). *Shaded areas* represent the normal ranges. **D.** In measuring degrees of flexion and extension on radiographs, reference lines through the teeth and the mastoid processes may be used. **E.** Clinical evaluation of range of motion. **F.** Ideally, range of motion should be determined through the use of a goniometer. (Adapted from Kapandji IA: The vertebral column as a whole. In: *The Physiology of the Joints,* vol 3: *The Trunk and the Vertebral Column.* New York, Churchill Livingstone, 1974, pp 215 and 247.)

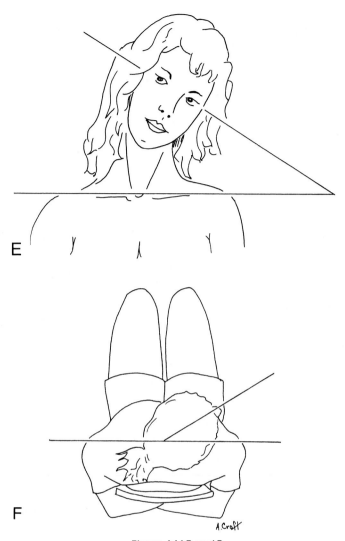

E

F

A.Croft

Figure 1.14 E and F.

range of cervical spine motion expressed as a mean value for all age groups are presented in Table 1.5, and their correlation for age and sex are presented in Table 1.6. These ranges are illustrated in Figure 1.14.

Intersegmental motion has also been studied in detail. Representative values for the upper cervical spine (which by definition includes the occiput, atlas, and axis) are listed in Table 1.7, and those values for the lower cervical spine are listed in Table 1.8.

Coupling

In the cervical spine, the movement of rotation is not a pure one. It is always accompanied by lateral flexion. Conversely, lateral flexion is always accompanied by some degree of rotation. These complex dual motions, which occur simultaneously, are said to be "coupled" motions. As is discussed later, certain compensatory mechanisms help to stabilize and coordinate these motions through agonist and

Table 1.6.
Cervical Spine Range of Motion (in Degrees) Correlated by Age and Sex[a, b]

Age	15–24 years	25–34 years	35–44 years	45–54 years	55–64 years	65–74 years
Total no. of subjects	65	59	38	15	16	6
No. of males	31	34	22	5	10	3
No. of females	34	25	16	10	6	3
Mean FE ± SD	139 ± 19	127 ± 21.5	120 ± 19	120 ± 15	116 ± 22	113 ± 18
Mean FE in males	133	129	115	120	117	101
Mean FE in females	148	129	121	115	115	123
Range of FE	90–185	95–180	70–155	100–155	80–165	95–125
Mean LF ± SD	81 ± 17	74 ± 14.5	67 ± 13.5	68 ± 18	62 ± 13	53 ± 24
Mean LF in males	80	76	62	63	64	43
Mean LF in females	82	72	74	71	61	70
Range of LF	40–120	45–105	30–120	45–120	45–85	30–90
Mean ROT ± SD	150 ± 18	143 ± 20	136 ± 15	138 ± 13	128 ± 12	116 ± 21
Mean ROT in males	147	143	132	138	125	101
Mean ROT in females	154	141	141	138	133	130
Range of ROT	105–185	105–195	100–170	125–165	103–145	80–140

[a]Adapted from Ferlic D: The range of motion of the "normal" cervical spine. *Johns Hopkins Hosp Bull* 110:59–65, 1962.
[b]Abbreviations: FE, flexion/extension; LF, lateral flexion; ROT, rotation.

Table 1.7.
Range of Motion of the Occiput-C1-C2 Complex[a]

Motor Unit	Type of Motion	Range of Motion[b]
Occipitoatlantal joint (occiput-C1)	Flexion/extension ($\pm \theta x$)	13
	Lateral flexion ($\pm \theta z$)	8
	Rotation ($\pm \theta y$)	0
Atlantoaxial joint (C1-C2)	Flexion/extension ($\pm \theta x$)	10
	Lateral flexion ($\pm \theta z$)	0
	Rotaion ($\pm \theta y$)	47

[a]Adapted from Panjabi MM, White AA: Physical properties and functional biomechanics of the spine. In White AA, Panjabi MM (eds): *Clinical Biomechanics of the Spine*. Philadelphia, JB Lippincott, 1978, p 65.
[b]Values are in degrees.

Table 1.8.
Range of Motion in the Lower Cervical Spine[a, b]

Motor Unit	Flexion/Extension ($\pm \theta x$)[b]		Lateral Flexion ($\pm \theta z$)[b]		Rotation ($\pm \theta y$)[b]	
	Limits of Range	Representative Angle	Limits of Range	Representative Angle	Limits of Range	Representative Angle
C2-C3	5–23	8	11–20	10	6–28	9
C3-C4	7–38	13	9–15	11	10–28	11
C4-C5	8–39	12	0–16	11	10–26	12
C5-C6	4–34	17	0–16	8	8–34	10
C6-C7	1–29	16	0–17	7	6–15	9
C7-T1	4–17	9	0–17	4	5–13	8

[a]Adapted from White AA, Panjabi MM: The basic kinematics of the human spine. *Spine* 3:12, 1978.
[b]Values are in degrees.

antagonist muscular activity, so that pure lateral flexion or rotation appears to occur in spite of this physiological coupling.

Instantaneous Axis of Rotation

At any given time, there exists a point about which some body or mass pivots such that this point or hypothetical point does not vary. This is known as the instantaneous axis of rotation (IAR), which is illustrated in Figure 1.15. Depending upon the plane of movement, there is an IAR for all vertebrae.

Helical Axis of Motion

Whereas IAR describes motion in a uniplanar sense, helical axis of motion describes motion in three-dimensional space, so that a moving body can be said to rotate about an axis that encompasses the resultant movement of the three rotations, i.e., those about the axes x, y, and z. This screw motion is a superimposition of rotation and translation along or around the same axis (Fig. 1.16).

Kinematics

"Kinematics," a word derived from the Greek *kinema* (motion), refers to the phase of mechanics that deals with the possible motions of a material body. It classically does not consider the driving forces behind this motion, i.e., the muscles.

Kinetics

"Kinetics," a word derived from the Greek *kinetikos* (of or for putting in motion), is the branch of dynamics concerned with the rate of change or movement of a body or structure. In this text, kinetics is considered the study of the forces that cause motion in the cervical spine.

KINEMATICS OF THE UPPER CERVICAL SPINE (OCCIPUT-C1-C2)

Occiput-Atlas Articulation

The normal physiological range of motion between the atlas and occiput is 13° for flexion-extension and 8° for lateral flexion. There is essentially no rotation possible at this level (Table 1.7). The integrity of the articulation depends upon the capsular ligaments between the lateral masses of the atlas and the occipital condyles as well as upon the other ligamentous connections that connect these two structures.

Flexion is limited by bony contact

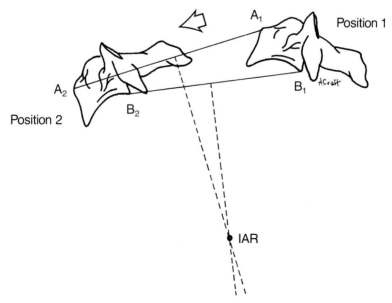

Figure 1.15. Method of determining the IAR in uniplanar motion. The IAR is defined as the point of intersection of the perpendicular bisectors of *lines A_1–A_2* and *B_1–B_2*. (Adapted from White AA III, Panjabi MM: *Spinal Kinematics. The Research Status of Spinal Manipulative Therapy,* NINCDS Monograph no 15. Washington, DC, United States Department of Health, Education and Welfare, 1975, p 93.)

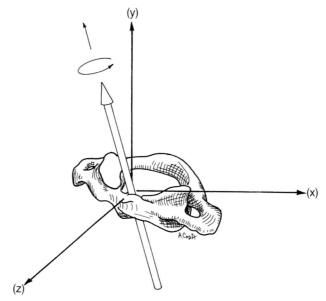

Figure 1.16. Method of determining the helical axis of motion in a three-dimensional space.

between the odontoid and the anterior margin of the foramen magnum as well as by the taughtness of the articular capsular ligaments and the nuchal ligament. Extension is limited by bony contact between the occiput, posterior arch of C1, and the spinous process of C2 (Fig. 1.17) and by the tectorial membrane.

Lateral flexion occurs in the upper cervical spine between the occiput and the atlas (8°) and between the axis and C3. There is no lateral flexion between the atlas and the axis. Left lateral flexion at the occiput-atlas articulation is resisted by the right alar ligament and by both articular capsules. The average range of motion between the occiput and C3 in this plane is 18° (8° and 10°) (Fig. 1.18).

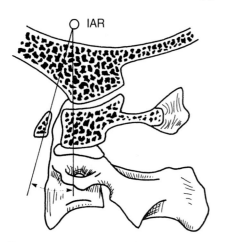
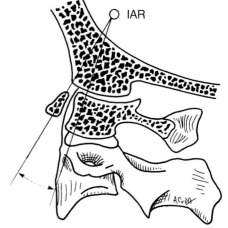

Figure 1.17. Flexion and extension of the occiput-atlas complex. The total range of motion is normally about 13°. The IAR is thought to occur at the *circle*. In some instances, the posterior arch of the atlas will appear closer to the occiput in flexion radiographs than in neutral lateral radiographs. This paradoxic motion may represent a normal variant but is often associated with myospasm of the suboccipital muscles (especially the rectus capitis posterior minor and the obliquus capitis superior). (Adapted from Kapandji IA: The vertebral column as a whole. In: *The Physiology of the Joints*, vol 3: *The Trunk and the Vertebral Column.* New York, Churchill Livingstone, 1974, p 185.)

There is no rotational motion between the occiput and the atlas. There also is no real coupling activity at this level. The instantaneous axes of rotation (IARs) for flexion/extension and lateral flexion are illustrated in Figures 1.17 and 1.18.

Atlantoaxial Articulation

The normal physiological range of motion at the atlantoaxial articulation is 10° for flexion/extension and 47° for rotation. There is essentially no lateral flexion at this joint (Table 1.8). The primary function of this complex is to allow for rotation, and about 50% of all cervical rotation occurs at this level. The remainder occurs from C2 to C7. When the head and neck are rotated, the first 40–50° of rotation occur at C1-C2 before the lower cervical spine begins to rotate.

A marked coupling motion occurs at this level, in that the axial rotation of C1 is asso-

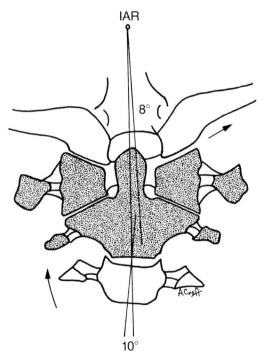

IAR

8°

10°

Figure 1.18. The normal physiological range of motion between the occiput and the atlas in lateral flexion is 8°. Between the axis and C3, the average is 10°. There is no lateral flexion motion between the atlas and the axis. The IAR is thought to occur at the *dot*. (Adapted from Kapandji IA: The vertebral column as a whole. In: *The Physiology of the Joints*, vol 3: *The Trunk and the Vertebral Column*. New York, Churchill Livingstone, 1974, p 185.)

ciated with a vertical translation. This is due to the biconcave surfaces of the articulations between the atlas and the axis (Fig. 1.19).

Whether axial rotation is a normal roentgen variant or a positioning artifact has been a source of debate. In general, it may be said that up to 4 mm of apparent lateral displacement of the atlas on the axis as seen on anteroposterior (AP) open mouth x-rays of the cervical spine may be due to positioning error whereby the patient had his or her head turned slightly at the time the x-ray was taken (61) (Fig. 1.20). In the case of trauma, however, this variation should not be casually dismissed as a mirage, and a rotary subluxation and possible disruption of the transverse ligament must be ruled out. Cineradiography in conjunction with other studies should be performed in order to define the lesion. (See Chapter 3 for more detail on the use of cineradiography.)

Another phenomenon that occurs exclusively at the C1-C2 articulation and that may have clinical significance is the stretching or kinking of the vertebral artery upon extremes of rotational range of motion. When the neck is extended and the head is rotated to the right, the contralateral vertebral artery may become stretched or kinked to such an extent that flow through the vessel is temporarily impeded (50). This may give rise to a temporary vertebrobasilar syndrome consisting of vertigo, nausea, tinnitus, or visual disturbances (62). In some cases, the patient may complain of retroocular pain (60). When extension and rotation are performed clinically, this maneuver is referred to as the Barré-Lieou test. This test should always be performed when patients are to be selected for cervical manipulation. The presence of any of the aforementioned symptoms during this test is a strong contraindication to rotary manipulation. The course of the vertebral artery is illustrated in Figures 7.36, 7.41, and 7.42.

The transverse ligament holds the odontoid firmly against the posterior aspect of the anterior arch of the atlas. Disruption of this ligament would allow a forward subluxation or dislocation of the atlas on the axis, which would, in turn, result in serious neurological consequence as the odontoid was pressed into the spinal medulla. Between

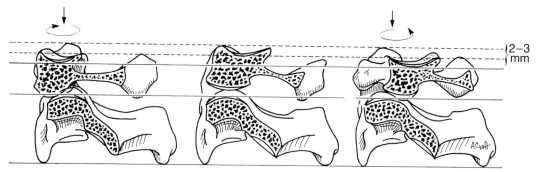

Figure 1.19.   The coupling motions between C1 and C2 result in a vertical translation along the y axis when rotation occurs around this y axis. This is due to the biconcave surfaces of the articulating facets and results in a motion that is actually helical. (Adapted from Kapandji IA: The vertebral column as a whole. In: *The Physiology of the Joints,* vol 3: *The Trunk and the Vertebral Column.* New York, Churchill Livingstone, 1974, pp 177 and 179.)

the anterior arch of the atlas and the dens is found a true synovial joint complex. This is seen on lateral x-ray as a radiolucent space known as the atlantodental interval (ADI), and its significance has often been misunderstood. In infants and children, the nor-

mal ligamentous laxity may allow up to 5 mm of separation at the ADI (63). This maximal separation occurs during flexion. Jackson (64) has suggested that 2.5 mm be set as the upper limits of normal for adults and 4.5 mm be set as the upper limits of normal for

Neutral

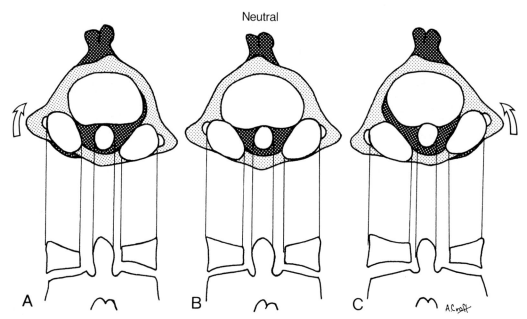

A   B   C

Figure 1.20.   The appearance of rotary subluxation of the atlas may be simulated by slight malpositioning of the patient prior to exposing an x-ray. In **A**, the head is turned slightly to the right. In **B**, there is no rotation and the normal interspaces are illustrated below. In **C**, the head is rotated to the left. In the space formed by the dens of the axis and the lateral mass of the atlas, up to 4 mm of disparity between the two slides may occur as a result of simple malpositioning. Greater disparity, however, may indicate rotary subluxation, ligamentous instability, or other pathology. (Adapted from Shapiro R, Youngberg AS, Rothman SLG: The differential diagnosis of traumatic lesions of the occipitoatlantoaxial segment. *Radiol Clin North Am* 11:505, 1973.)

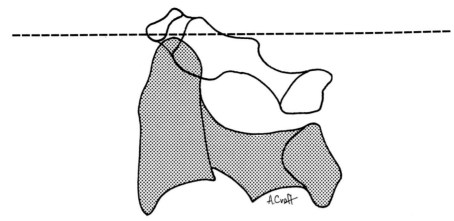

Figure 1.21. In 20% of normal children under the age of 8 years, more than two thirds of the anterior arch of the atlas may be seen above the level of the dens upon extension of the neck.

children, although according to Caffey (65), Locke et al. found that the most frequent measurement in adults was 2 mm and that in 92–97% of 200 children studied, the ADI was not more than 3 mm. Fielding et al. (66) tested the strength of the transverse ligament, describing it as a primary stabilizing component with very little elasticity. The secondary stabilizing component is the alar ligament which is weaker and more easily stretched, especially when the transverse ligament is ruptured. These ligaments are unable to prevent anterior displacement of the atlas. Fielding et al. noted that the ligament always ruptured before the dens fractured and that in some individuals this ligament was surprisingly weak.

Cattell and Filtzer (67) have reported that in 20% of normal children under the age of 8 years, more than two thirds of the anterior arch of the atlas may be found above the dens in extension (Fig. 1.21).

Axial rotation between C1 and C2 is limited by alar or check (these terms are synonymous) ligaments. Right rotation is checked by the left alar ligament, and left rotation is checked by the right alar ligament. The IAR is considered to occur in the center of the dens (Fig. 1.19).

KINEMATICS OF THE LOWER CERVICAL SPINE (C3–C7)

The range of motion for the cervical spine is listed in Table 1.8. It is tempting to speculate that the large amount of motion between C5 and C7 in flexion/extension may predispose this region to greater injury from acceleration/deceleration trauma. It is also tempting to suggest that there is some correlation between this finding and the high incidence of cervical spondylosis found at this level (60, 68). It has been shown by Hohl (69) that the incidence of cervical spondylosis occurring within 7 years following a whiplash injury is 39%, compared with 6% in age-matched healthy controls.

Anterior translation along the z axis is considered normal under physiological loads. This has been measured by White and Panjabi, and the maximum normal translation was said to be 2.7 mm (70). When this measurement is taken directly from radiographs, they recommend using 3.5 mm, as this measurement accounts for radiographic magnification. A value greater than this may indicate damage to the posterior ligamentous complex (defined as the nuchal ligament, interspinous ligament, capsular ligaments, ligamentum flavum, posterior longitudinal ligament and, included by some authors, the intervertebral disc). This abnormal motion is described as anterior subluxation. White and Panjabi's work was carried out on cadaver specimens, so I along with others believe that 1–2 mm should be considered subluxation (71, 72). This clinical condition is considered highly unstable (73).

The great range of motion in the cervical spine is partly accounted for by the size and shape of the discs. In general, a disc with a

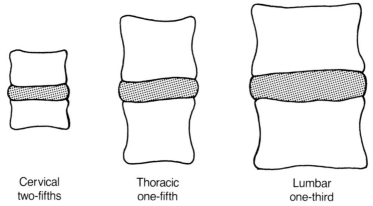

Cervical
two-fifths

Thoracic
one-fifth

Lumbar
one-third

Figure 1.22. Relative height ratios of disc to vertebra. The higher the ratio, the greater the mobility of that motor unit. The cervical spine has the greatest disc to vertebral height ratio and, therefore, is the most mobile section of the spine. (Adapted from Kapandji IA: The vertebral column as a whole. In: *The Physiology of the Joints*, vol 3: *The Trunk and the Vertebral Column*. New York, Churchill Livingstone, 1974, p 39.)

greater altitude allows greater rotation about all axes. Perhaps even more important is the ratio of the disc to the vertebral height. This is largest in the cervical spine (74) (Fig. 1.22). Similarly, a disc that is shorter in sagittal and coronal planes also lends mobility to a spinal segment.

Macnab (60) states that as degeneration of the disc proceeds, the vertical height is lost, and the first motion to be lost is extension. Flexion and extension occurring about an IAR have been variously described by different authors. There is little agreement on this subject, and further research is needed to accurately describe what actually happens. In extension, the superior vertebra slides posteriorly, putting tension on the anterior part of the disc. Motion is limited by the anterior longitudinal ligament, the joint capsules, contact between the posterior arches and ligaments, and the superior facet of the vertebra below. The nucleus pulposus is said to move slightly anteriorly within the disc. There is also a slight gapping of the facet joints.

In flexion, the reverse of the above occurs, although there is probably less posterior translation than anterior translation, in that the uncinate processes limit this motion and lateral flexion. As with extension, because the IAR is located somewhere anterior to the facet joint, there is transla-

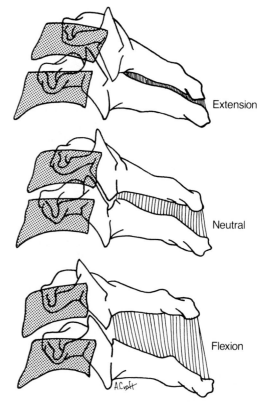

Extension

Neutral

Flexion

Figure 1.23. Kinematics of the lower cervical spine in flexion and extension. The neutral position and extremes of flexion and extension are illustrated. (Adapted from Kapandji IA: The vertebral column as a whole. In: *The Physiology of the Joints*, vol 3: *The Trunk and the Vertebral Column*. New York, Churchill Livingstone, 1974, p 197.)

tion and gapping at this articulation. There is a slight posterior displacement of the nucleus pulposus within the disc. Flexion is limited only by the intact posterior ligamentous complex. Damage to this complex permits an abnormal excursion, resulting in anterior subluxation. This can be visualized on x-ray as a forward angulation or kyphosis equal to or more than 11°, a loss of parallelism at the facet joints, a "perching" of facet joints (whereby the inferior surface of the inferior facet of the vertebra above appears to be perched atop the superior angle of the superior facet of the vertebra below), a "fanning" of the spinous processes posteriorly, and an anterior translation more than 1–2 mm (71, 72). (This subject is explored in greater detail later in this chapter.)

The normal kinematics of the lower cervical spine in flexion and extension are illustrated in Figure 1.23. Coupling motions are significant in the lower cervical spine. Lysell (75) noted a gradual change in the coupling ratio at subsequent lower levels in the cervical spine. At C2, there are 2° of coupled axial rotation for every 3° of lateral flexion (ratio of 0.67). At C7, there is 1° of coupled axial rotation for every 7.5° of lateral flexion (ration of 0.13).

Kapandji (76) in his excellent treatise on biomechanics describes the mechanism of this coupling action. Using the midcervical spine (C5) as an example (see Fig. 1.24), the facet joints lie at an angle of about 45°. Flexion and extension produce a symmetrical movement around an IAR probably located in the vertebral body. The facet joint movement indicated in this figure is similar to that shown in Figure 1.23. With a differential or relative movement of the facet joints such that one joint effectively extends while the other moves either in the opposite direction or not at all, both lateral flexion and axial rotation result. In other words, there is a

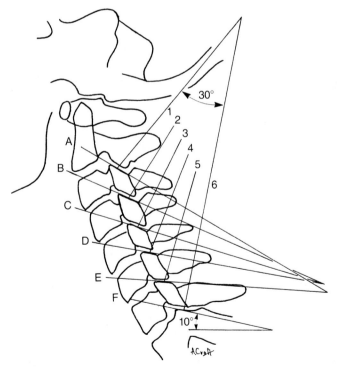

Figure 1.24. The coupled action of lateral flexion and axial rotation is due to the oblique orientation of the facet joints. (Adapted from Kapandji IA: The vertebral column as a whole. In: *The Physiology of the Joints*, vol 3: *The Trunk and the Vertebral Column*. New York, Churchill Livingstone, 1974, p 201.)

helical axis of motion. It is clear from Figure 1.24 that as one proceeds inferiorly through the cervical spine, the obliquity decreases such that at C2-C3 the angle formed by the facets is 40–45°, whereas at C7-T1 the angle formed is only 10°, giving a net change of 30–35°. The planes, however, do not change uniformly. *Lines A, B,* and *C* are more oblique, while *lines D, E,* and *F* are nearly parallel. When lines are drawn perpendicular to those of *A–F* and are labeled *1–6, line 6* is nearly vertical and almost pure rotation would be expected at that level, whereas *line 1* is at 40–45° and lateral flexion and rotation would be expected to be nearly equal.

Finally, one more component needs to be added to this model—extension. The cervical spine can only perform stereotyped movements which include lateral flexion, rotation, and extension. This extension component is automatically compensated for by flexion at the lower cervical spine. This coupled motion is illustrated schemat-

ically in Figures 1.25 and 1.26. The unique engineering system of the upper cervical spine, however, must compensate for the other unwanted coupled movements.

This works in the following way: With a primary intended movement of right lateral flexion, a certain degree of rotation must occur, and this movement occurs to the right. This unwanted rotation, however, is fully compensated for by left counterrotation that occurs at the atlantoaxial articulation. The resultant movement appears to be pure lateral flexion and illustrates the functional synergism found between the biomechanically distinct upper and lower cervical spines.

Unilateral facet dislocation, when trauma occurs during an oblique vector of hyperextension and/or hyperflexion, may result from this coupling activity in the neck. To a lesser degree, ligamentous or capsular damage more commonly results from these forces and may not be severe enough to be

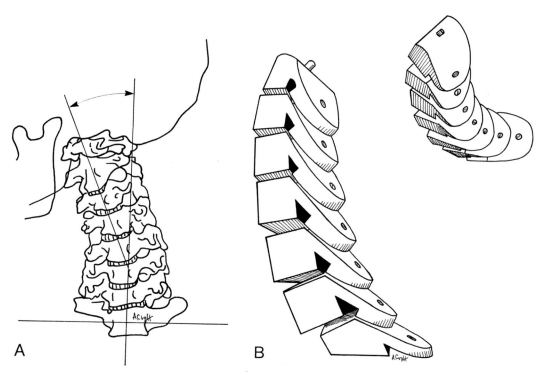

Figure 1.25. **A.** Coupled motions of rotation and lateral flexion. **B.** This same motion illustrated schematically. The third component (extension) as described by Kapandji cannot be appreciated with this mechanical model, however. (Adapted from Kapandji IA: The vertebral column as a whole. In: *The Physiology of the Joints*, vol 3: *The Trunk and the Vertebral Column.* New York, Churchill Livingstone, 1974, pp 209 and 211.)

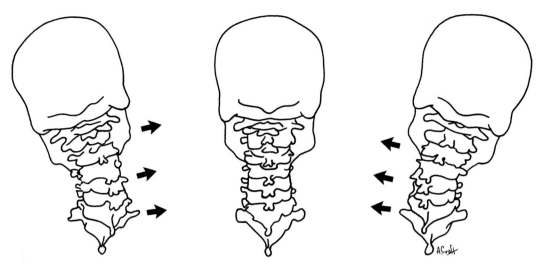

Figure 1.26.   Lateral flexion results in a coupled motion of axial rotation so that the spinous processes rotate toward the convexity. (Adapted from Panjabi MM, White AA: Physical properties and functional biomechanics of the spine. In White AA, Panjabi MM (eds): *Clinical Biomechanics of the Spine*. Philadelphia, JB Lippincott, 1978, p 73.)

grossly detectable with standard radiographic technique.

The uncinate processes and the vertebral body make up the uncovertebral joints (also known as the joints of Luschka). These joints, which are truly synovial in nature, were previously believed to be degenerative in origin. They are now considered to be a normal developmental process that begins in the late first decade and becomes fully mature at about 18 years of age. They are

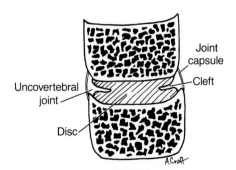

Figure 1.27.   The uncovertebral joint (also known as the joint of Luschka) is the result of a normal developmental process that begins in the late first decade and becomes mature at about 18 years of age. These joints are synovial in nature and are associated with clefts in the lateral margins of the intervertebral disc.

associated with a cleft that develops in the lateral margin of the intervertebral disc (77, 78) (Fig. 1.27). The uncinate processes are cartilage-lined facets that face superiorly and medially. These oppose the cartilage-lined semilunar facets of the corresponding upper vertebra that face inferiorly and laterally. During flexion and extension of the lower cervical vertebrae, the coupled translational movement that occurs (along the z axis) is facilitated by these uncovertebral joints which act as a guide for smooth gliding motion. They also act to limit lateral flexion and to some extent perhaps, posterior translation (77). This movement is illustrated schematically in Figure 1.28.

KINETICS OF THE UPPER CERVICAL SPINE

The combined movements of the upper and the lower cervical spine are the most complex in the entire body. The importance of ligamentous integrity of the spine cannot be overstated, and yet these structures serve only to stabilize and to protect the joints from trauma. The term "stability" is a relative one, however. It has been shown that the intact human spine with ligaments attached but devoid of rib cage and stripped of its muscles can withstand very little in the way of a vertical force. It buckles under a

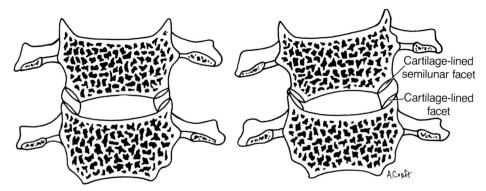

Figure 1.28.   The paired uncovertebral joints allow a gliding motion in forward translation along the z axis. This occurs during flexion and extension. They also limit lateral flexion and, to some extent, posterior translation along the −z axis. (Adapted from Kapandji IA: The vertebral column as a whole. In: *The Physiology of the Joints,* vol 3: *The Trunk and the Vertebral Column.* New York, Churchill Livingstone, 1974, p 199.)

load of only 20 N (4 lbf) (79). The intricate coupled movements of the neck are facilitated by a combined effort of the short intersegmental and suboccipital muscles and the longer and more powerful paraspinal muscles.

Intrinsic Muscles of the Upper Cervical Spine

Intrinsic muscles of the upper cervical spine are referred to as such (i.e., as intrinsic) because they have both origin and insertion on the skull and the cervical spine. The anterior portion includes the *rectus capitis anterior,* the *rectus capitis lateralis,* and the *longus capitis* muscles (in some literature, the rectus capitis anterior is referred to as the *rectus capitis anterior minor,* and the longus capitis is referred to as the *rectus capitis anterior major*) (80).

Bilateral contraction of the longus capitis results in flexion of the head on the neck with a flattening of the upper part of the cervical lordosis. Unilateral contraction produces forward and lateral flexion of the head on the ipsilateral side.

Bilateral contraction of the rectus capitis anterior produces flexion of the head at the atlantooccipital level, while unilateral contraction results in forward flexion, rotation, and lateral flexion (again at the atlantooccipital level) on the ipsilateral side.

The rectus capitis lateralis muscle is

regarded as the upper cervical homolog to the posterior intertransverse muscles of the lower cervical spine. Bilateral contraction produces flexion of the head, while unilateral contraction results in some lateral flexion of the head to the ipsilateral side. These muscles are illustrated in Figure 1.29.

The suboccipital muscles comprise the posterior component of the upper cervical intrinsic musculature. These include the *rectus capitis posterior major* and *minor,* the *obliquus capitis inferior,* and the *obliquus capitis superior.* These muscles are illustrated in Figure 1.30.

The obliquus capitis inferior muscle stabilizes the atlantoaxial joint. When these muscles contract bilaterally, the atlas is extended on the axis. With unilateral contraction, the atlas rotates posteriorly on the ipsilateral side (Fig. 1.31).

When all four occipital muscles contract unilaterally, the head is laterally flexed to the ipsilateral side. This motion occurs primarily at the atlantooccipital articulation. The obliquus capitis superior muscle is the most efficient of the group. Effective movement, however, depends on both the proper function of the agonist and the reciprocal inhibition of the antagonist. In other words, as the suboccipital group on the right contracts, the group on the left must relax. Muscle spasm due to injury will effectively inhibit this normal agonist/antagonist relationship (Fig. 1.32). Bilateral simultaneous contraction of the suboccipital muscles

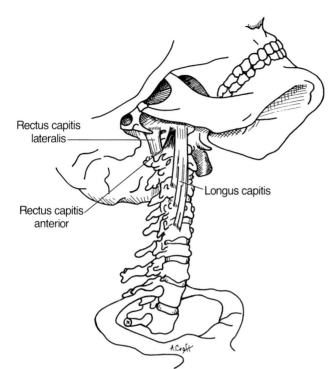

Figure 1.29. Deep intrinsic muscles of the anterior upper cervical spine. The longus capitis runs from the basiocciput to the anterior tubercles of C3–C6 (vertebral slips are variable). The rectus capitis lateralis is the upper cervical homolog to the intertransverse muscles in the lower cervical spine. The rectus capitis anterior runs from the anterior surface of the lateral mass of the atlas to the basiocciput. Note that the longus capitis and rectus capitis anterior are sometimes referred to as the rectus capitis anterior major and rectus capitis anterior minor, respectively. (Adapted from Kapandji IA: The vertebral column as a whole. In: *The Physiology of the Joints,* vol 3: *The Trunk and the Vertebral Column.* New York, Churchill Livingstone, 1974, p 223.)

results in extension of the head on the upper cervical spine.

Intrinsic Muscles of the Lower Cervical Spine

At the anterior aspect of the cervical spine is the *longus colli* (longus cervicis) muscle. It runs from the atlas to the third thoracic vertebra and can be divided into inferior oblique, superior oblique, and vertical parts.

Bilateral contraction of the longus colli results in flattening of the cervical spine and in flexion of the neck. These muscles are most important in straightening the cervical column and holding it rigid (81) (Fig. 1.33). The oblique portions produce lateral flexion. This has been confirmed by electromyography (82). The main antagonist of this muscle is the *longissimus cervicis* muscle (see Fig. 7.28).

At the posterior aspect of the cervical spine is the *transversospinalis group* consisting of the *semispinalis cervicis* and *capitis,* the *rotatores,* and the *multifidus* muscles. These are described in greater detail in Chapter 7.

With the exception of the semispinalis capitis, the fibers of these muscles run obliquely inferiorly, laterally, and slightly anteriorly. When they contract bilaterally and symmetrically, they accentuate the cervical lordotic curve and produce extension of the neck. When these muscles contract unilaterally, they produce lateral flexion ipsilaterally with contralateral rotation.

Accessory Muscles of Neck Movement

The *mylohyoid,* the *digastric (anterior belly section),* the *sternohyoid,* the *sternothyroid,* and the *omohyoid* muscles also act to flex the head on the neck and to straighten the cervical lordotic curve. These muscles, although not directly attached to the cervical vertebrae, act as powerful flexors of the neck (81). This is possible because their distance anterior to the spine produces a long lever arm (Fig. 1.34).

Large Flexors of the Cervical Spine

The longus colli muscle, an important flexor of the neck, is described on this page. The *sternocleidomastoid* muscle runs from the medial third of the clavicle and superior margin of the sternum to the mastoid pro-

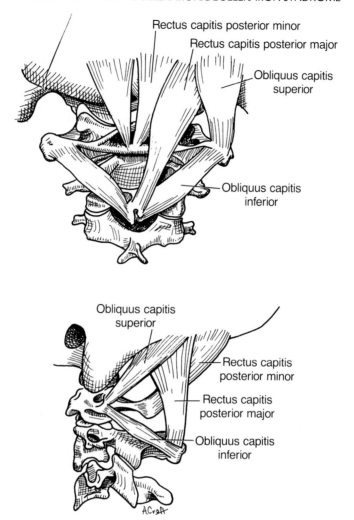

Figure 1.30.   The suboccipital muscles comprise the posterior component of the upper cervical intrinsic musculature. (Adapted from Kapandji IA: The vertebral column as a whole. In: *The Physiology of the Joints,* vol 3: *The Trunk and the Vertebral Column.* New York, Churchill Livingstone, 1974, p 233.)

cess and occiput. Unilateral contraction of this muscle results in contralateral rotation, ipsilateral lateral flexion, and extension of the head. Its action with regard to the head is analogous to the action of the suboccipital muscles with regard to the neck.

Bilateral contraction of the sternocleidomastoid muscles results in flexion of the head on the neck, when the cervical lordosis is held rigid, and in extension of the head on the neck, when the cervical spine is flexible (Fig. 1.35).

The *scalenus group* consists of the *anterior, middle,* and *posterior scalenus muscles.* A *scalenus minimus* muscle is occasionally present also. These muscles span from the first two ribs to the transverse processes of the cervical vertebrae. Their detailed anatomy is discussed in Chapter 7.

The scalenus muscles are tighteners of the spinal column. They are clinically important primarily because the brachial plexus and subclavian artery pass between the anterior and the medial muscles and injury to these muscles often results in the scalenus anticus syndrome which is one of the many forms of thoracic outlet syndrome (Fig. 1.36). This condition, because of its similar clinical presentation, is commonly misdiagnosed as a primary nerve root disorder.

As with bilateral contraction of the ster-

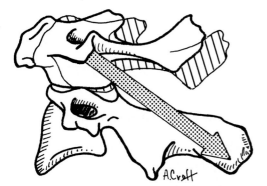

Figure 1.31. The obliquus capitis inferior (*arrow*) produces extension of the atlas upon the axis and serves to stabilize the atlantoaxial joint. Unilateral contraction results in posterior rotation of the atlas to the ipsilateral side. (Adapted from Kapandji IA: The vertebral column as a whole. In: *The Physiology of the Joints,* vol 3: *The Trunk and the Vertebral Column.* New York, Churchill Livingstone, 1974, p 235.)

nocleidomastoid muscles, the effects of bilateral contraction of the scalenus muscles depend upon the rigidity of the cervical spine. When the spine is flexible, bilateral scalene contraction results in flexion of the neck and accentuation of the lordotic curve. When the spine is held rigid by the longus colli muscles, bilateral contraction of the scalenes produces only flexion of the neck. Unilateral contraction of the scalenes results in lateral flexion and rotation of the neck ipsilaterally.

Large Extensors of the Cervical Spine

The larger muscles and muscle groups of the cervical spine act as extenders of the head. They are discussed only briefly here, however, since they are discussed more fully in Chapter 7.

The *trapezius* muscle acts as a powerful extensor when the scapula is fixed. Bilateral contraction results in extension of the head and accentuation of the cervical lordosis, while unilateral contraction produces both of these actions along with ipsilateral lateral flexion and contralateral rotation similar to that seen with the sternocleidomastoid muscle (Fig. 1.37).

The *splenius group* consisting of the *splenius capitis* and *cervicis* muscles are illustrated in Figure 7.30. Bilateral contraction of these muscles produces extension of the head and

neck with accentuation of the cervical lordotic curve, whereas unilateral contraction results in extension, lateral flexion, and rotation to the ipsilateral side. The *levator scapulae* muscle (see Fig. 7.29) produces essentially the same movements as the splenius group.

The *semispinalis* muscle is primarily an extender of the spine. The *capitis* portion also acts to accentuate the cervical lordosis. Lateral flexion is minimal (see Fig. 7.30).

The *longissimus* muscle (Fig. 7.30) also exends the head. Unilateral contraction produces ipsilateral lateral flexion and rotation.

With bilateral contraction, the *iliocostalis cervicis* muscles (Fig. 7.30) act as extenders of the lower cervical spine. With unilateral

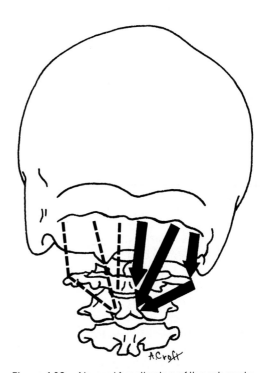

Figure 1.32. Normal functioning of the suboccipital group depends upon a properly functioning agonist/antagonist relationship. In this instance, right lateral flexion of the head by contraction of the right four suboccipital muscles (*arrows*) is dependent upon the normal physiological reciprocal inhibition and relaxation of the left four suboccipital muscles (*dashed lines*). (Adapted from Kapandji IA: The vertebral column as a whole. In: *The Physiology of the Joints,* vol 3: *The Trunk and the Vertebral Column.* New York, Churchill Livingstone, 1974, p 235.)

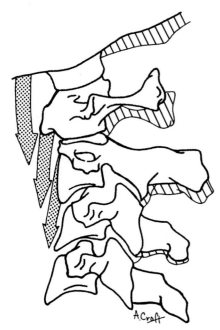

Figure 1.33. The longus colli (*arrows*) is most important in straightening the cervical lordotic curve and holding the cervical spine rigid. (Adapted from Kapandji IA: The vertebral column as a whole. In: *The Physiology of the Joints*, vol 3: *The Trunk and the Vertebral Column.* New York, Churchill Livingstone, 1974, p 229.)

contraction, this muscle acts as an ipsilateral lateral flexor and rotator.

When contraction of these long extensors is counterbalanced by equal contraction of the major flexor muscles, the net effect is tightening of the neck.

Reflexes and Muscle Strength

Foust et al. (83) have studied relative muscular strength and reflex time of the cervical musculature in volunteers of differing ages, sexes, and statures. They found that men tend to be stronger in middle age and that females decrease in strength gradually with age. Taller men are stronger in their youth, and both sexes of short stature are generally weaker throughout life.

They also found that although extensor muscles have faster stretch reflexes than flexor muscles (11% faster), they take longer to activate probably due to their greater complexity. Because of their mechanical advantage, the extensors are about 35% stronger than the flexors. A stretch reflex is

initiated with a G force of about one third to one half.

When reflexes and muscle strength between males and females were compared, it was seen that the reflex time of the female is about 11% faster than that of the male but that the strength of the female is about 60% that of the male.

Trauma and Instability of the Upper Cervical Spine (Occiput-C1-C2)

Trauma of the cervical spine may result from numerous types of injuries. Motor vehicle accidents, fist fights, falls, sports injuries, and accidents occurring from diving in shallow water all produce characteristic lesions.

It has recently been reported by Walter et al. (84) that 80% of all cervical spine fractures are the result of motor vehicle accidents. Hadley et al. (85) found that 68% of

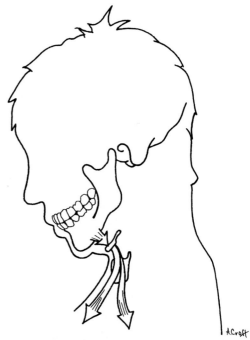

Figure 1.34 With the jaw clenched, the suprahyoid and infrahyoid muscles because of their distance anterior to the spine and the resulting long lever arm act as relatively strong flexors of the neck. (Adapted from Kapandji IA: The vertebral column as a whole. In: *The Physiology of the Joints*, vol 3: *The Trunk and the Vertebral Column.* New York, Churchill Livingstone, 1974, p 229.)

107 axis fractures that they reviewed were the result of motor vehicle accidents. In this chapter, only those injuries and instabilities resulting from this type of trauma are discussed, and although fractures and dis-

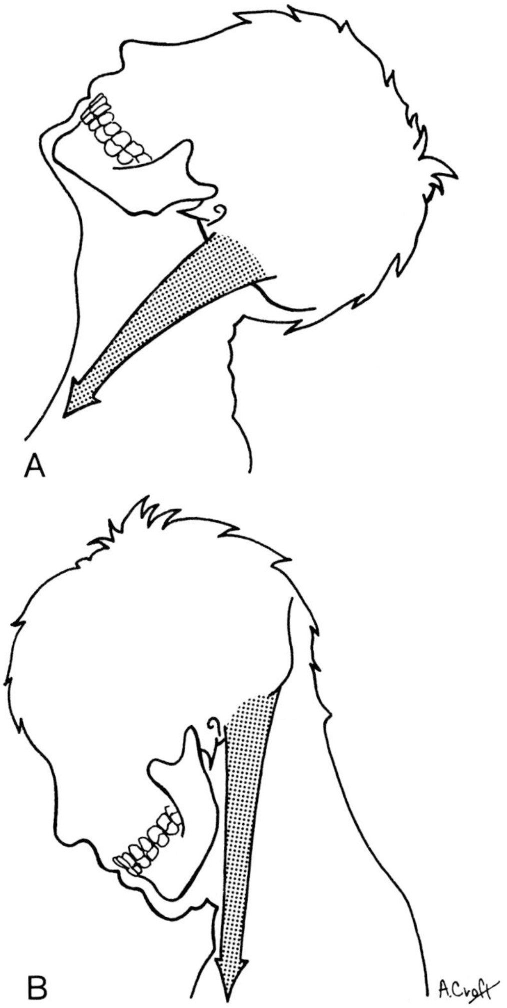

Figure 1.35. The effect of bilateral contraction of the sternocleidomastoid varies depending upon the relative rigidity of the cervical spine. **A.** When the spine is flexible, bilateral contraction of the sternocleidomastoid results in extension of the head. **B.** The increased tone of the intrinsic anterior cervical musculature (most notably the longus colli) renders the cervical spine relatively inflexible, and bilateral contraction of the sternocleidomastoid now results in flexion of the head. (Adapted from Kapandji IA: The vertebral column as a whole. In: *The Physiology of the Joints,* vol 3: *The Trunk and the Vertebral Column.* New York, Churchill Livingstone, 1974, pp 243 and 245.)

locations are covered, they are discussed in more detail in Chapter 6.

FRACTURE

Very little has been written on the subject of isolated occipital condyle fracture. There have been fewer than 10 reported cases since 1816. Except for the first reported cases, all have been the result of motor vehicle trauma. The incidence of this lesion is low probably because the occiput and its condyles are relatively strong and vertebral fractures will usually occur first and also because this type of fracture is usually associated with severe brain and spinal cord injury not compatible with life. Thomas and Jessop (86) have produced basiocciput fractures in primates subjected to acceleration/deceleration forces.

Two major types of fracture are seen in the atlas. The first occurs through the posterior arch just behind the lateral masses where the arch is grooved by the vertebral artery. Because of the groove, this is the weakest spot in the arch. This fracture is thought to be the result of hyperextension of the head and neck such that the posterior arch is forced caudally by the occiput (Fig. 1.38). Nondisplaced or only moderately displaced simple fractures are usually stable, but stability should be assessed with flexion/extension films and cineradiography. If the fracture is not stable, it should be treated with either a Minerva cast, halo plaster fixation, or surgical fusion from the occiput to C2.

The second type is the so-called Jefferson fracture consisting of a four-part comminution at the ring of the atlas. This injury results from a vertical load directed in the −y axis (Fig. 1.39). This vector of injury may occur (*a*) during roll-over accidents in which the occupant's head strikes the roof of the vehicle, (*b*) in accidents in which the occupant's head strikes the windshield or dashboard directly, and (*c*) in accidents in which the occupants are thrown free from the vehicle.

Fractures of the axis frequently fall into one of two categories: hangman's fracture or traumatic spondylolisthesis and the dens or odontoid fracture. Hangman's fracture (traumatic spondylolisthesis), so named because of its common association with judicial hanging, is a misnomer, since it is not the hangman whose neck is fractured, and White and Panjabi have suggested the term "hanged person fracture."

This fracture is often seen in motor vehicle accidents, although the outcome is usually less final than in judicial hanging. This is because the sustained load applied by the noose stretches and damages the spinal cord, resulting in neurological death (with strangulation, of course, as the added, definitive factor producing death). In traumatic spondylolisthesis from motor vehicle trauma, however, the cord is often not damaged because of the instantaneous decompression that results from the fracture. These injuries usually result from the occupant's forehead striking the windshield or dashboard or during roll-over accidents in which there is some extension component associated with a vertical load (Fig. 1.40).

These fractures are usually treated by immobilization. In more severe injuries in which anterior elements such as the disc and anterior longitudinal ligament are injured, the lack of stability that results may not be adequately treated with immobilization alone, and surgical fusion may be necessary.

The second kind of fracture of the axis is that of the dens or odontoid, and these have been classified into three distinct types (Fig. 1.41). Type I consists usually of an oblique fracture through the upper part of the dens well above the transverse ligament. Stability even in the case of non-union, therefore, is not compromised.

Type II fracture consists of a linear horizontal fracture through the base of the dens and is generally thought to be unstable. Movements of the head and neck in this condition can have disastrous neurological consequence. Management of this type is difficult, in that there is a very high rate of non-union. In spite of this, I recommend rigid immobilization for several months.

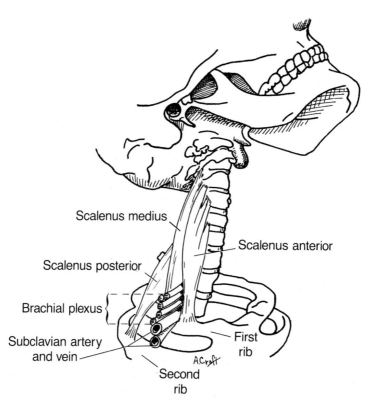

Figure 1.36. Roots of the brachial plexus along with the subclavian vessels pass between the scalenus anterior and the scalenus medius. These muscles along with the scalenus posterior facilitate both flexion and lateral flexion of the neck.

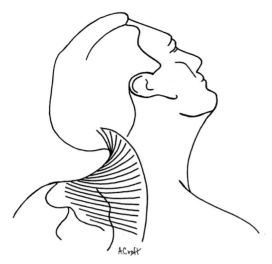

Figure 1.37.   Bilateral contraction of the trapezius produces extension and accentuation of the cervical lordotic curve. Unilateral contraction (illustrated) results in extension, accentuation of the curve, lateral flexion ipsilaterally, and contralateral rotation in the same manner as the sternocleidomastoid.

Surgical fusion may be resorted to if, after immobilization, there is failure of union.

Type III fracture occurs downward through the body of the axis and is generally more stable. It is usually nondisplaced or only minimally displaced and can be treated by immobilization with a 90% success rate (89). After fusion of this or the other types of dens fractures, stability should be evaluated with flexion/extension views as well as cineradiography.

All of these fractures may be seen in association with the hangman's fracture and may result from a similar type of injury vector. The force is directed from the anterior arch of the atlas through the dens (Fig.1.42).

Other less commonly seen fractures include fractures of the transverse processes of the atlas and axis and fractures of the body and spinous process of the axis. Small avulsion injuries of C2 have also been described.

DISLOCATION

Complete dislocation at the occiput-C1 level is rarely compatible with life, although I recently reviewed the case of a man who while crossing the street had been struck by a motor vehicle and thrown some 20 feet. His injury was initially not appreciated by the radiologist, but the patient was admitted to the hospital for observation. On the next day, a stress test was performed (described later in this chapter), and complete separation of occiput-C1 was shown to have occurred, along with transient neurological symptoms. Some disruption could be seen, in retrospect, on the admitting crosstable lateral film.

Atlantoaxial dislocations may be anterior, posterior, or rotatory depending upon the injury vector. Anterior dislocation is the result of a ruptured transverse ligament. Posterior dislocation of the atlas may occur as a result of a blow to the chin such as would occur from impact with a steering wheel, dashboard, or seatback. Usually, the transverse ligament is intact, and these patients can be treated with traction, with the dislocation manually reduced. Anterior dislocation is highly unstable, is often associated with a dens fracture, and is often a fatal injury.

INSTABILITY

White and Panjabi (88) define "clinical instability" as "the loss of the ability of the spine under *physiologic loads* to maintain relationships between vertebrae in such a way that there is neither damage nor *subsequent* irritation to the spinal cord or nerve roots, and, in addition, there is no development of *incapacitating deformity* or *pain* due to structural changes [*italics* mine]."

And Scher (72) defines instability as "abnormal mobility between any pair of vertebrae, with or without pain or other clinical manifestation." Certainly this is true. Instability may not always result in incapacitating pain, at least not in its early stages.

Instability is usually the result of fracture of bone and/or disruption of ligaments. Muscular injury usually does not result in instability as defined; thus this injury is discussed more fully in Chapter 8.

In the determination of clinical instability, x-rays and fluoroscopic cineradiography are most useful. One of the difficulties encountered when the measurement of x-rays is used in the evaluation is the magnification factor (88). The source-to-film distance is standardized at 72 inches (1.83 m) for the cervical spine. The factor that varies is the object-to-film distance. The greater this distance, the greater the magnification. Thus

$$M = \left(\frac{100 \times D_2}{D_1 - D_2}\right)\% \qquad \text{(Eq. 1.3)}$$

where M equals magnification in percentage of increase, D_1 equals the source (x-ray)-to-film distance, and D_2 equals the object (spine)-to-film distance.

Certainly, the spine of a man with wide shoulders will be magnified much more than that of a woman with slender shoulders. The difference in magnification may be as much as 15%. At a distance of 14 inches (D_2), the object will be magnified by 24% at a source-to-film distance (D_1) of 72 inches.

Powers et al. (89) uses a ratio of the distances between the basion/posterior arch of atlas and the opisthion/anterior arch of atlas to determine occipitoatlantal dislocations. A

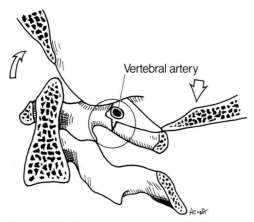

Figure 1.38. Hyperextension injuries may result in fracture of the posterior arch of the atlas. This occurs when the occiput is moved caudally against the posterior arch with great force. That part of the posterior arch that is grooved by the vertebral artery is the weakest (*circled area*) and, consequently, the most common site of fracture. (Adapted from Panjabi MM, White AA: Physical properties and functional biomechanics of the spine. In White AA, Panjabi MM (eds): *Clinical Biomechanics of the Spine.* Philadelphia, JB Lippincott, 1978, p 125.)

ratio of less than 1 is normal. The test is not valid if fracture is present (Fig. 1.43.)

The *posterior cervical line* that runs along the anterior cortex of the posterior arch of C1 and the spinous processes of C2 and C3 has been described by Swischuk (92). In the adult spine, the anterior cortex of the spinous process of C2 normally lies just posterior to this line. If it lies more than 2 mm behind this line, a hangman's fracture may be presumed. In children and adolescents, however, a pseudosubluxation may occur at C2 such that this line may pass through the cortex or lie 1.5–2.0 mm anterior to it (91) (Fig. 1.44). It has been shown that in the normal cervical spine of a child, an anterior pseudosubluxation of up to 4 mm can occur at other levels (92).

The ADI has long been a subject of controversy. Normally, this space is maintained by the taut transverse ligament of the atlas. Damage to this ligament allows forward translation of the anterior arch of the atlas relative to the anterior aspect of the dens, resulting in an increased ADI. The controversy revolves around the subject of normal measurements. Some have stated that in children the normal physiological ligamentous laxity allows an ADI of up to 5 mm (93). Most children display an ADI of less than 3 mm, however, and most adults display an ADI of 2 mm or less (94).

There are only a few reports of survival after complete rupture of the transverse ligament (66).

The rotary subluxation of the atlas on the axis is often traumatically induced by the acceleration/deceleration injury, especially when the victim's head is turned at the time of impact. This condition may be difficult to diagnose clinically. In more severe cases, the patient may present with a torticollis and a "Cock Robin" appearance when the head is held in slight lateral flexion and contralateral rotation.

Radiographically, this may be seen on the AP open mouth view as a disparity between the lateral masses of the atlas and the dens. This space will be wider on the side of posterior atlas rotation. The shadow of the lateral mass will be narrower on this side (Fig. 1.20). White and Panjabi (73) suggest that in order to diagnose a true rotary subluxation, there must also be an increase in the ADI seen on lateral films. This occurs, I believe,

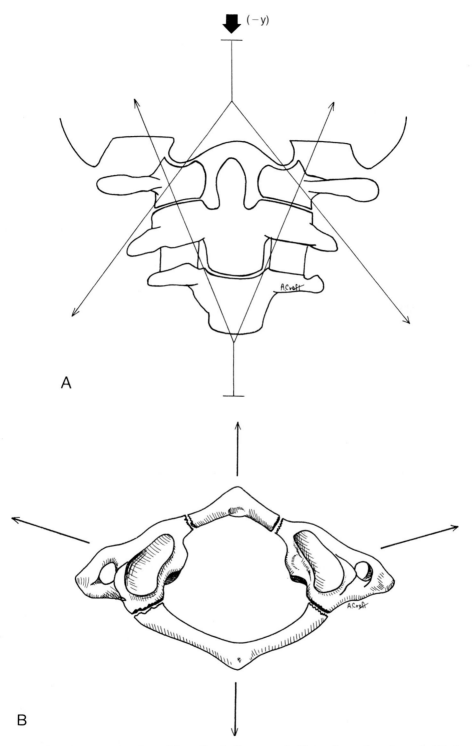

Figure 1.39.   Direct vertical loading of the atlas in the −y axis (**A**) produces the characteristic four-part Jefferson fracture (**B**). (Adapted from Panjabi MM, White AA: Physical properties and functional biomechanics of the spine. In White AA, Panjabi MM (eds): *Clinical Biomechanics of the Spine.* Philadelphia, WB Saunders, 1978, p 127; and Harris JH Jr: The normal cervical spine. In: *The Radiology of Acute Cervical Spine Trauma.* Baltimore, Williams & Wilkins, 1978, p 76.)

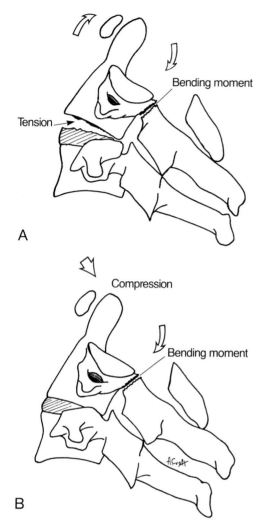

Figure 1.40. **A.** Typical forces encountered with judicial hanging. These forces result in traumatic spondylolisthesis or the so-called hangman's fracture. **B.** The hangman's fracture, which is produced by the typical rear-end impact motor vehicle accident, results from a similar bending moment, but instead of tension at the anterior aspect of the axis there is compression. (Adapted from Panjabi MM, White AA: Physical properties and functional biomechanics of the spine. In White AA, Panjabi MM (eds): *Clinical Biomechanics of the Spine.* Philadelphia, WB Saunders, 1978, p 139.)

only in extremes of subluxation, and the diagnosis should, therefore, be one of degree. The ADI may, in fact, be normal.

Several types of subluxation have been described by Fielding and Hawkins (98). These are defined in terms of relationship of the atlas upon the axis and include: type I, rotary fixation with no anterior displace-

ment (the odontoid acts as a pivot); type II, rotary fixation with an anterior displacement of 3–5 mm (one lateral articular process acts as a pivot); type III, rotary fixation with an anterior displacement of more than 5 mm; and type IV, rotary fixation with posterior displacement (Fig. 1.45). With the exception of the bilateral posterior subluxation that usually results from hypoplasia, absence, or fracture of the dens, all are clinically stable in the absence of neurological deficit. When neurological symptoms are present, however, this lesion should be considered clinically unstable until proven otherwise.

Rotary subluxation can generally be treated conservatively, with manipulation and other noninvasive measures. In all cases of trauma, however, the degree of instability must be carefully evaluated. Lateral flexion AP open mouth views and rotation AP open mouth views can be taken with standard x-ray equipment, but cineradiography should also be used. Both plain film radiography and cineradiography are useful in evaluating the dynamics of the lesion. Computed tomography (CT) scanning, as well as providing more detailed information about bony and soft tissue structures, allows more precise evaluation of the static lesion. Instability may be a contraindication to manipulation. Rotary subluxation without instability is not.

Trauma and Instability of the Lower Cervical Spine (C3–C7)

As in the case of the upper cervical spine, the more severe acceleration/deceleration-related trauma may result in vertebral fracture. The degree of injury may not be clinically apparent, and correlation between clinical findings and x-ray examination is crucial. Many times, a fracture is not readily visualized on standard cervical x-ray studies, and special views are necessary. In some cases of fracture, the only easily visible finding may be retropharyngeal space widening from extravasation of blood.

Fracture, dislocation, and radiographic technique are discussed in greater detail in Chapter 6. The discussion here is limited to

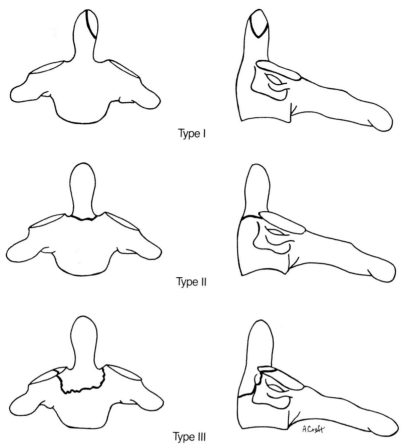

Type I

Type II

Type III

A.Craft

Figure 1.41. Three types of dens fracture. All may result from hyperextension injuries to the neck. Type II fractures may be difficult to distinguish because of the so-called "mach" effect produced by the shadow of the superimposed arch of the atlas.

the biomechanics that produce the lesion and to the biomechanics and instability that result from it.

FRACTURE

A forceful hyperflexion or deceleration injury, whether the primary trauma to the neck or the secondary phase of an injury (i.e., following the hyperextension phase), may result in a *wedge fracture* of the vertebral body. This is generally seen on AP and lateral radiographs as a loss of anterior body height (Fig. 1.46) and is generally considered a stable fracture. The use of the term "stable" is often misleading, however. Most often, a spinal fracture is said to be stable if it does not pose a serious neurological threat to the spinal cord or nerve roots. It also usu-ally implies that the fracture can be treated with halo traction, a Minerva jacket, or cervical collar immobilization and that surgical decompression or fusion may not be necessary, at least not until conservative measures have failed and/or the lesion has proved to be unstable.

In truth, however, the forces resulting from moderate acceleration and decelera-tion of the neck in vehicular accidents can be great, and the clinician should assume that significant injury to the invertebral disc and the posterior ligamentous complex has occurred when a wedge fracture is seen on x-ray.

Ligamentous instability results in bio-mechanical instability, and this equates to clinical instability. Therefore, a stable frac-ture in no way connotes clinical stability; to

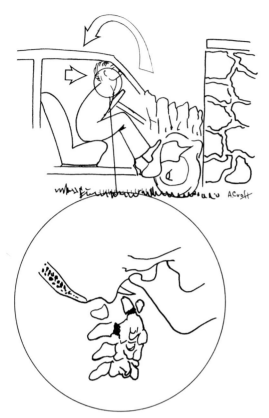

Figure 1.42. The same injury vector that produces the hangman's fracture also produces the various types of dens fracture. Illustrated is a type II dens fracture and a hangman's fracture. (Adapted from Sances A Jr, Mykelbust JB, Maiman DJ, Larson SJ, Cusick JF, Jodat RW: The biomechanics of spinal injuries. *CRC Crit Rev Biomed Eng* 11(1):1–76, 1984 (review).)

the contrary, forces severe enough to fracture bone are usually adequate enough to damage ligaments and muscles.

The *clay shoveler's fracture* is seen, in order of frequency, at the spinous process of C7, C6, or T1 (96). It results from sudden or unexpected muscular contractions such as those seen in the neck and upper back of a man shoveling clay. He is biomechanically prepared to sling the weight of a shovel full of clay over his shoulder and then return the unladen shovel to its previous position. When the clay is wet, however, it sticks to the shovel and does not release when he throws it over his shoulder. This produces severe compensatory muscular contraction and results in the fracture. The same type of

phenomenon occurs in motor vehicle trauma but as a result of pulls in different vectors and may be seen in whiplash trauma (97).

The clay shoveler's fracture can occur at multiple levels, but this is uncommon. It is a stable fracture but may signify ligamentous injury. Some suggest early surgical removal of the fragment (98), whereas others treat the patient with this lesion with a cervical orthosis (99, 100). I recommend immobilization in a cervical orthosis such as is seen in Figure 8.31*E–H*, for up to 6 weeks, followed by range of motion and rehabilitative exercises. Large amounts of soft tissue imposition between fracture surfaces will prevent union, however, and may ultimately necessitate surgical removal of the fragment.

The most severe flexion forces produce the comminuted *flexion teardrop fracture* of the anterior aspect of the vertebral body. Commonly associated with the anterior cervical cord syndrome (see Chapter 9), this fracture also signifies significant disruption of the posterior ligamentous complex and intervertebral disc, as well as the anterior longitudinal ligament (97), and is highly unstable (Fig. 1.47).

Fractures of the *articular pillar* may occur with a combined motion of hyperextension and rotation. When this occurs, the vertical compressive load results in a vertical fracture through the pillar.

On the lateral cervical x-ray, this fracture may be seen as a "double outline" sign (101), while on the AP cervical x-ray, a disruption of the normally smooth and wavy cortical line may be seen (Fig. 1.48). Often, however, the pillar fracture is not appreciated in these views or in the oblique views, and special pillar views should be taken (Chapter 4).

When isolated, fracture of the articular pillar is stable in spite of radicular symptoms resulting from local swelling, hemorrhage, or displaced fracture fragments. Discovery of this fracture, as with discovery of any other type of fracture, should prompt a search for other injuries, and CT scanning is most useful in this regard. Fractures of the lamina are also seen with this type of injury.

The *compression fracture* is the result of a vertical force directed along the −y axis. The

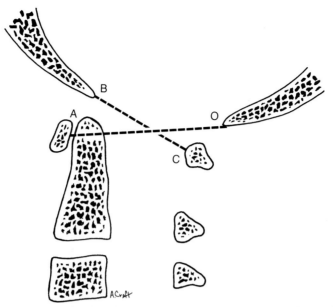

Figure 1.43. The ratio of the distances between the basion/posterior arch of atlas (*BC*) and the opisthion/anterior arch of atlas (*OA*) is normally less than 1. In cases of atlantooccipital dislocation, the ratio may be more than 1. (Adapted from Powers B, Miller MD, Kramer RS, Martinez S, Gehweiler JA Jr: Traumatic anterior atlantooccipital dislocation. *Neurosurgery* 4(1):12–17, 1979.)

vector of injury is essentially the same as that in the Jefferson fracture. Moderate compressive forces produce minimal compression. With greater force, however, the endplates tend to rupture into the vertebral body, and vertical trabeculation collapses. The intervertebral disc is frequently torn or ruptured, although posterior herniation of nuclear material is unlikely with pure vertical compression alone.

When the force of injury is very great, the nucleus pulposus is imploded into the body of the vertebra through the endplate. This causes the vertebra to explode from within (35). Frequently, the posterior displacement of bone fragments results in the acute anterior cervical cord syndrome due to cord contusion (Chapter 9), although these fragments may spontaneously reduce such that the amount of neurological damage appears way out of proportion to the injury as it appears on x-ray (Fig. 1.47). This injury is less severe than the flexion teardrop fracture and is considered stable, although ligamentous injuries should be ruled out.

These fractures can usually be managed with rest and a semirigid orthosis (preferably one that stabilizes the upper thoracic spine as well). The orthosis should be worn 4–8 weeks, depending on the rate of healing as evidenced by follow-up radiographic evaluation. In all cases of fracture, those patients who smoke should be encouraged to quit, at least until bony union has occurred. Brown et al. (102) recently studied the relationship of cigarette smoking to the incidence of failure to fuse after posterior lateral lumbar fusion. After subjects in this study had been matched for age, gender, and race, it was noted that those in the nonsmoking group had a failure rate of 8%, whereas those in the smoking group had a failure rate of 40%.

In more severe comminuted fractures, small fragments of bone may penetrate the posterior longitudinal ligament and injure the cord. These may not be visible on standard x-ray views and may require CT evaluation. CT scanning should be performed routinely when fracture is present or in the presence of moderate to severe neurological injury.

The *extension teardrop fracture* has been described by Holdsworth (103, 104) as a triangle-shaped fracture of the anterior inferior body of the axis. This injury is the result

Figure 1.44. Posterior cervical line as described by Swischuk (92). The normal relationship is illustrated in the *unshaded area.* In children, the anterior cortex of the spinous process of C2 may be posteriorly displaced up to 2 mm—a condition known as "pseudosubluxation." A disparity of more than 2 mm, however, should be assumed to be pathological until proven otherwise. In adults, a displacement of more than 2 mm may indicate a hangman's fracture.

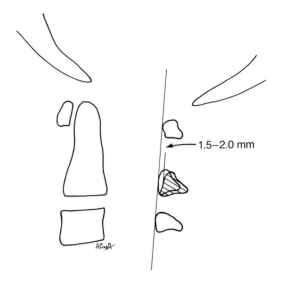

of severe hyperextension forces that rupture the anterior longitudinal ligament and fracture the bone. Anterior ligamentous damage results in a spinal segment that is stable in flexion but unstable in extension (Fig. 1.49).

Stability of the injury must be evaluated following bony union. This fracture should be treated the same as with compression fracture. In some instances, surgical stabilization may ultimately be necessary. In an older less active adult with minimal instability, surgery is probably not indicated.

Other fractures seen in whiplash trauma include those of the articulating facets and of the uncinate processes. Occasionally, a fractured superior facet will move anteriorly and encroach upon the neuroforamina. This is usually seen clinically as a monoradiculopathy. Although from a neurological standpoint both types of fractures are stable, clinical stability must be assessed as soon as healing is complete.

Treatment should consist of semirigid immobilization for 3–6 weeks, followed by passive and active range of motion exercises, appropriate manipulation to restore normal biomechanical function, and appropriate physical therapy modalities to aid in the rehabilitation process. The latter should include cervical traction. This postfracture healing protocol should be part of the man-

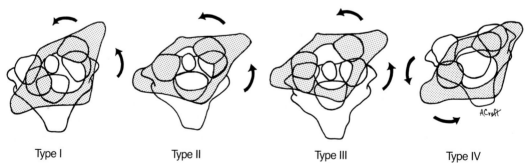

| Type I | Type II | Type III | Type IV |

Figure 1.45. Various types of rotary fixation or subluxation of the atlas. In type I rotary fixation, there is no anterior displacement and the odontoid acts as a pivot. In type II rotary fixation, there is 3–5 mm of anterior displacement, and one articular process acts as a pivot. In the type III rotary fixation, anterior displacement exceeds 5 mm; and in the type IV rotary fixation, there is posterior displacement. (Adapted from Fielding JW, Hawkins RJ: Atlanto-axial rotatory fixation: fixed rotatory subluxation of the atlanto-axial, joint. *J Bone Joint Surg* 59A(1):37–44, 1977.)

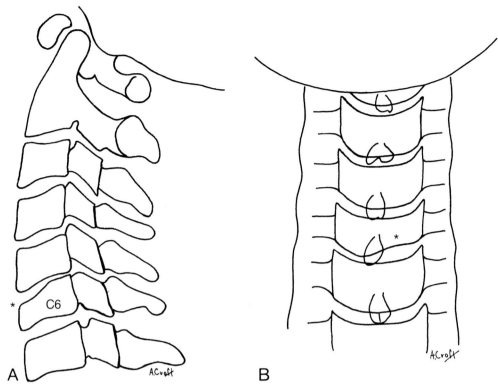

Figure 1.46. Typical wedge fracture from severe hyperflexion trauma. This may be a primary injury or the secondary (flexion) phase of an acceleration/deceleration injury. Usually, it is visible on the neutral lateral radiograph (illustrated in **A** at *asterisk*) as a loss in the anterior vertical height of the vertebral body (shown at C6). Its presence can sometimes also be detected on the AP radiograph (illustrated in **B** at *asterisk*).

agement of *all* fractures and generally will result in a shorter convalescence and a more favorable long-term prognosis.

Table 1.9 depicts the mechanism of injury of some of the fractures discussed. A more complete review of mechanisms is found in Chapter 6. The degree of stability for various cervical spine fractures is outlined in Table 1.10.

DISLOCATION

In the cervical spine, as in other parts of the body, dislocations are frequently associated with fractures and are best described as fracture dislocations. In the lower cervical spine, these frequently go unrecognized (105). Another consideration in the evaluation of the trauma patient is the fact that although biomechanical forces were severe enough to cause a dislocation, it may have reduced spontaneously and x-ray appearances may be perfectly normal.

Complete dislocation of a spinal segment is the result of severe trauma in which all ligamentous structures are disrupted and the spinal cord is usually critically damaged. Steele's rule of thirds provides a method of approach in the evaluation of upper cervical spinal trauma (106). According to this rule, the inside AP diameter of the atlas can be divided into thirds: One third is taken up by the dens, one third is taken up by the spinal cord, and the last third is potential space. This and the normal AP diameters at other spinal levels are indicated in Figure 1.50.

Unilateral facet dislocations can usually be recognized on plain lateral x-ray films as an overriding of one vertebra on another equivalent to one half or less of the AP diameter of the body of the vertebra. On oblique films, this dislocation may be recognized as a disruption of the normal stacked appearance of facets and laminae

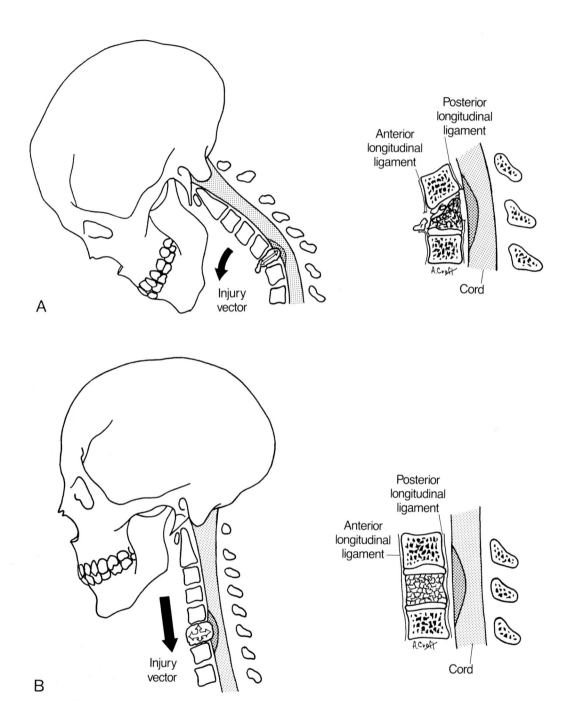

Figure 1.47.   A. Flexion teardrop fracture. **B.** Burst fracture. Both fractures may be associated with severe anterior cord injury. Flexion teardrop fractures are highly unstable, whereas burst fractures are considered stable. In both cases, the cord may be severely contused and/or lacerated. *Heavily stippled areas* represent the area of cord damage. In the flexion teardrop fracture, there is often complete disruption of the anterior and posterior longitudinal ligaments, whereas in the burst fracture, these structures are usually intact.

Table 1.9.
Mechanism of Injury in Cervical Spine Fractures[a]

Type	Mechanism of Injury
Simple wedge fracture	Flexion
Clay shoveler's fracture	Flexion
Flexion teardrop fracture	Flexion
Pillar fracture	Extension/rotation
Bursting fracture (Jefferson fracture of the atlas) (burst fracture of lower cervical vertebrae)	Vertical compression
Extension teardrop fracture	Extension
Posterior neural arch fracture (atlas)	Extension
Hangman's fracture	Extension
Facet fracture	Extension, Lateral flexion
Uncinate process fracture	Lateral Flexion

[a]Adapted from Harris JH Jr: *The Radiology of Acute Cervical Spine Trauma.* Baltimore, Williams & Wilkins, 1978, p 29.

(Fig. 1.51). This injury is usually the result of a combined injury vector of flexion and rotation. Stability depends upon the severity of the trauma. White and Panjabi (107) have stated that when the initial trauma is significant enough to produce neurological injury, the segment should be considered clinically unstable. Most reports have indicated that these injuries can be treated conservatively, with there being a low incidence of late instability (108), but in experimental studies Beatson (109) has shown that when unilateral facet dislocation occurs, there is a rupture of the interspinous ligament and the involved joint capsule with some damage to the disc and posterior longitudinal ligament. The disparity in these and other reports is usually in the definition of "late instability." As is discussed later in this chapter, this diagnosis is based upon x-ray criteria about which there has been general agreement. These x-ray criteria, however, are based upon plain films alone, do not include the evaluation of fluorovideo motion studies, and do not encompass clinical evaluation. Fluorovideo (cineradiography) has been shown to detect abnormal motion in cases in which plain films were evaluated as "normal," and plain films have been shown to detect abnormality in cases in which fluorovideo was evaluated as "normal" (110, 111) (see Chapter 3).

Correlation between clinical, radiographic, and cineradiographic presenta-

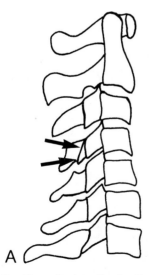
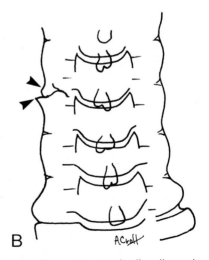

Figure 1.48. The articular pillar fracture is often missed on routine x-ray examination. It may be seen in the lateral view (illustrated in **A**) as a "double outline" sign. This is formed by the posteriorly displaced articular pillar fragment (*arrows*). On the AP lower cervical view (illustrated in **B**), there may be an interruption of the normally smooth, undulating lateral cortical margin (*arrowheads*). These fractures are better appreciated on oblique and pillar views.

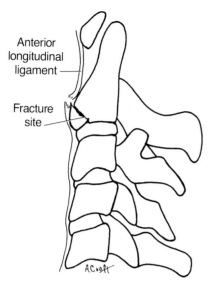

Figure 1.49. The extension teardrop fracture is seen following severe hyperextension injuries. Because the anterior longitudinal ligament is ruptured, this injury is stable in flexion but unstable in extension.

tion, force and vector of injury, and prognosis is an area in which further research is needed. This lesion should be considered clinically unstable, and the patient with this lesion should be treated with a flexible cervical orthosis and the appropriate physical therapy modality for 3–6 weeks. Later on, mild traction should be instituted along with light manipulation to reduce scar formation and restore normal spinal biomechanics. This should be accompanied by muscle strengthening and range of motion exercises.

Bilateral facet dislocation is the result of severe hyperflexion of the neck and is a highly unstable condition even after reduction. It has been shown that in order for this amount of displacement to occur, all of the following must be ruptured: both facet joint capsules, the posterior longitudinal ligament, the interspinous ligament, and the disc (109). Surgical stabilization is usually necessary to achieve ultimate stability.

SUBLUXATION

Subluxation is a term that defies casual explanation and precise definition. Its use, therefore, is highly controversial and hotly debated and probably will remain so. In medical dictionaries, subluxation is defined as, simply, "less than a luxation," but in chiropractic, its very essence perhaps encompasses one of the most fundamental principles of chiropractic theory. By most conventional schools of thought, it is considered not so much a static finding on x-ray but rather a dynamic joint dysrelationship usually requiring manual manipulation for reduction.

Several definitions have been adopted; perhaps none are universally acceptable. Thus for discussions of clinical instability in this text, *subluxation* is defined as a state of dysrelationship between contiguous vertebrae, due to either disease, injury, or both, that is demonstrable on plain film radiography of the cervical spine. (This x-ray evaluation must include flexion and extension views.) Subluxation is not the result of fracture but rather is the result of joint laxity which, in turn, may be the consequence of degenerative or other disease or traumatic ligamentous stretching or rupture. Both can and often do coexist.

In speaking of subluxation of the spine, the usual convention is to describe the upper vertebral unit and its relationship to the vertebral unit immediately below it. For

Table 1.10.
Stability in Cervical Spine Fractures[a]

Stable	Unstable
Simple wedge fracture	Flexion teardrop fracture
Posterior neural arch fracture (atlas)	Extension teardrop fracture (stable in flexion, unstable in extension)
Pillar fracture	Hangman's fracture
Uncinate process fracture	Jefferson fracture of atlas
Clay shoveler's fracture	Type II dens fracture
Transverse process fracture	
Type I dens fracture	
Type III dens fracture	

[a]Adapted from Harris JH Jr: *The Radiology of Acute Cervical Spine Trauma.* Baltimore, Williams & Wilkins, 1978, p 41.

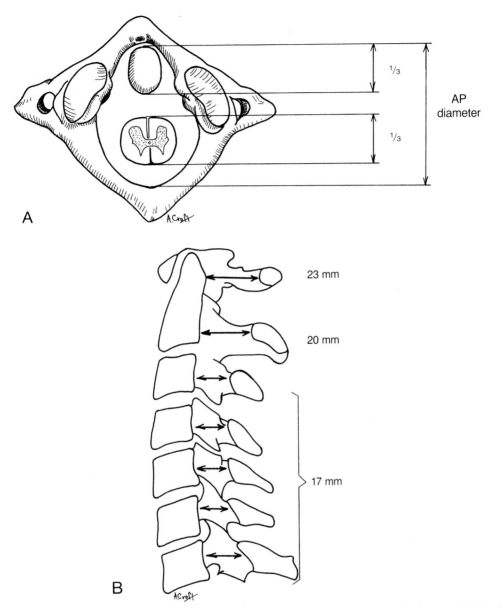

Figure 1.50. **A.** Steele's rule of thirds. One third of the AP inside diameter of the atlas is occupied by the cord, one third is occupied by the dens, and the remaining third is potential space. **B.** Average AP inside diameters at subsequent cervical levels when films are exposed at the standard distance of 72 inches. (Actual measurements are slightly less when adjusted for geometric distortion.) (Adapted from Panjabi MM, White AA: Physical properties and function biomechanics of the spine. In White AA, Panjabi MM (eds): *Clinical Biomechanics of the Spine.* Philadelphia, JB Lippincott, 1978, pp 132 and 199.)

example, the condition in which C2 has moved forward in relationship to C3 (+z axis) is described as an anterior subluxation of C2 on C3 or, simply, anterior subluxation C2-C3. Other forms of subluxation have been described in chiropractic and medical literature, but the description and management of these are beyond the scope of this textbook.

The amount or degree of subluxation is significant. I have stated that subluxation may be a normal finding in children (pseu-

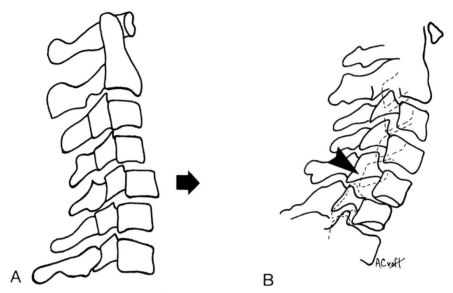

Figure 1.51. Illustrated appearance of unilateral facet dislocation on x-ray. **A.** Anterior translation equal to or less than one half of the AP diameter of the vertebral body is suggestive of unilateral facet dislocation (*arrow*). **B.** Unilateral facet dislocation may be seen as an overriding or disrelationship of normal facet overlapping (*arrowhead*). (Adapted from Harris JH Jr: The normal cervical spine. In: *The Radiology of Acute Cervical Spine Trauma.* Baltimore, Williams & Wilkins, 1978, p 63.)

dosubluxation) which may, in fact, be a contradiction in terms and all the more reason to define the word in a dynamic rather than a static sense. I, therefore, discuss the criteria for anterior subluxation only as it relates to trauma and posttraumatic sequelae.

INSTABILITY

In general, clinical instability in addition to other clinical findings is manifested by subluxation. I define clinical instability as any interruption in the normal smooth transitional vertebral biomechanics as evidenced by incomplete, jerky, or excessive spinal movements. This may be demonstrated by flexion and extension x-rays, cineradiography, or both and is often (but not always) associated with chronic or intractable pain syndromes and neurological symptomatology. Clinical instability usually precedes the subsequent accelerated development of spondylosis or degenerative disc disease at the same levels. These findings must occur during passive movements within normal physiological ranges of motion and under normal physiological loading (Table 1.11).

Radiographic Evidence of Instability

Instability of the upper cervical spine may be appreciated on plain films or by cineradiography of the neck, usually by ranges of motion that when adjusted for the age of the patient may be considered excessive (see Tables 1.7 and 1.8). The most reliable x-ray evidence of instability in the lower cervical spine is the anterior subluxation. Its presence is significant because the incidence of delayed instability is said to be 21% (112). This condition is severe and may require surgical stabilization. When anterior subluxation does not increase when there is change from the neutral to the flexion position, however, the amount of soft tissue damage and the likelihood of delayed instability are less (113).

The x-ray findings associated with anterior subluxation include: (*a*) a fanning of the spinous processes from damage to the posterior element, (*b*) a narrowing of the anterior disc space and a widening of the posterior disc space, (*c*) a loss of cervical lordosis or a kyphotic angulation at the level of the lesion equal to or more than 11° more than that found at adjacent levels, (*d*) a lack of parallelism of the facet joints, and (*e*) a

Table 1.11.
Score Card for Clinical Instability of the Cervical Spine

Findings	Point Value[a]
Positive stretch test	20
Spondylosis or degenerative disc disease developing within 3 years of injury	20
Plain x-ray evidence of instability	15
Cineradiographic (fluorovideo) evidence of instability	15
Any documented cervical spine fracture (not counting healed fractures)	15
Spinal cord or nerve root irritation subsequent to injury (especially with progressive worsening)	15
Initial neurological symptoms lasting longer than 1 week	5
Intractable pain resulting from injury	5
Spondylosis or degenerative disc disease present at the time of injury	5

[a] $\geq$30 means definite clinical instability; $\geq$20 means clinical instability probable; 10–15 means clinical instability possible; and $\leq$5 means clinical instability unlikely.

forward translation of one vertebra over another. These do not all need to be present, especially the last. White and Panjabi (70), using motion segments from cadavers, have conducted experiments on the stability of the cervical spine. They have suggested that 2.7 mm (3.5 mm on lateral x-ray) is the upper limit of the normal translational movement. Green et al. (71) have

Table 1.12.
X-ray Findings in Anterior Subluxation

Decreased anterior disc height (at involved segment)

Increased posterior disc height (at involved segment)

Nonparallel facet planes (at involved segment)

Fanning of spinous processes (at involved segment)

Kyphotic angulation of $\geq$ 11° (at involed segment)

Anterior translation of superior segment over inferior segment of 1–2 mm (at involved segment) (measured from the posterior inferior corner of the body of the superior vertebra to the posterior superior corner of the inferior vertebra)

stated that 1–3 mm of movement should be considered subluxation and that 3.5 mm or more is only seen in frank dislocation, fracture, or pseudosubluxation. Others have suggested 1–2 mm as indicating subluxation. Scher (72) studied normal cervical spine x-rays and found that in none had there been seen more that 1 mm in translation. He stated that the 3.5 mm criterion suggested by White and Panjabi is seldom seen clinically. Figure 1.52 illustrates these x-ray findings which are summarized in Table 1.12.

I have stated that cineradiography is important in the evaluation of ligamentous instability. Although several studies have indicated the importance and sensitivity of cineradiography in the evaluation of soft tissue lesions of the neck. I am unaware of any published accounts of specific normal fluoroscopic biomechanics of the cervical spine and am currently engaged in this research. Until more data are available, I believe that the protocol described in Table 1.13 should be followed.

Table 1.13.
Protocol for Cineradrographic (Fluorovideo) Analysis of the Cervical Spine

AP view

Cone in on upper cervical spine
   Nodding (flexion and extension) with mouth open and closed
   Rotation to left and right with mouth open and closed
   Lateral flexion to left and right with mouth open and closed

Lower cervical spine
   Rotation to left and right
   Lateral flexion to left and right

Lateral view

Cone in on upper cervical spine
   Nodding (flexion and extension)
   Rotation to left and right

Lower cervical spine
   Flexion and extension
   Rotation to left and right

Oblique view

Cone in on upper cervical spine
   Nodding (flexion and extension)

Lower cervical spine
   Flexion and extension

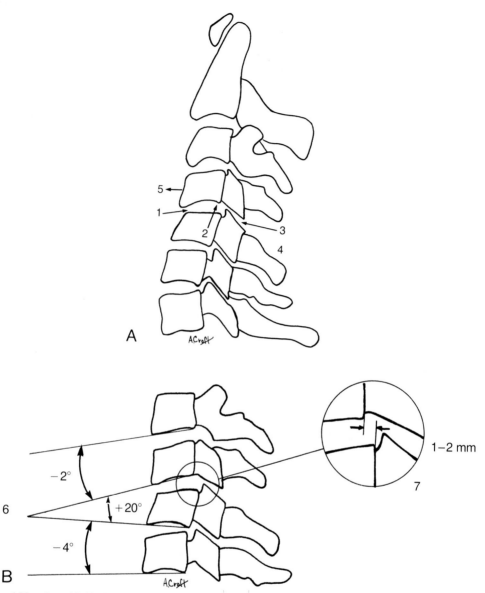

Figure 1.52.   A and B. Illustrated common x-ray findings in anterior subluxation of the lower cervical spine. These include: (*1*) decreased anterior disc height, (*2*) increased posterior disc height, (*3*) nonparallel facet surfaces, (*4*) fanning of adjacent spinous processes, (*5*) anterior translation of the superior vertebra, (*6*) kyphotic angulation equal to or more than 11°, and (*7*) anterior displacement of 1–2 mm or more measured between the posterior inferior corner of the superior vertebra and the posterior superior corner of the vertebra below. **B.** To determine kyphotic angulation, the angle between adjacent subluxated segments is first measured by drawing lines parallel with their inferior surfaces. Similar measurements are then obtained one level above and one level below. Convergent angles are designated by a positive number, and divergent angles are assigned a negative number. These second measurements are then subtracted from that of the primary angle (subluxated segment). The final figure must be equal to or more than 11° in either case. Thus,

$$20 - (-2) = 22$$

both are more than 11

$$20 - (-4) = 24$$

(Adapted from White AA, Johnson RM, Panjabi MM, Southwich WO: Biomechanical analysis of clinical stability in the cervical spine. *Clin Orthop* 109:85, 1975.)

Stretch Test

White and Panjabi (114, 115) have demonstrated experimentally that axial traction along the y axis will abnormally distract an intervertebral space when either all of the anterior structures or all of the posterior structures have been transected. The stretch test has been used under careful clinical supervision to detect areas of instability that were difficult to appreciate in other ways. Because the spinal cord and nerve roots can safely be stretched a short distance in this axis, it is considered a safe test when performed under the protocol to be described. The test is intended to find lesions of the lower cervical spine, although I have observed one case of occipitoatlantal separation with the use of this test.

The stretch test indicates abnormality when either an interspace separation of more than 1.7 mm or a change in angle between vertebrae of more than 7.5° is found when the neutral nonstretched spine is compared with one under axial traction equivalent to one third of the body weight. Table 1.14 is an outline of the procedure for this test which is illustrated in Figure 1.53.

Evolution of Current Thinking on the Forces Generated in and the Results of Rear-End Impact Collisions

Severy et al. (116) experimented with anthropomorphic dummies and human volunteers in the 1950's. They found that initially the torso was being accelerated underneath the unrestrained head. The head then accelerated secondarily at a greater rate than the torso. They found that an 8-mile/hour rear-end collision produced a 2-G acceleration of the vehicle and a 5-G acceleration of the head. This occurred within a span of 300 msec or less and is shown graphically in Figure 1.54. It can be

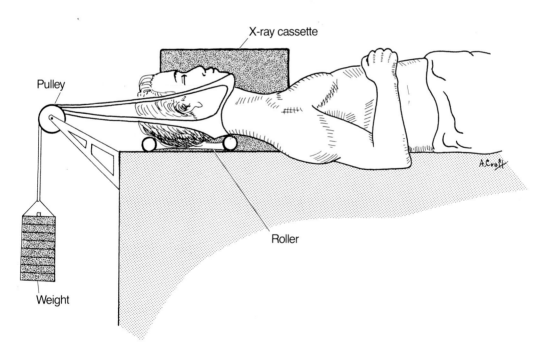

Figure 1.53. Stretch test. Traction is induced by the gradual stepwise addition of weight. Serial cross-table lateral x-rays are taken as incremental loads up to 33% of body weight (or 65 lb) are applied. At the first sign of neurological involvement, intervertebral joint widening of more than 1.7 mm or intervertebral angulation of more than 7.5°, the test is concluded. See Table 1.14. (Adapted from Panjabi MM, White AA: Physical properties and functional biomechanics of the spine. In White AA, Panjabi MM (eds): *Clinical Biomechanics of the Spine.* Philadelphia, JB Lippincott, 1978, p 229.)

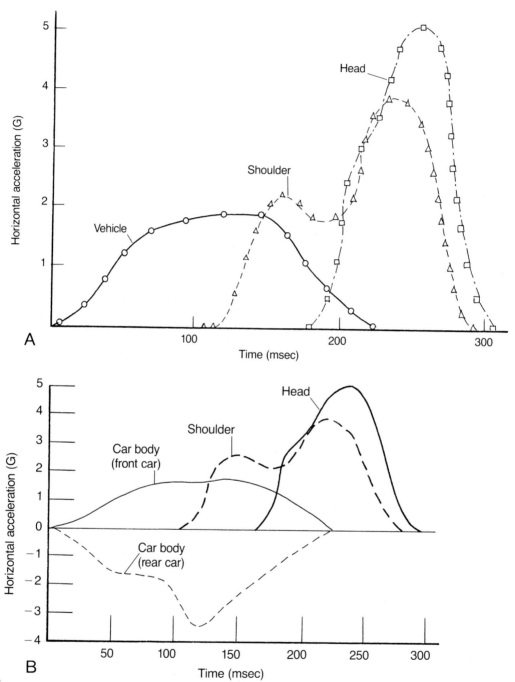

Figure 1.54. **A** and **B**. Experimental results of Severy et al. (123) and Severy and Mathewson (116), respectively. These early studies pointed to several important facts regarding rear-end automobile collisions: The acceleration of the body of the occupant occurs more than 100 msec after the collision, and the resulting G forces measured at the occupant's head are much greater than that of the vehicle itself. **C–E.** Sets of acceleration time, velocity/time, and displacement/time curves, respectively, calculated from a 5-G peak, half-sine pulse 200 msec in duration, as described by Martinez and Garcia (125). Most notable is the head rotation, relative to the torso, occurring from acceleration and velocity and the overall displacement of the head.

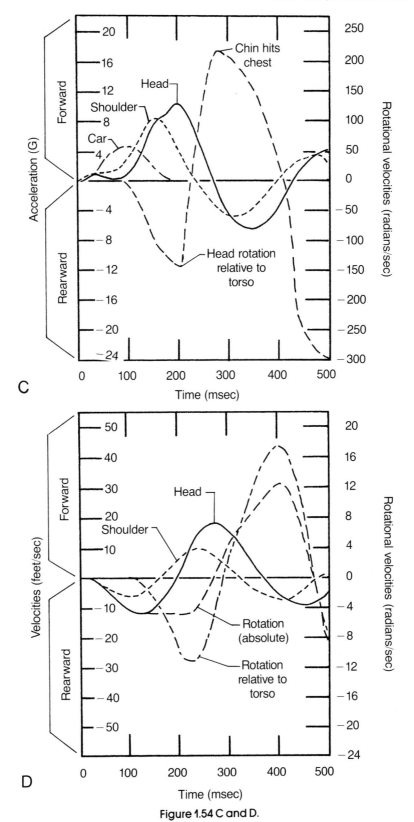

Figure 1.54 C and D.

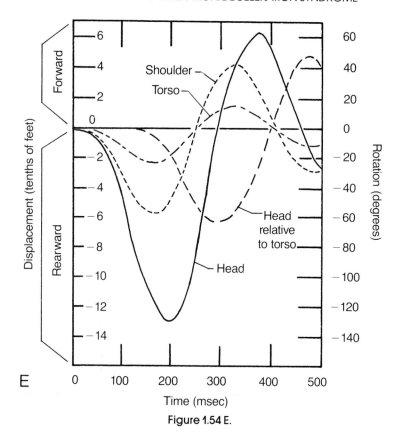

Figure 1.54 E.

seen here that the forces occurring in the head are 2–2.5 times those occurring in the vehicles themselves. In 1958, Severy and Mathewson (117) reported some of the data obtained from car-to-car rear-end collisions. Table 1.15 contains additional data from car-to-car rear-end collisions collected after Severy and Mathewson's report.

Since that time, researchers have continued to experiment with anthropomorphic dummies, animals, cadavers, and, to a limited extent, human volunteers. The shortcomings with all of these tests have been described. Anthropomorphic dummies have undergone continuous evolution through the years and today provide a fairly well representative model of human reactions to trauma. It can be argued, however, that certain of the human variables cannot be controlled for with dummies. This is especially true of the neuromuscular reflex action and the ability to consciously brace for impact.

Animal models often pose the same problem. Most of the experiments have used primates that were sedated with short-acting barbiturates. These animals can only represent those individuals who are caught totally unaware of the impending collision. It has also been fairly argued that the anatomical and physiological differences between primates and humans make interpretation of data somewhat unreliable.

The shortcomings of cadavers as models are plentiful. Some studies have used embalmed cadavers, while others have used fresh specimens (118, 119). Many times, these cadavers have been dissected to varying degrees. Often, they have been sectioned through the torso and mounted to a plate (119). In some cases, the heads or parts of the head have been replaced with accelerometers or other electronic equipment. In addition, most of the spines from these cadavers were quite old, with advanced stages of degenerative disease represented.

Table 1.14.
Guidelines and Protocol for the Cervical Stretch Test[a]

1. Test is performed under the close clinical supervision of the physician.

2. Traction is applied with skeletal fixation or a head halter. If traction is used later, a gauze sponge is placed between the molars.

3. A roller is placed under the head to reduce friction.

4. Target-to-film distance is 14 inches; source-to-film distance is 72 inches.

5. Initial lateral x-ray is taken (without traction) and developed.

6. Traction of 15 lb is applied.

7. Lateral films are taken and developed after addition of initial traction weight, and after each sequential 10-lb increment, the patient should be allowed to equilibrate to each phase of traction for at least 5 minutes before more weight is added.

8. Weight is added in 10-lb increments, as explained in step 7, until either 65 lb or one third of body weight has been reached.

9. After each addition of weight, the patient's neurological status is checked.

10. The test is considered positive and is concluded after any one of the following conditions is achieved:
   Change in neurological status;
   Intersegmental separation of >1.7 mm;
   Change in angulation between adjacent vertebrae of >7.5° (compared with that in the film taken in step 5).[b]

---

[a]Adapted from Panjabi MM, White AA: Physical properties and functional biomechanics of the spine. In White AA, Panjabi MM (eds): *Clinical Biomechanics of the Spine.* Philadelphia, JB Lippincott, 1978, p 229.

[b]This test is contraindicated in cases of obvious clinical instability.

Other factors such as storage time and temperature are important variables that are difficult to define. Some researchers have not allowed their cadavers to equilibrate to room temperature after being stored at $-20°$ Celsius. All of this makes it difficult to extrapolate data and to compare the results of one experiment with those of another.

After Severy's original work in 1955 (116), several investigators have set out to create a mathematical model that would allow them to estimate the severity and type of injury that would result from acceleration/deceleration trauma. In 1966, McHenry and Naab (120) developed an 11° of freedom, lumped parameter model for front-end collisions. This model proved to be inaccurate, however, because it represented the neck as a simple pivot type joint with constant rotational stiffness (120). At about the same time, Garcia (121) developed a series of linear and nonlinear lumped parameter models which were evaluated by Martinez et al. (122) on experimental animals. These latter investigators found that by using the acceleration parameters described by Severy et al. (123), resultant acceleration patterns of the head and shoulders, as determined by a set of linearized equations describing the system, resembled those found by Severy. The shortcoming of this model, however, was that it did not precisely depict the dynamic characteristics of the human body exposed to trauma (124).

This shortcoming was overcome with development of a nonlinear mathematical model describing head motion as made up of two elements: translation relative to the shoulder, causing a shearing action in the neck, and rotation of the head about the top of the cervical spine. This model was described by Martinez and Garcia in 1968 (125). More recently (1984), Merrill et al. (126) have extended the lumped parameter head-neck model to allow study of various types of neck trauma (specifically, whiplash and sidelash) with a three-dimensional response. This study was designed not only to account for a normal head-neck motion, as described previously, but also to consider the mechanical response of each intervertebral joint, which was then lumped into a single force-deformation relation. This model was then evaluated on the basis of various mechanical properties determined by other investigators. Agreement between the kinematic variables and the results of both the previous two-dimensional whiplash analysis and the experimental data obtained from a human volunteer was considered satisfactory. Because of differences attributable to higher facet stiffness/separation of the model relative to the volunteer, insufficient damping, and substantial differences in the me-

Table 1.15.
Kinematic Parameters from Rear-End Collisions[a]

Striking Car	Struck Car	Impact Velocity (miles/hour)	Kinematics of Struck Car			
			Change in Velocity (miles/hour)	Pulse Time (msec)	Peak Acceleration (G)	Acceleration Distance (cm)
1955 Hudson	1956 Olds	10	9.1	135	5.9	27.4
1955 Hudson	1956 Olds	23	14.8	132	10.0	43.7
1955 Hudson	1955 Nash	23	15.2	135	10.3	46.0

[a]Adapted from Mertz HJ Jr, Patrick LM: Investigation of the kinematics and kinetics of whiplash. In: *Proceedings, 11th Stapp Car Crash Conference*, SAE 670919. Detroit, MI, Society of Automotive Engineers, 1967; and based on data from Severy and Mathewson (117).

chanical deformation characteristics of the prototype components and numerical model, however, correspondence between the three-dimensional predictions and the reactions of the volunteer was poorer.

Clearly, no single method of evaluation—be it anthropomorphic dummy, rhesus monkey, cadaver, or mathematical finite element analysis—can account for all of the myriad variables occurring in acceleration/deceleration trauma. All methods of evaluation, however, have contributed greatly to the pool of knowledge that now exists.

SEQUENCE OF EVENTS

The whiplash phenomenon causes high rotational and translational accelerations of the victim's head that are much greater than that of the vehicle itself. Examination of the sequence of events following the rear-end impact collision facilitates a better understanding of the complex dynamics involved.

Initially, as the vehicle in front is struck from the rear by another vehicle, the two quickly attain a common velocity (Fig. 1.54), as is typical for a nonelastic collision. The greater the impact speed, the greater the deformation of the vehicles and, therefore, the more plastic the collision.

The torso, which is the first part of the victim's body to be affected by whiplash in a rear-end impact collision, is forced backward into the seatback. The head and neck initially remain fixed while the vehicle moves forward underneath; then, at the end of this rearward translation, the head and

neck begin to extend. At this time, the neck is subjected to very high tensile forces, which equates essentially to axial stretching. These are the same forces that Clemens and Burow (119) observed in experimental acceleration/deceleration whiplash simulation of cadavers. These investigators found fissures or ruptures in 80% of the discs studied.

After deflecting off the seatback or the head restraint, the head rebounds at about the same time as the vehicle's acceleration pulse tapers off and ends. This forward flexion continues, carrying the head, neck, and shoulders over the torso. In midphase when the head and neck are in about the neutral position, the chin is held high, indicating that forward angular acceleration of the head occurs late (125). The resulting hyperflexion may result in the so-called second collision in which the occupant comes into contact with part of the vehicle, such as the steering wheel, dashboard, or windshield. This may occur even if seat belts and shoulder harnesses are used (especially when there is appreciable slack in this restraint system).

In this simple description of the chain of events occurring after the rear-end collision, there are a great many variables; only the most important are covered here. In this description, extension preceded flexion of the neck. This may not be the case, however. McKenzie and Williams (124), using a discrete parameter mathematical model of the head, neck, and torso patterned after the work of Orne and Liu (127), have predicted that some degree of initial flexion of the head relative to the torso occurs prior to rapid hyperextension. This brief low-amplitude initial flexion is predicted to be related to the dynamics of the seatback stiffness such that a decreasing stiffness is associated with an increase in initial flexion. Unterharnscheidt (10), upon exposing rhesus monkeys to varying degrees of acceleration forces, observed that in some cases, these monkeys died shortly after + Gx vector injuries in which the peak head angular velocity was unusually low. He found that the position of the head at the beginning of impact was of most significance. When the initial position was slight flexion of the neck, the following sequence of events occurred after acceleration: (*a*) compression of the entire cervical spine, followed by (*b*) marked flexion of the cervical spine in the second phase and (*c*) rotation of the head in the forward direction. He termed this phenomenon the "concertina effect." This initial sequence absorbs or damps a substantial amount of kinetic energy and is then followed by hyperextension. In a pure + Gx vector acceleration, the hyperextension phase begins immediately after acceleration begins.

FORCES GENERATED

In speaking of the forces generated in the head and neck as a result of whiplash, the convention is to use the term G. One G is the acceleration due to the earth's gravity, typically 9.81 m/sec^2 (32.2 feet/sec^2). I have stated that the forces that develop in the head are 2–2.5 times that of the struck vehi-

cle. Ewing et al. (128) measured the maximum peak acceleration of the head of human volunteers exposed to nominal 10-G, 250-G/sec runs and found the surprisingly high force of 47.8 G. Thus in some cases the head may accelerate at up to 5 times the input acceleration.

Clemens and Burow (119) measured cranial (vertical) accelerations of 40–50 G and tractional forces at C1 of 1600–2000 N (350–440 lb) in cadavers exposed to acceleration equivalent to about 10 miles/hour. McKenzie and Williams (129) in their mathematical model have predicted that at higher impacts the resulting tensile loads on the cervical spine reach values much higher than would seem reasonable to expect. For example, in a rear-end impact collision that produces an acceleration of 12 G, the resulting horizontal acceleration of the head is greater than 50 G for a period of about 40 msec. For a 20-G acceleration, the maximum tensile load on the cervical spine may exceed 700 lbf which is far in excess of the numbers quoted by Yamada (130) for the average tensile breaking load of cervical vertebrae (224 lbf) and cervical intervertebral discs (194 lbf). Table 1.16 provides examples of acceleration parameters and their resulting G forces.

The linear velocity developed after a rear-end impact collision is usually expressed in feet per second (feet/sec) or as meters per second (m/sec). Angular velocity is expressed in radians per second (radians/sec). To understand forces that develop in the head and neck it would seem more appropriate to describe the angular acceleration that results. This is expressed in radians

Table 1.16.
Range of Input Acceleration Parameters^a

Code	Amplitude (G)	Duration (msec)	Maximum Jerk (G/sec)
S	5	200	78.5
T	20	200	314.0
U	30	200	471.0
V	12	120	314.0
W	15	100	471.0
X	20	120	524.0

^{a}Adapted from McKenzie JA, Williams JF: The effect of collision severity on the motion of the head and neck during 'whiplash'. *J Biomech* 8:257–259, 1975 (technical notes).

per second per second (radians/sec²). Both measurements are to be found in the literature, however. For example, Martinez and Garcia (125), using their mathematical model for an input of a 5-G peak, half-sine pulse 200/msec in duration, predicted a forward (linear) velocity of 20 feet/sec for the head and rotational (angular) velocities of 20 radians/sec in flexion and 12 radians/sec in extension.

Ommaya and Hirsch (131) studied the tolerances of subhuman primates to whiplash injuries. They predicted that head rotations of 1800 radians/sec² would result in cerebral concussion in humans about 50% of the time. This angular acceleration of 1800 radians/sec² (100,000°/sec) is reached when a car is struck from behind and accelerated horizontally by 5 G. Stated another way, if a car is hit in the rear and accelerated to a speed of 10.8 miles/hour within the time span of 100 msec, the occupants stand a 50/50 chance of sustaining a cerebral concussion.

McKenzie and Williams (129) have predicted much higher angular accelerations.

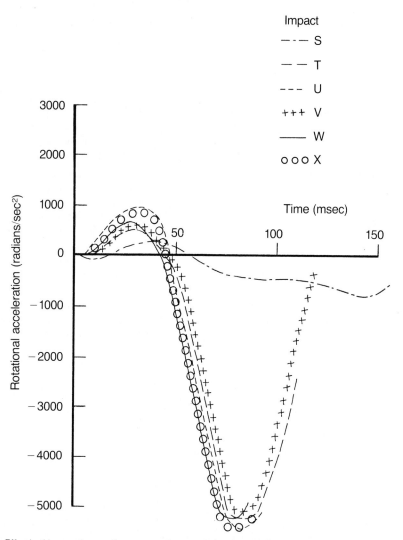

Figure 1.55.   Effect of impact severity on angular acceleration of the head, relative to the torso, resulting from impact parameters described in Table 1.16. (Adapted from McKenzie JA, Williams JF: The effect of collision severity on the motion of the head during 'whiplash'. *J Biomech* 8:257–259, 1975 (technical notes).)

The information presented in Table 1.16 is derived from six tests from their study. Figure 1.55 illustrates the resulting rotational accelerations, most of which far exceed the 50% concussion threshold predicted by Ommaya and Hirsch.

The positive bending moment that occurs in the hyperextension phase produces high compressive loading on the articular pillars, which may result in failure (124). The threshold for this load, however, and the early motion in the neck have been predicted. Most of the early motion in the neck (which occurs as the torso is accelerating underneath) is translational. This produces a shearing type of displacement of the neck, followed by the beginning of head rotation at the top of the spine. In extremes of hyperextension, this rotation may exceed 120° (125). It is at this point that shear forces and bending moments become maximum.

McKenzie and Williams (129) report high tensile loading in all regions of the cervical spine, combined with negative shear and negative bending in the upper cervical spine

and negative shear and positive bending in the lower cervical spine. It has been postulated, however, that head torque (rotational accelerations) rather than shear or axial forces is the major factor in neck injury resulting from whiplash (132). Some have argued that the hyperextension phase of the injury accounts for the major part of the damage to soft tissues (124), while others believe that the flexion phase does this (119). Most have not speculated. It has been argued that because flexion is ultimately limited by chin on chest contact, there is less likelihood of exceeding the limits of the soft tissue with this motion. Most people, however, do not easily touch their chin to their chest with their mouth closed. Also, it is known that the deceleration forces of hyperflexion are greater than the acceleration forces of hyperextension (125); it cannot be assumed, however, that a head and neck flexing at an angular velocity of 20 radians/sec, especially without normal neuromuscular control, are following a normal arc of physiological motion.

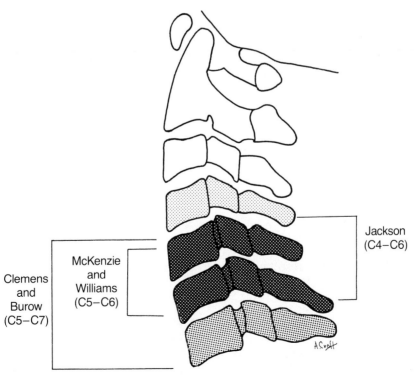

Figure 1.56.   Most researchers have found that the lower cervical spine sustains the greatest amount of damage in the acceleration/deceleration injury.

It must also be appreciated that much writing on this subject predates the common use of head restraints and most cars are now equipped with these. Without them, only the seat back itself limited the hyperextension phase. Even when these safety devices are adjusted improperly, they limit extension. It should also be pointed out that the study suggesting extension as the major injury vector was based upon a mathematical model, whereas the one postulating flexion as the major injury vector involved actual dissection of cadaveric materials.

Other confounding variables, such as the use of the shoulder harness, second collisions with vehicles in front, and individual physiological variances, reduce the issue of flexion versus extension as the major injury vector to one of academics. These variables are discussed later.

AREA OF INJURY

In general, it can be said that in this form of injury, the lower segments receive the brunt of the damage. Jackson (133) has stated that C4-C5 is the region of greatest strain and stress in hyperextension and C5-C6 is the area of greatest strain in hyperflexion. McKenzie and Williams (124) have stated that C5-C6 is the most highly stressed segment. Clemens and Burow (119) studied cadavers subjected to whiplash and found that most injuries occurred at C5-C6 and C6-C7. They found only disc injuries in the middle cervical spine and almost no injury to the upper cervical spine (Fig. 1.56).

VELOCITY AND ACCELERATION

The notion that one can calculate or predict the type or extent of soft tissue damage sustained by the occupants of a vehicle merely by calculating the G forces produced in the vehicle by the resultant collision should clearly be laid to rest. The practice of calculating bodily injury to the victim by estimating the cost of auto damage is naive at best and should be condemned.

When a moving vehicle collides with a nonmoving vehicle, both vehicles will attain a common velocity. This usually occurs in about 160 msec in light to moderate impacts.

If the masses and initial velocities of the two vehicles are known, the law of conservation of linear momentum can be used to calculate this final velocity. The coefficient of restitution can be calculated as

$$e = \frac{(U_1 - U_2)}{(V_2 - V_1)} \qquad \text{(Eq. 1.4)}$$

where U_1 and U_2 equal the velocities of the striking and struck cars, respectively, after impact, and V_1 and V_2 equal the velocities of the striking and struck cars, respectively, before impact. For a perfectly elastic impact, e equals 1, whereas for a perfectly plastic impact, e equals 0.

Ommaya and Hirsch (131) have described a case in which a large subdural hematoma resulted from a motor vehicle accident. This probably represents an injury within the range of threshold for concussion. In this instance, the masses and velocities were known, and the common velocity was calculated as 32.7 feet/sec (approximately 22 miles/hour).

If it is assumed that the peak velocity (V_f) of the combined masses is reached about 0.16 sec (160 msec) (T_t) after the collision and that the time to each peak acceleration (A_f) is half this value, then

$$A_f = \frac{V_f/T_t}{2} = \frac{32.7}{0.08} = 409 \text{ feet/sec}^2 \quad \text{(Eq. 1.5)}$$

If it is assumed that 1 G is equal to 32.2 feet/sec², then the resulting acceleration was equivalent to 12.7 G. I have stated, however, that the G forces generated at the occupant's head may be 2–4 times that of the struck vehicle. At 5 G this amplification factor is about 2–2.5, whereas at 12 G it may be as high as 4 (129).

Based upon the experimental results of Severy and Mathewson (117, 123), a crude graph of estimated acceleration forces (Fig. 1.57) can be constructed. This graph is based upon data obtained in rear-end impact collisions of like-sized vehicles in which no brakes were applied. In most cases, it is impractical to attempt to calculate the G forces involved in a rear-end collision, simply because the velocity of the striking car is seldom known and because there are a large number of mechanical variables that affect this force and that are very difficult to account for in a practical sense.

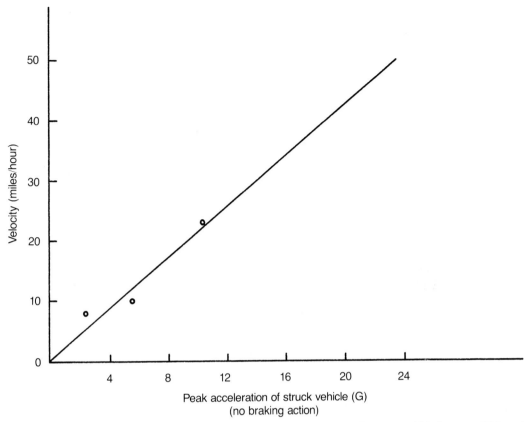

Figure 1.57. Velocity-acceleration curve based on data reported by Severy and Mathewson (117) and described in Table 1.15. This graph assumes no braking action in the struck vehicle.

OTHER VARIABLES

Although the G forces produced for a given collision between vehicles of known size and velocity can be calculated, the large number of physical (vehicle) and physiological (human) parameters that come into play introduce a great deal of variance in this calculation. Following is a discussion of both groups of known and proposed parameters.

Vehicle Parameters

I have stated that the relative sizes of colliding vehicles as well as their relative velocities are important known variables in determining the outcome of the crash. For example, a streetcar traveling at a speed of 3 miles/hour will produce the same amount of damage and acceleration force as a compact car traveling at 40 miles/hour (134).

Head restraints are designed to limit the backward displacement of the head during the acceleration phase of the whiplash injury. By limiting this motion, some or all of the shear and tensile loading of the cervical spine is eliminated. When the hyperextension phase is reduced, so too will be the resulting hyperflexion phase.

In 1969, head restraints became mandatory standard equipment in all cars sold in the United States. Although their design was originally for safety purposes, they soon became known as "headrests," clearly indicating the general misconception of their real function by the driving public. When these restraints are adjusted so that the head can be comfortably cradled by the restraint, it is not likely to provide any appreciable protection against whiplash. In fact, when the head restraint is adjusted in a low position, it may make the injury even more severe than it would have been without the restraint at all. In this down-adjusted position, it actually acts as a fulcrum over

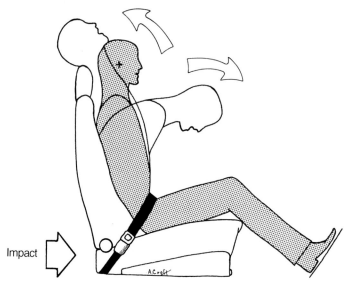

Figure 1.58. After rear-end impact collision, the vehicle accelerates forward, forcing the occupant backward into the seatback. At the same time, some vertical motion may also occur. This phenomenon, known as "ramping," reduces the effectiveness of the head restraint by allowing the head to rotate backward and over the top of the restraint.

which the cervical spine pivots. This is especially likely with tall drivers (135).

Two types of restraint systems are currently in use: the integral system, which is actually built onto or is part of the seatback, and the adjustable head restraint. Integral systems have been shown to be less expensive and more effective at reducing injury (17% versus 10% effective for adjustable restraints) (136). This is largely because most adjustable restraints are improperly adjusted. In one study, 74% of male drivers in Los Angeles, California, and 90% of male drivers in Washington, DC, had their restraints improperly adjusted (too low) (136).

Ideally, head restraints should be adjusted so that the center is at least at the level of the ears. This is about the center of gravity of the head. In a practical sense this may be understated, however, because of the phenomenon of *ramping*. During the acceleration phase of the whiplash, the torso is forced backward against the seatback and, at the same time, may undergo some vertical displacement as well, depending upon the degree of inclination of the seatback and the amount of friction between seatback and driver. This is known as ramping. I have also

stated that a great deal of tensile force occurs as the torso moves forward in relation to the neck. Both of these phenomena may cause the head to move up and back over a properly adjusted head restraint (Fig. 1.58).

One of the problems with seat safety engineering is that seats are designed for males in the 50th percentile for height. This provides reasonable safety and protection for the average-sized male without creating visibility problems for a small female. For the tall driver, however, seatbacks are too short and head restraints are too low to provide reasonable protection against whiplash. This is illustrated in Figure 1.59.

Another important parameter regarding head restraints is the distance between the occupant's head and the restraint at the time of impact. The restraint works by allowing the head to be accelerated at the same time as the torso is accelerated by the seatback. An increase in this distance results in a proportionate decrease in the effectiveness of the restraint. This has been demonstrated by Mertz and Patrick (132). This distance can be affected by the posture of the occupant and by the degree of seatback inclination (Fig. 1.60).

Severy et al. (116) have suggested that by

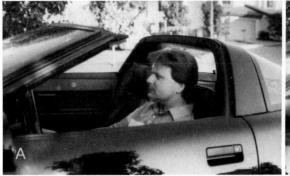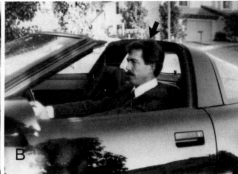

Figure 1.59. Most seatbacks are designed for the 50th pecentile male body size. This allows reasonable safety for average-sized male drivers without hindering visibility for smaller drivers. **A.** A 50th percentile man (5 feet 10 inches tall) fits this seatback properly. **B.** A 95th percentile man (6 feet 2 inches tall) does not fit this seatback properly. The center of gravity of the head is well above the top of the integral head restraint. Aside from being somewhat uncomfortable, this seat does not adequately protect this man from rear-end collision. Also note the dangerous proximity of the metal bar above the head (*arrow*).

increasing seatback stiffness, the peak translational head acceleration can be decreased. This would presumably reduce the potential for neck injury. McKenzie and Williams (124) have predicted that low seatback stiffness could result in high tensile loading with positive bending in the lower cervical regions, which might result in tensile damage to anterior ligaments and associated structures. They point out, however, that with increasing seatback stiffness, the peak axial force in the lower cervical region becomes compressive, leaving open the possibility of articular pillar damage.

Martinez and Garcia (125) predicted that a seatback designed to allow a controlled backward collapse would provide fluid-damping characteristics that would mini-

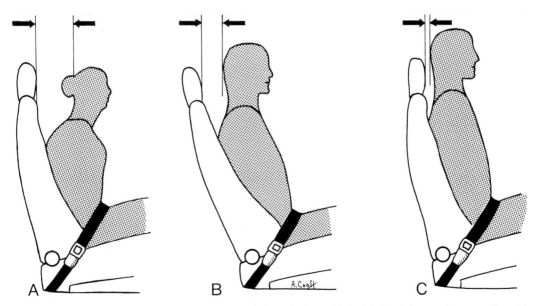

Figure 1.60. The effectiveness of head restraints in reducing whiplash injury is inversely proportional to the distance between the occupant's head and the head restraint. This can be affected by posture and seatback inclination. **A.** Kyphotic posture of the elderly. **B.** Excessive seatback inclination. **C.** Proper relationship of about 2 inches.

mize the forces acting on the head and neck. They also suggested the same fluid-damped system be incorporated into the seat belt and shoulder harness to reduce the forces seen in frontal impacts. This reasoning is in line with that of Macnab (134) who found that with seatbacks tilted back 30° at impact, the injuries received by primates exposed to acceleration trauma were significantly less. With the use of the system as described by Martinez and Garcia, no more than 5–10° of backward tilting would be necessary, and this would allow the driver to maintain control of the car after the collision. Mertz and Patrick (132) have also demonstrated that the injuries sustained will be less severe when seatback rigidity is decreased. In other words, a controlled seatback collapse reduced the severity of injury from rear-impact accidents. This was true for seats with and without head restraints. Seats should be designed, however, so that the deformation or backward rotation is not followed immediately by a forward counterrotation. In other words, seatbacks should behave in a plastic rather than an elastic manner. This is because if the latter occurred prior to the time for maximum hyperextension of the head and neck (i.e., before 200 msec), the corresponding increase in torso acceleration that would result would increase the tensile and shear loading in the neck during this phase of injury. On the other hand, if it occurred after maximum angular rotation of the head (i.e., after the first 200 msec) when the head and neck were beginning to accelerate, this forward spring-like action would likely amplify both linear and angular acceleration of the head. Stated another way, a seatback that reacted like a steel spring would result in a "diving board" action and intensify the injury, whereas a seatback with plastic deformability would dampen the whiplash and reduce the injury.

There is little question that seat belts and shoulder harnesses significantly reduce the number of deaths and injuries from auto accidents. It has been suggested that by restraining the chest with the shoulder harness the amount of inertial forces exerted on the cervical spine in a whiplash injury are reduced (135). The use of a shoulder harness system with fluid-damping characteristics would reduce these forces even more.

Some vehicles are equipped with shoulder harnesses that can be locked in position at a distance from the occupant's chest, thereby reducing the annoyance of constant harness pressure. In an impact, this slack may allow the victim's body to travel far enough to make contact with the steering wheel or other parts of the car's interior, and in this way the safety potential of the

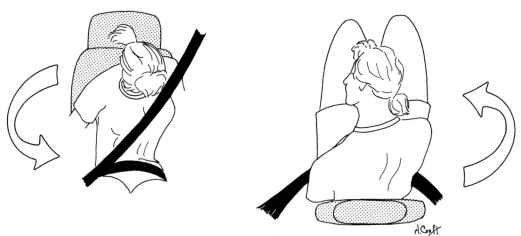

Figure 1.61. Asymmetric loading is produced by decelerating against a diagonal shoulder harness. This adds the component of rotation to the hyperflexion phase of a whiplash injury. When the shoulder harness is tight against the chest at the time of impact, this effect is probably nil but becomes more significant as the slack between the chest and the strap increase. Allowing slack in this way defeats some of the purpose of shoulder harnesses and reduces their overall effectiveness.

system is reduced. This slack could also potentiate the forward angular rotation $(+\theta x)$ of the cervical, thoracic, and lumbar spines and result in greater injury to these areas. In addition, a rotational component is added when a torso that is moving forward relative to the seatback is stopped abruptly with a diagonal strap. In this instance, instead of pure hyperflexion in the sagittal direction as would be seen with a symmetrical strap system (i.e., over both shoulders), the torso and the neck, as the torso decelerates against the shoulder harness, will actually pivot around the belt (i.e., around the y axis). This is due to the forward momentum of the free shoulder. The resulting motion is combined flexion and rotation toward the secured shoulder (Fig. 1.61). This rotational component may play a major role in soft tissue injuries.

Much of the energy that is transmitted from the striking vehicle to the struck vehicle is absorbed by the crumpling of the two cars. The more deformation of the cars, the more distribution and dispersion of forces. Many years ago, race car drivers drove heavy race cars at speeds that were not very impressive by today's standards. These cars, like their everyday counterparts of the time, were constructed of heavy gauge steel — much heavier than that used today. In spite of this heavy construction, race car driving was considered a very dangerous sport because of the high incidence of injury and death. Today's race cars travel around the track at average speeds above 200 miles/hour, yet race car driving is a safer sport today than it was 60 years ago. Why? Partly because of the way these races are managed and party because all of the various safety and support mechanisms that have evolved, but largely because of the design of the race cars themselves.

The safety concept of "building it like a tank" is no longer valid. Engineers now design sophisticated lightweight race cars capable of great speeds that, when they crash into the retaining wall (at 200 miles/hour), nearly disintegrate piece by piece, very often after flipping end over end and rolling over and over before finally coming to rest. And the driver climbs out of the wreckage with only minor injuries. The secret to this incredible crashworthiness is built into the car—this intentional piecemeal disintegration absorbs nearly all the energy of the crash.

Thus a car that is built to collapse with impact (within safe limits) is safer than one that is not. Offsetting this effect, however, is the fact that heavier built cars also have greater mass and, therefore, will be accelerated at lower rates than smaller lighter cars.

Human Parameters

Certain physiological variances in people will significantly affect the amount of damage they sustain in a collision. This is why, as is often seen in practice, one occupant in a crash may be injured, while another may escape with no apparent injury.

With an increase in age, the elasticity of tissues decreases. Range of motion in the cervical spine also decreases. In both cases, the potential for injury is increased because the neck is less resilient. The strength of neck musculature diminishes with age. Over the adult life span, cervical range of motion is reduced by an average of nearly 40%, cervical muscle reflexes slow by 23%, and voluntary strength capability diminishes by 25% (83).

It has been suggested that in a suprise rear-end collision, neuromuscular reflexes may come into play and perhaps help to mitigate some of the injury (116, 132). Foust et al. (83) have shown that the average reflex time for muscles of the cervical spine is slightly more than 60 msec. Full activation of muscles requires about another 60 msec. If the head does not reach full acceleration until about 200 msec, it is possible that activation of muscles could attenuate some of the damaging acceleration forces. In older people, however, even at low-speed impacts, this is unlikely. And in moderate- to high-speed impacts, even in young people, this attenuation is also unlikely (83, 137).

Sex seems to play a part in this injury, in that women seem to be injured more seriously than men (138) (see Chapter 8). Other physiological variances that may have a negative affect on acceleration/deceleration injuries include congenital anomalies of the spine, previous surgeries of the spine, previous spinal injuries, osteoporosis, osteoarthritis, rheumatic disorders, metabolic disorders affecting bone, primary or metastatic neoplasia, or infection of bone.

I have stated that the likelihood of injury is greater when nonsymmetrical loads are applied to the spine. This can occur with oblique collisions, such as those that would occur when a vehicle was struck in the left rear corner as it was turning left. This type of collision may also occur when the occupant's head is turned during a rear-end collision. When the head is rotated 45°, the amount of extension that the spine is capable of is decreased by 50%. This results in increased compressive loads at the facet joint and articular pillar on the ipsilateral side and increased tensile loads at the facet joint on the contralateral side. The intervertebral foramen is also smaller on the side of rotation and lateral flexion, and its contents are more vulnerable to injury.

There will usually be a larger number of and more serious injuries in surprise rear-end collisions, i.e., those in which an occupant is unaware of the impending crash, than in those rear-end collisions in which the occupant is braced for the impending crash. This is true even in normal healthy young people whose generally quicker neuromuscular reflexes have a negligible affect in a moderate to severe crash.

The acceleration of a car that is struck from behind can be calculated as previously shown. To appreciate the true acceleration, however, several other factors must be taken into account. For example, the ability of a car to roll after impact will directly affect acceleration. If the brakes are on at the time of impact, it will accelerate less. If the car is on ice, however, it will accelerate rapidly and the corresponding soft tissue injury will be greater. The same is true if the car is moving forward at the time it is struck.

Apologia for Change in Automotive Safety Engineering

In 1971, the National Safety Council estimated that there are nearly 4 million rear-end collisions in the United States and that this results in as many as 1 million reported injuries every year. (139). Because of the increase in the number of cars on the road today, these figures are probably a conservative estimate.

It has also been estimated that 86% of all neck injuries seen clinically result from auto accidents and that 85% of these injuries are the result of rear-end collisions (i.e., acceleration/deceleration injuries) (140–142). Macnab (2) has conservatively estimated that 45% of those suffering whiplash injuries to the neck will continue to be symptomatic for at least 2 years.

Each year, more than 30,000 men, women, and children are killed on United States highways, and millions more are permanently disfigured or disabled. Auto accidents are the leading cause of death for young Americans under age 35, the major source of paraplegia and quadriplegia, and a significant cause of epilepsy and brain damage. This is one of the major public health problems in the United States, and the cost in human suffering and expense to society is second only to that from cancer (143). The National Coalition to Reduce Car Crash Injuries has stated that proper crash protection in automobiles would mean savings of more than $25 billion each year in the United States alone.

Surprisingly, even with mandatory use laws, fewer than 50% of drivers wear seat belts and shoulder harnesses. The United States Department of Transportation has stated that a seat belt use rate of 50% would reduce the number of annual vehicle deaths by 4400 and that with air bags the savings would be almost 9000 lives.

In 1986, consumer protection agencies rated several American cars "unsafe" in collision speeds of only 21 miles/hour. This seems grossly unacceptable with the maximum speed limit in most states at 55 miles/hour.

Many, if not most, injuries would be prevented or reduced with the incorporation of several relatively simple safety design changes including:

1. Energy absorbing front and rear vehicle components.
2. Seatbacks designed to absorb acceleration forces by incorporating a system that

would allow a limited slow collapse of the seatback with fluid-damping characteristics.

3. Shoulder harnesses with the same fluid-damping characteristics to allow a controlled limited forward motion of the torso during deceleration forces.
4. Adequate seatback height to protect tall drivers (which may require dealer adjustment).
5. Air bags as standard equipment for both front seats.
6. Integral rigid, padded (nonadjustable) head restraints that extend above the center of gravity of the occupant's head (the distance between the back of the head and the restraint should not exceed 2.5 inches).

Due to politics and the economics of big business, changes in safety laws come very slowly. Automobile manufacturers generally respond only to changes in the law and, not surprisingly, are represented by a very large lobby in Washington, DC.

Largely due to the efforts of physicians to educate the public to the dangers of cigarette smoking, the incidence of smoking is down significantly from that of the 1960's. It seems only natural, therefore, that we who deal daily with the pain and the suffering from motor vehicle trauma attempt to educate the public at every opportunity on the importance of automotive safety.

References

1. Crowe HE: Injuries to the cervical spine. Paper presented at the meeting of the Western Orthopaedic Association, San Francisco, 1928.
2. Macnab I: Acceleration extension injuries of the cervical spine. In Rothman RH, Simeone FA (eds): *The Spine*, ed 2. Philadelphia, WB Saunders, 1982, vol 2, p 654.
3. Ebbs SR, Beckly DE, Hammonds JC, Teasdale C: Incidence and duration of neck pain among patients injured in car accidents. *Br Med J* 292:94–95, 1986.
4. Norris SH, Watt I: The prognosis of neck injuries resulting from rear-end vehicle collisions. *J Bone Joint Surg* 65B (5):608–611, 1983.
5. Ommaya AK, Hirsch AE, Martinez JL: The role of whiplash in cerebral concussion. In: *Proceedings, 10th Stapp Car Crash Conference*, SAE 660804. Detroit, MI, Society of Automotive Engineers, 1966.
6. Ommaya AK, Hirsch AE, Flamm ES, Mohone RH: An experimental model for cerebral concussion in the monkeys. *Science* 153(3732):211, 1966.
7. Russell WR: Cerebral involvement in head injuries; a study of 200 cases. *Brain* 55:549, 1932.
8. Denker PG, Perry GF: Postconcussion syndrome in compensation and litigation: analysis of 95 cases with electroencephalographic correlations. *Neurology* 4:912–918, 1954.
9. Glasser MA, Shafer FP: Skull and brain trauma. *JAMA* 98:27, 1932.
10. Unterharnscheidt F: Pathological and neuropathological findings in rhesus monkeys subjected to −Gx and +Gx indirect impact acceleration. In Sances A, Thomas DJ, Ewing CL, Larson SJ, Unterharnscheidt F (eds): *Mechanisms of Head and Spine Trauma*. Goshen, NY, Aloray, 1986.
11. Wickstrom J, Martinez J, Rodrigues R: Cervical spine syndrome: experimental acceleration injuries of the head and neck. In: *Proceedings, Prevention of Highway Injury*. Ann Arbor, MI, Highway Safety Research Institute, University of Michigan, Ann Arbor, 1967, pp 182-187.
12. Macnab I: Acceleration extension injuries of the cervical spine. In Rothman RH, Simeone FA (eds): *The Spine*, ed 2. Philadelphia, WB Saunders, 1982, vol 2, p 650.
13. Panjabi MM, White AA: Physical properties and functional biomechanics of the spine. In White AA, Panjabi MM (eds): *Clinical Biomechanics of the Spine*. Philadelphia, JB Lippincott, 1978, p 25.
14. Messerer O: *Über Elasticität and Festigkeit der Menschlichen Knochen*. Stuttgart, JG Cottaschen Buchhandlungen, 1880.
15. Pintar FA, Mykebust JB, Yoganandan N, Maiman DJ, Sances A: Biomechanics of human spinal ligaments. In Sances A, Thomas DJ, Ewing CL, Larson SJ, Unterharnscheidt F (eds): *Mechanisms of Head and Spine Trauma*. Goshen, NY, Aloray, 1986, p 520.
16. Bell GH, Dunbar O, Beck JS, Gibb A: Variation in strength of vertebrae with age and their relation to osteoporosis. *Calcif Tissue Res* 1:75, 1967.
17. Rockoff SD, Sweet E, Blenstein J: The relative contribution of trabecular and cortical bone to the strength of human lumbar vertebrae. *Calcif Tissue Res* 3:163, 1969.
18. Farfan HF: Torsion and compression. In: *Mechanical Disorders of the Low Back*. Philadelphia, Lea & Febiger, 1973, p 68.
19. Farfan HF: Torsion and compression. In: *Mechanical Disorders of the Low Back*. Philadelphia, Lea & Febiger, 1973, p 78.
20. Hayes WC, Carter DR: The effect of marrow on energy absorption of trabecular bone. Paper presented at the 22nd Annual Meeting of Orthopaedic Research Society, New Orleans, 1976.
21. Perry O: Fracture of the vertebral end plate in the lumbar spine. *Acta Orthop Scand* 25 (Suppl), 1957.
22. Panjabi MM, White AA: Physical properties and functional biomechanics of the spine. In White AA, Panjabi MM (eds): *Clinical Biomechanics of the Spine*. Philadelphia, JB Lippincott, 1978, p 30.
23. Panjabi MM, White AA: Physical properties and functional biomechanics of the spine. In White AA, Panjabi MM (eds): *Clinical Biomechanics of the Spine*. Philadelphia, JB Lippincott, 1978, p 34.
24. Farfan HF: Anatomy of the lumbar spine. In: *Mechanical Disorders of the Low Back*. Philadelphia, Lea & Febiger, 1973, p 24.
25. Panjabi MM, White AA: Physical properties and functional biomechanics of the spine. In White AA, Panjabi MM (eds): *Clinical Biomechanics of the Spine*. Philadelphia, JB Lippincott, 1978, p 4.
26. Harris RI, Macnab I: Structural changes in the lumbar intervertebral disc. Their relationship to low back pain and sciatica. *J Bone Joint Surg* 36B:304, 1954.
27. Hassler O: The human intervertebral disc: a microangiographical study on its vascular supply at various ages. *Acta Orthop Scand* 40:765, 1970.
28. Roffe PG Innovation of annulus fibrosus and posterior longitudinal ligaments. *Arch Neurol Psychiatry* 44:100, 1940.
29. Markolf KL: Stiffness and damping characteristics of the thoracic-lumbar spine. In: *Proceedings of Workshop on Bioengineering Approaches to the Problems of the Spine*. Washington, DC, National Institutes of Health, 1970.

30. Panjabi MM, White AA: Physical properties and functional biomechanics of the spine. In White AA, Panjabi MM (eds): *Clinical Biomechanics of the Spine.* Philadelphia, JB Lippincott, 1978, p 9.
31. Virgin W: Experimental investigations into physical properties of intervertebral disc. *J Bone Joint Surg* 33B:607, 1951.
32. Markolf KL, Morris JM: The structural components of the intervertebral disc. *J Bone Joint Surg* 56A:675, 1974.
33. Hirsch C: The reaction of intervertebral discs to compression forces. *J Bone Joint Surg* 37A:1188, 1955.
34. Farfan HF Hypothesis of degenerative process. In: *Mechanical Disorders of the Low Back.* Philadelphia, Lea & Febiger, 1973, p 201.
35. Roaf R: A study of the mechanics of spinal injuries. *J Bone Joint Surg* 42B:810, 1960.
36. Farfan HF: Torsion and compression. In: *Mechanical Disorders of the Low Back.* Philadelphia, Lea & Febiger, 1973, p 82.
37. Lin HS, Liu YK, Adams KH: Mechanical response of the lumbar intervertebral joint under physiological (complex) loadings. *J Bone Joint Surg* 60A:41–55, 1978.
38. Liu YK, Ray G, Hirsch C: The resistance of the lumbar spine to direct shear. *Orthop Clin North Am* 6:33–48, 1975.
39. Farfan HF, Sullivan JD: The relation of facet orientation to intervertebral disc failure. *Can J Surg* 10:179, 1967.
40. Farfan HF: The effect of torsion on the intervertebral joints. *Can J Surg* 12:336, 1969.
41. Farfan HF, Cossette JW, Robertson GH, Wells RV Kraus H: The effects of torsion on the lumbar intervertebral joints: the role of torsion in the production of disc degeneration. *J Bone Joint Surg* 52A:468, 1970.
42. Panjabi MM, White AA: Physical properties and functional biomechanics of the spine. In White AA, Panjabi MM (eds): *Clinical Biomechanics of the Spine.* Philadelphia, JB Lippincott, 1978, pp 14–15.
43. Lafferty JF, Kahler RL: Viscoelastic properties of intervertebral discs. In Sances A, Thomas DJ, Ewing CL, Larson SJ, Unterharnscheidt F (eds): *Mechanisms of Head and Spine Trauma.* Goshen, NY, Aloray, 1986.
44. Panjabi MM, White AA: Physical properties and functional biomechanics of the spine. In White AA, Panjabi MM (eds): *Clinical Biomechanics of the Spine.* Philadelphia, JB Lippincott, 1978, p 17.
45. Arutynow AJ: Basic problems of the pathology and surgical treatment of prolapsed intervertebral discs. *Vopr Neirokhir* 4:21, 1962.
46. Pintar FA, Mykebust JB, Yoganandan N, Maiman DJ, Sances A: Biomechanics of human spinal ligaments. In Sances A, Thomas DJ, Ewing CL, Larson SJ, Unterharnscheidt F (eds): *Mechanisms of Head and Spine Trauma.* Goshen, NY, Aloray, 1986, p 505.
47. Nachemson A, Morris JM: In vivo measurements of intradiscal pressure. *J Bone Joint Surg* 46:1077, 1964.
48. Nachemson A, Evans J: Some mechanical properties of the third lumbar inter-laminar ligament (ligamentum flavum). *J Biomech* 1:211, 1968.
49. Panjabi MM, White AA: Physical properties and functional biomechanics of the spine. In White AA, Panjabi MM (eds): *Clinical Biomechanics of the Spine.* Philadelphia, JB Lippincott, 1978, p 25.
50. Noyes FR, DeLucas JL, Torvik PJ: Biomechanics of anterior cruciate ligament failure: an analysis of strain-rate sensitivity and mechanisms of failure in primates. *J Bone Joint Surg* 56A:236, 1974.
51. Panjabi MM, White AA, Southwick WO: Mechanical properties of bone as a function of rate of deformation. *J Bone Joint Surg* 55A:322, 1973.
52. Breig A: *Biomechanics of the Central Nervous System: Some Basic Normal and Pathological Phenomena.* Stockholm, Almqvist & Wiksell, 1960.
53. White AA, Panjabi MM: Kinematics of the spine. In White AA, Panjabi MM (eds): *Clinical Biomechanics of the Spine.* Philadelphia, JB Lippincott, 1978, p 62.
54. Ewing CL, Thomas DJ: Human head and neck response to impact acceleration. *Naval Aerospace Med Res Lab Monogr* 21, August 1972.
55. Gell DF: Table of equivalents for acceleration terminology: recommended for general international use by the Acceleration Committee of the Aerospace Medical Panel. *AGARD Aerospace Med* 32:1109–1111, 1961.
56. Snyder RG: Impact. In Parker VR, West VR (eds): *Bioastronautics Data Book,* ed 2. Washington, DC, National Aeronautics and Space Administration, 1973, pp 221–295.
57. Thomas DJ, Robbins DH, Eppinger RH, King AL, Hubbard RP: *Guidelines for the Comparison of Human Analogue Biomechanical Data. Report of an Ad-Hoc Committee.* Ann Arbor, MI, University of Michigan, 1974.
58. Ferlic D: The range of motion of the "normal" cervical spine. *Johns Hopkins Hosp Bull* 110:59–65, 1962.
59. Hunt WE: Cervical spondylosis: natural history and rare indications for surgical decompression. *Clin Neurosurg* 27:466–480, 1980.
60. Macnab I: Cervical spondylosis. *Clin Orthop* 109:69–77, 1975.
61. Gibb A: Appendix. In Bell GH, Dunbar O, Beck JS, Gibb A: Variation in strength of vertebrae with age and their relationship to osteoporosis. *Calcif Tissue Res* 1:75, 1967.
62. Anderson GBJ, Ortengren R, Herberts P: Quantitative electromyographic studies of back muscle activity related to posture and loading. *Orthop Clin North Am* 8:85, 1977.
63. Harris JH Jr: The normal cervical spine. In: *The Radiology of Acute Cervical Spine Trauma.* Baltimore, Williams & Wilkins, 1978, p 2.
64. Jackson H: The diagnosis of minimal atlanto-axial subluxation. *Br J Radiol* 23:672, 1950.
65. Caffey J: *Pediatric X-ray Diagnosis,* ed 6. Chicago, Year Book, 1972.
66. Fielding JM, Cochran GVB, Lawsing JF III, Hohl M: Tears of the transverse ligament of the atlas. *J Bone Joint Surg* 56A(8):1683–1691, 1974.
67. Cattell HS, Filtzer DC: Pseudosubluxation and other normal variations of the cervical spine in children. *J Bone Joint Surg* 47A:1295, 1965.
68. Prasad P, King AI, Ewing, CL: The role of articular facets during +Gx acceleration. *J Appl Mech* 41: 321, 1974.
69. Hohl M: Soft-tissue injuries of the neck in automobile accidents. *J Bone Joint Surg* 56A(8):1675–1682, 1974.
70. White AA, Johnson RM, Panjabi MM, Southwick WO: Biomechanical analysis of clinical stability in the cervical spine. *Clin Orthop* 109:85, 1975.
71. Green JD, Hare TS, Harris JH: Anterior subluxation of the cervical spine. *AJNR* 2:243–250, 1981.
72. Scher AT: Anterior cervical subluxation: an unstable position. *AJR* 133:275–280, 1979.
73. White AA, Panjabi MM: The problem of clinical instability in the human spine: a systematic approach. In White AA, Panjabi MM (eds): *Clinical Biomechanics of the Spine.* Philadelphia, JB Lippincott, 1978, p 207.
74. Kapandji IA: The vertebral column as a whole. In: *The Physiology of the Joints,* vol 3: *The Trunk and the Vertebral Column.* New York, Churchill Livingstone, 1974, p 38.
75. Lysell E: Motion in the cervical spine. *Acta Orthop Scand* 123 (Suppl), 1969.
76. Kapandji IA: The cervical vertebral column. In: *The Physiology of the Joints,* vol 3: *The Trunk and the Vertebral Column.* New York, Churchill Livingstone, 1974, p 200.
77. White AA, Panjabi MM: Kinematics of the spine. In White AA, Panjabi MM (eds): *Clinical Biomechanics of the Spine.* Philadelphia, JB Lippincott, 1978, p 74.
78. Sherk HH, Parke WW: Developmental anatomy. In Bailey RW, Sherk HH, Dunn EJ, Fielding JW, Long DM, Ono K, Penning L, Stauffer ES (eds): *The Cervical Spine,* a publication of the Cervical Spine Research Society. Philadelphia, JB Lippincott, 1983, p 8.
79. Lucas D, Bresler B: Stability of ligamentous spine. In:

Biomechanics Lab Report 40. San Francisco, University of California, San Francisco, 1961.

80. Kapandji IA: The cervical vertebral column. In: *The Physiology of the Joints,* vol 3: *The Trunk and the Vertebral Column.* New York, Churchill Livingstone, 1974, p 222.

81. Kapandji IA: The cervical vertebral column. In: *The Physiology of the Joints,* vol 3: *The Trunk and the Vertebral Column.* New York, Churchill Livingstone, 1974, p 228.

82. Fountain FP, Minear WL, Allison RD: Functions of longus colli and longissimus cervicis muscles in man. *Arch Phys Med* 47:665–669, 1966.

83. Foust DR, Chaffin DB, Snyder RF, Baum JK: Cervical range of motion and dynamic response and strength of cervical muscles. In: *Proceedings, 17th Stapp Car Crash Conference,* SAE 730975. Detroit, MI, Society of Automotive Engineers, 1973, p 285.

84. Walter J, Doris P, Shaffer M: Clinical presentation of patients with acute cervical spine injury. *Emerg Med Clin North Am* 13(7):512–515, 1984.

85. Hadley MN, Sonntag VKH, Grahm TW, Masferrer R, Browner C: Axis fractures resulting from motor vehicle accidents: the need for occupant restraints. *Spine* 11(9):861–864, 1986.

86. Thomas DJ, Jessop ME: Experimental head and neck injury from inertial forces. In Sances A, Thomas DJ, Ewing CL, Larson SJ, Unterharnscheidt F (eds): *Mechanisms of Head and Spine Trauma.* Goshen, NY, Aloray, 1986, p 373.

87. Anderson LD, D'Alonzo RT: Fractures of the odontoid process of the axis. *J Bone Joint Surg* 56A:1663, 1974.

88. White AA, Panjabi MM: The problem of clinical instability in the human spine: a systematic approach. In White AA, Panjabi MM (eds): *Clinical Biomechanics of the Spine.* Philadelphia, JB Lippincott, 1978, p 192.

89. Powers B, Miller MD, Kramer RS, Martinez S, Gehweiler JA Jr: Traumatic anterior atlanto-occipital dislocation. *Neurosurgery* 4(1):12–17, 1979.

90. Swischuk LE: Anterior dislocation of C2 in children: physiologic or pathologic? *Radiology* 122:759, 1977.

91. Cornish BL: Traumatic spondylolisthesis of the axis. *J Bone Joint Surg* 50B:31, 1968.

92. Sullivan CR, Bruwer AJ, Harris LE: Hypermobility of the cervical spine in children: a pitfall in the diagnosis of cervical dislocation. *Am Surg* 95:636–640, 1958.

93. Brocker JEW: *Die Occipital-Cervical-Gegend.* Stuttgart, Thieme, 1955, as cited in Harris (63).

94. Locke GR, Gardner JE, VanEpps EF: Atlas-dens interval (ADI) in children. *AJR* 97:135, 1966.

95. Fielding JW, Hawkins RJ: Atlanto-axial rotatory fixation: fixed rotatory subluxation of the atlanto-axial joint. *J Bone Joint Surg* 59A(1):37–44, 1977.

96. Harris JH Jr: Flexion injuries. In: *The Radiology of Acute Cervical Spine Trauma.* Baltimore, Williams & Wilkins 1978, p 58.

97. Gershon-Cohen J, Glauser F: Whiplash fracture of cervicodorsal spinous process. *JAMA* 155:560–561, 1954.

98. Hall RD: Clay-shoveler's fracture. *J Bone Joint Surg* 12:63, 1940.

99. Annan JH: Shoveler's fracture. *Lancet* 1:174, 1945.

100. Watson-Jones R: *Fractures and Joint Injuries,* ed 3. Edinburgh, E & S Livingstone, 1943.

101. Harris JH Jr: Flexion- and extension-rotation injuries. In: *The Radiology of Acute Cervical Spine Trauma.* Baltimore, Williams & Wilkins, 1978, p 71.

102. Brown CW, Orme TJ, Richardson HD: The rate of pseudoarthrosis (surgical nonunion) in patients who are smokers and patients who are non-smokers: a comparison study. *Spine* 11(9):942–943, 1986.

103. Holdsworth FW: Early orthopaedic treatment of patients with spinal injuries. In Harris P (ed): *Spinal Injuries.* London, Morrison & Gibb, 1963.

104. Holdsworth FW: Fractures, dislocations and fracture-dislocations of the spine. *J Bone Joint Surg* 52A:1534, 1970.

105. Marar BC: Hyperextension injuries of the cervical spine: the pathogenesis of damage to the spinal cord. *J Bone Joint Surg* 56A:1655, 1974.

106. Steele HH: Anatomical and mechanical considerations of the atlanto-axial articulation. *J Bone Joint Surg* 50A:1481, 1968.

107. White AA, Panjabi MM: The problem of clinical instability in the human spine: a systematic approach. In White AA, Panjabi MM (eds): *Clinical Biomechanics of the Spine.* Philadelphia, JB Lippincott, 1978, p 215.

108. Braakman R, Vinken PF: Unilateral facet interlocking in the lower cervical spine. *J Bone Joint Surg* 40B:249, 1967.

109. Beatson TR: Fractures and dislocations of the cervical spine. *J Bone Joint Surg* 45B:21, 1963.

110. Buonocore E, Hartman JT, Nelson CL: Cineradiograms of the cervical spine in diagnosis of soft-tissue injuries. *JAMA* 198(1):143–147, 1966.

111. Woesner ME, Mitts MG: The evaluation of cervical spine motion below C2: a comparison of cineroentgenographic and conventional radiographic methods. *AJR* 115(1):148–154, 1972.

112. Cheshire DJE: The stability of the cervical spine following conservative treatment of fractures and fracture-dislocations. *Paraplegia* 7:193, 1969.

113. Webb JK, Broughton RBK, McSweeney T, Park W: Hidden flexion injury of the cervical spine. *J Bone Joint Surg* 58B:322-327, 1976.

114. Panjabi MM, White AA, Keller D, Southwick WO, Friedlaender G: *Clinical Biomechanics of the Cervical Spine,* 75-WA/B10-7. New York, American Society of Mechanical Engineers, 1975.

115. Panjabi MM, White AA, Johnson RM: Cervical spine mechanics as a function of transection of components. *J Biomech* 8:327, 1975.

116. Severy DM, Mathewson JH, Bechtol CP: Controlled automobile rear-end collisions, an investigation of related engineering and mechanical phenomenon. *Can Services Med J* 11:727, 1955.

117. Severy DM, Mathewson JH: Automobile barrier and rear-end collision performance. Paper presented at the Society of Automotive Engineers summer meeting, Atlantic City, NJ, June 8–13, 1958.

118. Kabo JM, Goldsmith W, Harris NM: In-vitro head and neck response to impact. *Trans ASME* 105:316–320, 1983.

119. Clemens HJ, Burow K: Experimental investigation on injury mechanisms of cervical spine at frontal and rear-front vehicle impacts. In: *Proceedings, 16th Stapp Car Crash Conference,* SAE 720960. Detroit, MI, Society of Automotive Engineers, 1972.

120. McHenry RR, Naab KN: *Computer Simulation of Automobile Crash Victim in a Frontal Collision,* validation study report YB-2126-V-1. New York, Cornell Aeronautical Laboratory, 1966.

121. Garcia DJ: Investigation of non-linearities in the whiplash problem. PhD Thesis, Tulane University, New Orleans, LA, 1966.

122. Martinez JL, Wickstrom JK, Barcelo BT: *The Whiplash Injury—A Study of Head-Neck Action and Injuries in Animals,* ASME paper 65-WA/HVF-6. New York, American Society of Mechanical Engineers.

123. Severy DM, Mathewson JH, Bechtol CO: Controlled automobile rear end collisions—an investigation of related engineering and medical phenomena. In: *Medical Aspects of Traffic Accidents, Proceedings of the Montreal Conference,* 1955, pp 152–184.

124. McKenzie JA, Williams JF: The dynamic behaviour of the head and cervical spine during 'whiplash'. *J Biomech* 4(6):477-490, 1971.

125. Martinez JL, Garcia DJ: A model for whiplash. *J Biomech* 1:23-32, 1968.

126. Merril T, Goldsmith W, Deng YC: Three-dimensional response of a lumped parameter head-neck model due to impact and impulsive loading. *J Biomech* 17(2):81–95, 1984.

127. Orne D, Liu YK: A mathematical model of spinal response to impact. *J Biomech* 4:49–71, 1971.

128. Ewing CL, Thomas DH, Patrick LM, Beeler GW, Smith MJ: Living human dynamic response to −G impact acceleration: II. Accelerations measured on the head and neck. In: *Proceedings, 13th Stapp Car Crash Conference,* SAE 690817. Detroit, MI, Society of Automotive Engineers, 1968.

129. McKenzie JA, Williams JF: The effect of collision severity on the motion of the head and neck during 'whiplash'. *J Biomech* 8:257–259, 1975 (technical notes).

130. Yamada H: *Strength of Biological Materials.* Baltimore, Williams & Wilkins, 1970.

131. Ommaya AK, Hirsch AE: Tolerances for cerebral concussion from head impact and whiplash in primates. *J Biomech* 4:13–21, 1971.

132. Mertz HJ Jr, Patrick LM: Investigation of the kinematics and kinetics of whiplash. In: *Proceedings, 11th Stapp Car Crash Conference,* SAE 670919. Detroit, MI, Society of Automotive Engineers, 1967.

133. Jackson R: Anatomy. In Jackson R (ed): *The Cervical Syndrome.* Springfield, IL, Charles C Thomas, 1977, p 40.

134. Macnab I: Acceleration extension injuries of the cervical spine. In Rothman RH, Simeone FA (eds): *The Spine,* ed 2. Philadelphia, WB Saunders, 1982, vol 2, p 654.

135. Severy PM, Brink HM, Baird JD: Backrest and head restraint design for rear-end collision protection. Paper presented at the Automobile Engineering Congress, January 1968, SAE 680079, 114.

136. Kahane CJ: An evaluation of head restraints: federal motor vehicle safety standard 202. *NHTSA Tech Rep* DOT HS-806-108, February 1982.

137. Soechting JF, Paslay PR: A model for the human spine during impact including muscular influence. *J Biomech* 6:195–203, 1973.

138. Schutt CH, Dohan FC: Neck injury to women in auto accidents. *JAMA* 206(12):2689–2692, 1968.

139. National Safety Council: *Accident Facts.* Chicago, National Safety Council, 1971, p 47.

140. Jackson R: Crashes cause most neck pain. *Am Med New,* December 5, 1966.

141. Jackson R: The positive findings in alleged neck injuries. *Am J Orthop* 6:178–181, 184–187, 1964.

142. States JD, Korn MW, Masengill JB: The enigma of whiplash injuries. In: *Thirteenth Annual Conference Proceedings.* Rochester, NY, American Association for Automotive Medicine, 1969, pp 83–108.

143. National Coalition to Reduce Car Crash Injuries: *Statement of Purpose.* Washington, DC, National Coalition to Reduce Car Crash Injuries, July 1985.

144. Fleming A: *About Air Bags,* ed 3. Washington, DC, Insurance Institute for Highway Safety, 1985.

2

Physical Examination, Part 1

STEPHEN M. FOREMAN, DC, DABCO

The history and physical examination performed by the physician on the patient's initial office visit will usually "make or break" the future medicolegal case. Proper physical and radiological examination thus forms the basis for both the patient's care and the attorney's case.

The physical examination should be an area of primary consideration, and the time expended in the examination room, if used wisely, will eliminate hours of frustration in the future. First, the physical examination is critical in the assessment of an accurate clinical picture. What was the patient's condition before the injury? What amount of disability and pain is directly attributable to the injury? What is the most rational treatment plan? All of these questions must be considered and, if possible, answered during the physical examination.

Of legal importance is not only the physician's skill in physical examination but also his or her ability to document, inter-

pret, and convey the findings to an attorney, insurance carrier, and judge. In these litigious times, the physician is only effective if the needs of all parties are considered. Unfortunately, the best examination by any treating physician is legally worthless if the results are not documented. To put it simply, if it is not written down, it does not exist. All information, including findings that are within normal limits, must be reference or baseline. For example, a patient who suffers a severe hyperflexion-hyperextension injury can experience nerve root damage and develop a secondary atrophy of the shoulder girdle musculature. The treating physician, who may have observed that the muscles were weak but symmetrical in size on initial examination and that atrophy was manifested at 1-week follow-up and has remained as a permanent residual condition, will be faced with a problem at the end of the case. He or she will need to answer questions regarding the atrophy and its etiology, and his or her opinion will be questioned, since at the beginning of the case there was no recording of the patient's muscle size to serve as a reference point for the subsequent atrophy. In short, the physician must initially record all findings that may need to be reexamined later.

Since the topic of "physical examination" covers a wide area, only those in-office procedures that are usually indicated after trauma to the cervical spine are discussed.

History

Elicitation of an accurate history is a time-honored practice that no amount of technology will ever replace. It provides the foundation for an accurate diagnosis and the rationale for all tests. The "history" can be divided into four areas: past history, traumatic history, family history, and chief complaints.

PAST HISTORY

It is not unusual for patients to present with a complicated history of musculoskeletal injuries, especially previous incidents of cervical trauma. This problem would seem to be more common in heavily populated areas, in that in these areas there are an increased number of vehicles. For patients with a history of cervical trauma, it is vitally important for the examining physician to spend the necessary time to "sort out" the details of these specific injuries. The clinical significance of each incident must be evaluated. Documentation should include the date of injury, the treatment received, the status of the patient at discharge, the amount of permanent impairment (and, if appropriate, the amount of the award), and the patient's physical abilities after the accident. Some of this information may be obtained from a review of past medical records.

Some patients will avoid discussion of or deny previous episodes of trauma. This usually stems from fears or misconceptions about the legal system that have been instilled by family or friends. Encourage the patient to disclose all previous accidents and their clinical ramifications. Discovery of a previous accident at a later date by opposing counsel does little to enhance the patient's credibility. Some factions may even suggest that the treating physician was attempting to "hide" past episodes of trauma.

Among lawyers, there are two schools of thought concerning the importance of previous episodes of trauma. The position usually taken by the defense in a legal case is that the effects of prior episodes of trauma are cumulative in nature and are responsible for a majority of the patient's present symptoms. It is usually the defense's contention that posttraumatic changes are responsible for the present symptoms and that the most recent accident has very little to do with the present symptoms. The argument is obviously intended to reduce the legal liability of the defendant.

The other position, usually taken by the prosecution in a legal case, is that despite the previous accidents the patient was asymptomatic and the present complaints are all due to the latest injury. This position is designed to avoid "apportionment" of the award to previous accidents and is usually contended by the plaintiff's attorney.

The truth usually lies between these two positions. Most of these arguments take place at the end of the case, and the process is termed apportionment. The most important considerations of apportionment are the patient's condition at the time of release from treatment after the last injury, the length of time since that release, and the date of the most recent accident. A short asymptomatic period between two separate injuries is often a source of debate. It is contended that the current level of pain stems from both accidents. A long (more than 5 years) period tends to isolate the most recent accident as the chief cause of the patient's symptoms. In either case, it must be realized that every patient and every injury is unique and that the physician's opinion concerning apportionment must be justified.

Physicians should be as impartial as possible and "ride the fence" in decisions concerning apportionment. It is a temptation for some to favor the party who has engaged the physician's services, regardless of the facts. Physicians who take sides are quickly marked and lose their credibility in the legal system.

The past history also includes such usual items as previous surgeries, medications, and hospitalizations. Past surgeries and hospitalizations may indicate a metabolic or neoplastic condition that the patient did not relate. The use of medication is also important, in that the use of certain medications will not only help to reveal other physical conditions that the patient may have failed to mention but will also give the examiner an idea of the patient's pain threshold level.

Pain is a subjective symptom that is highly variable from patient to patient, and medications can alter the perception of pain. Aspirin and other such over-the-counter products can mask pain, and knowing that the patient has taken such drugs may alter the examiner's initial opinion.

A past history of joint disease must be evaluated. Conditions such as rheumatoid and other arthritides have been known to cause ankylosis and damage to the upper cervical ligaments that may complicate a "minor" accident (1).

FAMILY HISTORY

A complete family history, including all orthopaedic and rheumatological disorders, should be elicited and documented. Such hereditary disorders as multiple exostosis and some arthritides may affect the patient's family members, and the physician should be aware of these at the initial examination (2).

HISTORY OF ACCIDENT

Each patient should be questioned regarding the speed and direction of the vehicle in which the patient was riding and the road surface conditions at the time of the accident. This information is needed not to establish the fault or legal liability of the patient but to help the physician reconstruct the injury and apply the information to the patient's current clinical condition. The patient should also be questioned about the things that happened during the accident. Did the patient hit his or her head or lose consciousness? Were the patient's glasses knocked off or dentures knocked out? These objective findings are valuable when the examining physician attempts to communicate the severity of the accident to an attorney or insurance carrier.

The history must also include information concerning the environment within the vehicle. Was the patient or passenger wearing a seat belt? And if so, what type: shoulder or lap belt? Was the patient aware of the oncoming vehicle? These and other factors affect the biomechanics of the injury and should be documented by the examining physician. (See Chapter 1 for a discussion of the biomechanics of the cervical acceleration/deceleration syndrome).

CHIEF COMPLAINTS

Documentation of the patient's complaints should follow an established protocol. An accurate description will aid the physician in examining the areas that have been injured and will establish the reference point from which to judge improvement upon reevaluation.

Complaints should be recorded as the patient relates them; i.e., they should not be embellished by the examiner. The patient's description is often quite accurate and may give valuable clues as to the tissue causing pain. The medication used by the patient is a primary consideration during evaluation of the patient's complaints. The patient who is consuming medium to high levels of analgesics or antiinflammatory drugs will obviously have an altered sensitivity to pain.

Patient complaints that the examiner must specifically address during the examination include:

1. *Headache*. Headache is a common symptom that may arise after the trauma but could have been preexisting. The differentiation is complex and is discussed later in chapter eight.

2. *Seizures or Loss of Consciousness*. The character of each episode of syncope should be documented. The patient's loss of consciousness may be isolated, be related to a blow to the head, or have occurred as multiple episodes after the injury. Initial documentation of the symptoms is critical, in

that the condition of some patients may worsen and result in a posttraumatic epilepsy or other chronic condition. It is proper protocol to have each patient who presents with alterations in consciousness evaluated by a neurologist.

3. *Visual Disturbances.* Visual disturbances commonly occur in a patient who suffers head trauma during a vehicular accident. Diplopia, scotomas, field changes, loss of acuity, and progression of the symptoms are suggestive of a neurological insult and may often be seen in conjunction with increased intracranial pressure (3). These symptoms should be a "red flag" to the examiner and justify a complete neurological investigation.

4. *Pain.* Pain seems to be the most significant patient complaint. It can vary within the person and from person to person. Some individuals are hysteric and overexaggerate even the most minor complaint. Other patients are stoic and feel that it is a personal failure to admit to pain or impairment. The ultimate and final authority often rests with the examiner, and the courts rely on the examiner's opinion to categorize these patients so that just compensation may be awarded.

A general question that the examiner needs to determine is: "Does the clinical picture or history of trauma correlate with the symptomatic picture?" Clinical judgment comes into play when these two situations do not match.

Because there is variability in sensitivity to pain, it is important that the patient describe his or her own symptoms in an attempt to convey this severity to the physician. The physician can facilitate this process by asking specific, pointed questions. The mnemonic "O,P,Q,R,S,T" is suggested as a memory aid for the doctor that will allow for a thorough review of the patient's symptomatic picture:

O for Onset. The onset of a patient's symptoms is an important diagnostic clue. Patients with pain immediately after the accident may have suffered osseous damage. Gradual onset of pain after a whiplash injury may arise from muscles that are slowly swelling. Notations as to the pro-

gression of the symptoms from their onset to the time of examination should be made.

P for Provoking or Palliative Factors. Provoking activities are those that reproduce the patient's symptoms. The two major provoking factors are usually cervical motion and muscular contraction. Pain upon motion may indicate a joint problem, whereas pain upon isometric contraction is indicative of a muscle strain or tear.

Palliative factors are activities that alleviate the patient's symptoms. These factors may be physical, such as antalgia, or external, such as heat or cold.

Q for Quality. The quality of pain is the patient's description of that pain. The description will typically give the examiner clues regarding the structures that are causing the pain (Table 2.1).

R for Radiation. Radiation refers to pain that has been referred to another area. The pattern and quality of the pain must be established because different structures (such as nerves, muscles, and ligaments) will produce varied pain patterns. Nerve root or radicular pain follows specific myotome and dermatome patterns (Fig. 2.1). Pain arising from an injured muscle may also refer to peripheral areas. The distribution will follow specific patterns known as myotomes. Pain arising from injured ligaments may also refer pain into specific areas. The areas have been delineated into sclerotomes. Chapter 8 contains a more complete discussion of these pain referral patterns.

S for Severity. The severity of one's pain is difficult to assess. The patient should be asked to describe the level of pain on a 1–10 grading system. Grade 1 represents an annoyance, whereas grade 10 represents a severe, debilitating pain. The patient's nu-

Table 2.1.
Pain Description Chart[a]

Symptom	Structure
Deep, burning or dull pain	Bone
Crampy pain	Muscle
Sharp pain	Fracture
Throbbing pain	Vascular
Stabbing or lightning-like pain	Nerve

[a]These descriptions may appear vague, but they may help guide the examiner.

merical assessment should match his or her facial appearance and overall behavior. Is the patient currently taking pain medication? The patient's response should be noted, as it puts his or her numerical pain description into proper perspective.

T for Time The time or frequency of the pain should be noted. Is the pain constant or intermittent? Does the pain intensify during the night? Does the pain occur in cycles or wake the patient up at night?

Physical Examination

The term physical examination means different things to different people. Some examiners believe that a "complete" physical examination should take 6 hours and be concluded with a whole-body magnetic resonance scan just to make sure that nothing was missed. Others conclude their examination when they verify that the patient can see lightning and hear thunder. I believe that the areas outlined below fall somewhere in the middle and give the physician the basic information needed for the initiation of treatment or ordering tests.

VITAL SIGNS

A record of the patient's temperature, pulse rate, respiratory rate, and blood pressure should be routinely made. The implications of fever or hypertension are apparent and need not be discussed.

GENERAL APPEARANCE

The patient's general appearance is often ignored by many physicians. This is unfortunate because the patient may give clues about not only his or her physical condition but also his or her mental and social condition. Does the patient appear alert, depressed, in pain, or anxious? How does the patient dress? What style of clothing does the patient wear? Some patients wear loose or slip-on clothing because of pain in one area of the body. It is not uncommon to see a patient with low back pain wear sandals or leave his or her shoes untied. Take the time to observe these subtle clues and ask the patient for his or her reasons for a particular style of dress.

General Behavior

The patient's cooperation, speech, posture, and general attitude should be observed. Family and friends that come to the office with the patient may want to be questioned regarding the patient's behavior at home. Patients sometimes display behavioral changes after a severe cervical injury, especially after a head injury.

Does the patient's ability to communicate seem to be altered? Is the patient able to stay directed in his or her thought, or does the patient lose concentration easily and seem to "drift?" Answers to direct questions should be documented in the patient's chart, verbatim.

Mood

The patient's mood with respect to emotions such as fear, anxiety, aggression, and suspicion should be estimated and the estimate should be recorded. For example, does the patient seem cooperative, or is the patient indifferent?

Orientation

Some patients, particularly the elderly, may be disoriented to some extent for some time after an accident. Mild posttraumatic dementia may be responsible for the changes. Is the patient correct in his or her assessment of the day, date, time, and place? Does the patient know who the President is, and can the patient remember recent, current events? Questioning family members will often prove quite valuable in determining the onset of memory changes. If the patient's disorientation seems recent, a neurological consult should be sought.

Visual Inspection

Visual inspection of the patient should begin during the history. Does the patient appear to be under stress or in discomfort due to pain? Is the patient able to ambulate without a compensatory antalgia? Can the patient rise from a chair without support from a friend?

Postural analysis may reveal changes in spinal alignment secondary to either muscle spasm or idiopathic changes. External changes such as unusual head position, short neck, low hairline, or café au lait spots may indicate such underlying conditions as Klippel-Feil syndrome (Fig. 2.2), fibrous dysplasia, or neurofibromatosis.

Areas of muscle spasm or atrophy should be observed. Malingering or exaggeration should be suspected if the patient's actions and appearance do not correlate with his or her complaints.

PALPATION

The cervical spine should be palpated in each of four areas: anterior cervical musculature, posterior cervical musculature,

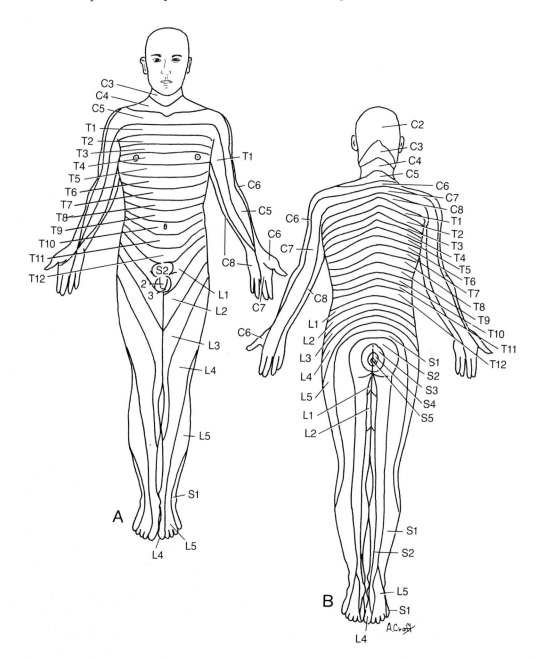

Figure 2.1. Dermatome chart depicting anterior and posterior levels. (Adapted from: *Ciba Collection of Medical Illustrations,* vol 1, *Nervous System.* New York, Colorpress, 1977.)

interspinous spaces, and related areas. Palpation should first be done lightly, and changes such as pain upon light touch, anesthesia, paresthesias, and differences in surface temperature and moisture should be noted.

Anterior Cervical Musculature

The anterior cervical area is usually damaged in the acceleration phase of the injury. Most of the damage results from the sudden stretching.

Palpation of muscles may reveal atrophy, swelling, tenderness, or asymmetry between the right and left sides. Spasm may be felt in either the superficial or the deeper muscles. The patient's ability to swallow in a smooth and pain-free manner should be noted. Dysphagia may be the result of either neurological, vascular, or soft tissue damage.

The lymph nodes, particularly the anterior cervical chain, and the supraclavicular nodes should be inspected for size, tenderness, and consistency. The thyroid

should be examined for size, tenderness, and the presence of nodules.

The carotid pulses should be evaluated for their rate, amplitude, and symmetry. Deep digital palpation over the intervertebral foramen may produce moderate pain if the nerve root at that level is irritated or inflamed.

Posterior Cervical Musculature

Deceleration injuries are sometimes less severe than acceleration injuries. The posterior musculature is protected by the strong ligamentum nuchae, and hyperflexion is sometimes limited by the patient's chin striking the chest. The damage done is usually limited to the musculature and to ligamentous and osseous areas.

The musculature may be torn and may exhibit pain, swelling, or spasticity upon palpation. The hyperflexion injury may have caused the majority of damage to the ligamentous attachments along the occiput and superior-medial border of the scapulae. Palpation of these areas may demonstrate marked tenderness. Chronic pain in these areas is often the result of long-term muscle spasm causing a reactive tenoperiostitis at the insertion. This may cause pain in the area for months, since tendons heal slowly.

Interspinous Spaces

On palpation, the interspinous spaces may be markedly tender due to hyperflexion and a subsequent stretching or tearing of the interspinous ligaments. Palpation is quite specific and may reproduce the patient's peripheral pain. The pain being produced in this manner should be documented and compared with the pain produced in sclerogenic areas. (See Chapter 8 for a full discussion.)

The interspinous tenderness may be accompanied by a palpable increase in the interspinous distance. The pain and the unusual distance between the interspinous spaces indicate a tear or stretch of the ligamentum nuchae and of the interspinous ligaments.

Pain upon direct palpation of the spinous process may be marked. This pain,

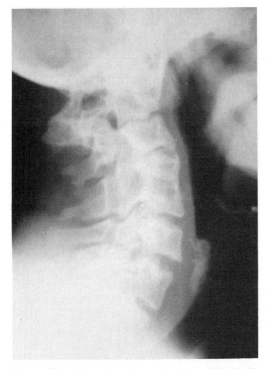

Figure 2.2. Lateral radiograph of a patient with Klippel-Feil syndrome.

combined with the history of trauma and a possible degree of aberrant movement, strongly suggests a clay shoveler's fracture.

Related Areas

Other areas should be included in the palpation phase of the physical examination. The peripheral support muscles of the back and upper chest should be inspected first. The trapezius and pectoral muscles may be swollen and tender after an accident. The suprascapular muscle and the rhomboids may be in spasm, resulting in referred pain to either the shoulder or the cervical area.

The inspection should then center around the temporomandibular joints. Palpation may reveal tenderness or asymmetry of mandibular motion. Pain upon chewing should be noted. Palpation of the masseter and buccinator muscles may reveal swelling and pain if these areas were damaged during the hyperextension phase of the injury. (See Chapter 10 for a detailed discussion of injury to the temporomandibular joints.)

PERCUSSION

Percussion plays a limited role in the evaluation. Its major function is to aid the palpation process in the localization of posterior arch fractures.

RANGE OF MOTION

"Normal" range of motion is a relative term, despite the multitude of charts and tables that are available on the subject. Some physicians compare the range of motion in all their patients, regardless of their age, with the range of motion considered normal in younger individuals. In a strict, academic view, this attitude may be justified. Other examiners view the patient's range of motion as they would blood pressure, i.e., something that changes with age. The latter attitude results in loss of some objective, ratable evidence that the patient may present at the initial evaluation.

A patient's range of motion is dependent upon osseous, ligamentous, and muscular integrity. Each component must function without restriction if motion is to be considered normal. Small aberrations in joint function or muscular contraction may disturb segmental motion. Spasticity of the paravertebral musculature has a "splinting" effect if the spasm involves multiple levels. The splinting can markedly reduce the range of motion of the entire cervical spine.

Osseous integrity may be acutely disrupted by both fractures and dislocations. Chronic degeneration of the osseous structures will take the form of osteoarthritis or of hyperostotic changes such as diffuse idiopathic skeletal hyperostosis. These conditions typically restrict the range of motion even before the patient's accident. Degenerative changes such as intervertebral osteochondrosis cause a primary and a secondary restriction as the progress of posterior joint degeneration is hastened.

Clinical differentiation of motion restriction secondary to muscular function may be achieved by using a combination of isometric contractions and assessment of the patient's active and passive range of motion. Muscular damage, such as a strain, is usually revealed by isometric contraction testing. The contraction of the muscles is likely to reproduce the patient's symptoms. The pain is usually not attributed to the joint complex because the area did not undergo movement.

Isometric contraction may cause pain in a facet joint even if the joint does not move. The facet joints in the lower cervical segments are compressed together and may cause pain when the muscles of the anterior cervical spine are contracted. To differentiate the pain arising from a joint from that arising from a muscle, simply repeat the test with the patient's neck in full flexion. The cervical flexion will reduce the compressive effects on the facets and thereby stop the pain.

Most patients with cervical muscle strain will present with pain on active movement. The majority of the pain disappears with passive or physician-assisted testing. The passive testing is less likely to produce pain because the muscles are allowed to rest during the testing.

The following is a summary of the differential diagnostic criteria used to determine the type of range of motion problem encountered:

1. *Osseous Problem Only.* The patient presents with a restricted active and passive range of motion. There is no pain on isometric contraction because the problem is isolated within the articular facets and the paravertebral muscles are not involved.

2. *Muscular Problem Only.* The patient presents with a restricted active range of motion. The patient's motion improves on passive testing. Pain will be produced, because of muscle injury, on isometric contraction.

3. *Combined Osseous and Muscular Problems.* Patients with combined osseous and muscular problems present with a restricted active and passive range of motion. This is due to osseous joint derangement. The muscular damage produces pain on isometric contraction.

The range of motion should not only be full but should also be smooth. Areas of restriction and crepitus should be noted.

"Normal" values may differ in various texts. Thurber (4) has suggested that "the examiner consider the age of the patient, his general physical condition, his stature, anomalies, or other abnormal conditions" and use these factors to determine the normal range of motion for that patient. The patient's range of motion should be rated as a percentage of normal for his or her age group. The following examples demonstrate application of this principle:

Example 1. PMS, a 26-year-old man, had had no previous episodes of neck pain or restricted motion. The patient's appearance was normal, and there were no visible signs of structural abnormalities such as scoliosis. The patient's hairline was located at the normal level, and the skin was free of café au lait spots. Goniometric measurement revealed restriction at 45° upon right rotation. A rotation of 90° would normally be expected, since there were no indications of underlying restrictive change. Therefore, the documentation should read: "range of motion: 45°, 50% of normal."

Example 2. RJB, a 72-year-old man, had had numerous episodes of cervical pain and stiffness over the past 20 years. His current complaint consisted of "pain," and although his neck was stiff, he reported it felt "no worse than always." Goniometric measurement revealed that both right and left rotations were limited at 45°. All other directions of motion were likewise restricted.

Radiography showed degenerative changes in the posterior facets and disc areas that were consistent with the patient's age. Documentation should, therefore, read: "right and left rotation: 45°, 100% of normal."

Neurological Examination___

Injuries arising from vehicular accidents may also damage the central or peripheral nervous system. These delicate structures are vulnerable to damage by both traction and compression. Traction injuries usually develop when the patient's head is thrown laterally. Compression injuries result from a sudden compression of the spinal nerve root. The compression may be caused by an intervertebral foramen compromised by hypertrophic bone formation. A normal intervertebral foramen may also cause nerve root damage if ligamentous damage allows instability within the canal.

The nervous system damage may result in damage to either motor or sensory units of the nerve root. The physical examination should allow an adequate exploration of motor and sensory functions. (See Chapter 9 for a complete discussion of damage to the central, peripheral, and autonomic nervous systems.)

The nervous system may be evaluated by various methods. Some physicians prefer to examine each nerve root level individually. I prefer to test for each function as a separate entity. This method increases the speed of the examination and assures that findings are not omitted.

TESTS FOR COORDINATION, GAIT, AND EQUILIBRIUM

Alterations in the patient's coordination and ambulatory abilities may arise from both trauma to and disease of the brain or spinal cord. Acceleration/deceleration injuries may result in a change in the patient's abilities either from increased intracranial pressure due to an intracranial hematoma or from spinal cord pressure. Spinal cord pressure may be applied via a herniated disc, via a hematoma, or directly via a fracture or dislocation.

A variety of tests may be employed to evaluate a patient's ambulatory skills. The following tests, most of which center around cerebellar dysfunction (5), should be employed in cervical injury cases in which injury to the brain or spinal cord must be ruled out:

1. *Walking Test.* Observation of the patient's ability to walk will reveal information about his or her coordination, gait, antalgia, and peripheral joint function. Is the patient able to walk smoothly and execute quick turns? Is the patient's stance normal or broad based for balance? Does the patient use his or her arms for balance, or does the patient swing his or her arms in a normal fashion at the side?

If the patient's walking pattern is normal, proceed onto more demanding tests. Is the patient able to walk heel-to-toe and maintain balance? This type of exercise requires a higher degree of function from the patient's dorsal columns and may indicate damage. Instructing the patient to close his or her eyes during this test eliminates a visual reference and further tests the functional ability of the balance system.

2. *Romberg's Test.* Romberg's test is performed by instructing the patient to place his or her feet together, close the eyes, and attempt to maintain a normal balance. This test is a variation of the walking tests previously described and is considered positive (Romberg's sign) if the patient sways excessively or falls down. A positive test indicates dysfunction of the dorsal columns.

3. *Finger Tests.* The finger (finger-to-finger and finger-to-nose) tests are cerebellar tests that aid in examining the patient's ability to move an extremity through space and to stop at a specific point. The finger-to-nose test requires the patient to close his or her eyes and touch the index fingers to the nose. The finger-to-finger test consists of the patient touching his or her fingers together with the arms extended and eyes closed. Cerebellar disease or dysfunction arising from increased intracranial pressure may cause the patient to develop dysmetria.

4. *Finger Movement Test.* Rapid movement of the fingers requires cerebellar control. Intracranial pressure or cerebellar disease prohibits rapid movement.

5. *Test for Rebound Phenomenon.* The previously described disease processes will depress the patient's ability to stop strong active movements. This can be recognized when the patient cannot avoid striking his or her shoulder when the doctor quickly releases the patient's strongly contracted arm. This is known as the rebound phenomenon or Holmes test.

MOTOR EXAMINATION

Integrity of the motor fibers in the cervicobrachial plexus is ascertained by testing the strength of the major muscle groups of the upper extremities. Each level, C5–T1, must be tested for strength as well as examined for the duration of time the strength is available.

Muscle strength is categorized by the following grades:

Grade 0. There is no evidence of muscle contraction. This would include evidence produced during electrodiagnostic testing.

Grade 1. There is palpable or visual evidence of muscle contraction, but the muscle is not strong enough to move the joint adjacent to the area.

Grade 2. There is poor muscle strength. The muscles are capable of moving the adjacent joint through a complete range of motion if gravity is removed.

Grade 3. There is fair muscle strength. The patient is capable of moving the area through a full range of motion against gravity. Any additional amount of imposed weight of resistance stops the patient's movement.

Grade 4. There is good muscle strength in the affected area. The patient's strength is not considered normal, however, as he or she is not able to move the area through its normal range of motion against partial resistance.

Grade 5. The patient's muscle strength is considered "normal." The patient is able to move the limb through a normal range of motion even against heavy resistance.

These grades (0–5) should be applied (*a*) to neurological levels if the nerve root is damaged and (*b*) to specific muscles when these are injured.

Grades 0–3 are most often seen in injuries that directly affect multiple nerve roots. Other injuries, such as crushing or tractional injuries, may damage the roots and produce grades 0–3. Atrophy may appear within 72 hours in the muscles directly supplied by the injured nerves. Grades 3 and 4 are more commonly encountered in ambulatory practice.

Duration or endurance of strength is often overlooked during the physical examination. Examiner-induced fatigue can reveal subclinical evidence of nerve root damage. Testing of a suspect neurological level by five or six consecutive muscle contractions of the innervated area may reveal an underlying weakness. The problem may be evident only after the repetitive movement induces ischemia in the damaged nerve root. These subtle changes must be verified by testing the uninvolved side in an identical manner. If, by chance, an identical weakness on the uninvolved side is discovered, these results should be compared with those tests of the surrounding levels.

A more objective method of testing the strength of the upper extremities is through the use of the Jaymar dynamometer. The dynamometer simply records the maximum effort of grip strength. Documentation should include the position of the adjustable grip. The examiner must state whether the patient exerted maximum effort. A patient who is suspected of using less than maximum effort automatically invalidates that portion of the examination. The procedure is performed three times on each extremity. Specific muscular actions in the upper extremities are then correlated with specific nerve root levels (Table 2.2).

Table 2.2.
Neurological Breakdown by Level, Nerve, and Muscle Affected

Level	Nerve	Muscle
C5	Axillary	Deltoid
C6	Musculocutaneous	Biceps
C7	Radial	Triceps
C8	Median	Finger flexors
T1	Ulnar	Finger abductors

SENSORY EXAMINATION

The sensory examination is an important aspect of the physical examination because many of the presenting symptoms will be alterations in the patient's sensory abilities. Many of these abnormalities will be described as areas of numbness that may be vague and difficult to localize for the patient. A complete sensory examination can be exhausting for both the physician and the patient. Each participant should be well rested and attempt to be cooperative.

Injuries to specific peripheral nerves or spinal nerve roots can cause sensory loss that may be traced to one specific area of the body known as a dermatome. Dermatome levels may vary from one individual to the next but will usually be fairly consistent. The examination should be conducted with the aid of Whartenberg pinwheel, and each arm should be tested independently. Each dermatome level should be compared with its adjacent level for similar loss of sensitivity. When sensory loss in several contiguous levels is noted, sensory examination of the other extremity should be carried out.

Areas of vague pain may present in an extremity and will not conform to a specific dermatomal pattern. These are often areas of referred pain from ligamentous structures. See Chapter 8 for complete discussion of the referral pattern from these structures.

Other sensory functions may be altered after cervical trauma. The following sensory functions should be tested as part of the regular physical examination:

1. *Pain Perception.* A patient's ability to perceive pain may be evaluated by use of a sharp pin. The amount of pressure needed to cause the patient pain may be compared with the amount of pressure needed to cause pain in the examiner's arm or in the patient's opposite extremity. Changes include:

A. Anesthesia—complete loss of sensation.
B. Hypesthesia—diminished sensation.
C. Hyperesthesia—increased tactile sensibility.
D. Hyperalgesia—increased sensibility to pain.

2. *Temperature Sensibility.* Damage to

either the peripheral nerves or lateral spinothalamic tract of the spinal cord may cause the patient to lose perception of hot and cold. Testing of these sensations may be accomplished by using test tubes, one filled with hot water and the other filled with cold, and applying them to the surface of the patient's skin to determine whether the patient can differentiate between the two.

Severe trauma to the spine may cause either a functional or an actual hemisection of the spinal cord. This injury will cause a loss of pain and temperature sensibility on the contralateral side and a loss of proprioception, vibratory perception, two-point discrimination, and joint position on the ipsilateral side. This phenomenon is clinically termed the Brown-Séquard syndrome (6).

3. *Two-Point Discrimination.* Two-point discrimination is a widely used method for testing the functional capacity of the dorsal columns and lemniscal system. The test is conducted by placing two pins closely together on the patient's skin and gradually

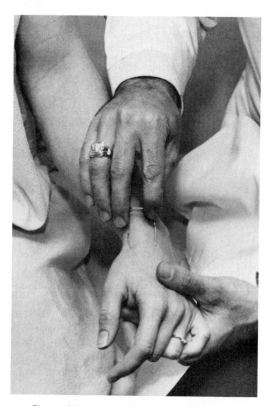

Figure 2.3. Two-point discrimination test.

moving them farther apart until two separate points are felt (Fig. 2.3). The fine discrimination of these stimuli depends on the amount and organization of the specialized tactile receptors in the skin. These receptors are more concentrated in the hairless areas of the skin, which explains why the normal two-point distance is 2–5 mm on the hands and as much as 30–70 mm on the back. Alterations in the perception of the two points may indicate damage to either the dorsal columns or the lemnisus. These results should be correlated with the results of other tests in order to confirm this diagnosis.

4. *Vibratory Perception.* The vibratory effect of a tuning fork can be perceived by Meissner and Pacini corpusles and transmitted only in the dorsal column of the spinal cord. Testing done with a 128-cycle/sec tuning fork is a valuable indicator of dorsal column disease. The fork should be placed over the bony prominences in the upper and lower extremities, and the quality and duration of the perception should be noted. It is not unusual for the geriatric patient to have little vibratory interpretation below the knee.

5. *Sense of Position.* Joint position can be categorized as both static and kinesthetic. The sense of static position is the conscious recognition of joint or extremity position in relation to the body. The sense of kinesthetic position is the recognition of the rate and direction of joint or extremity movement.

A variety of nerve endings are responsible for the detection and interpretation of joint movement. Ruffini endings, Golgi tendon receptors, and Pacini corpuscles are responsible for the majority of interpretive duties (7). The examiner may test for sense of position by holding the sides of the patient's great toe and bending the toe at the joint. The patient, with eyes closed, attempts to determine the direction of movement. Other joints may be tested in this same manner.

6. *Stereognosis.* Stereognosis is the interpretive ability of the brain to assess the weight and form of objects held in the hand. The patient, with eyes closed, is asked to identify and name common objects, such as a house key, coin, or comb, that are placed in his or her hand by the examiner.

7. *Light Touch.* The examiner may test the patient for the ability to perceive light touch by stroking the skin with cotton.

8. *Topognosis.* Topognosis is the ability to perceive and localize tactile stimulation. The examiner should have the patient close his or her eyes and then touch the person on the arm or leg. The patient (with eyes still closed) should then be able to point to the spot touched by the examiner.

TESTS FOR CIRCULATORY DISORDERS

Cervical acceleration/deceleration syndrome may cause the previously described sensory abnormalities, but areas of "numbness" and paresthesia may arise not only from neural damage but also from circulatory complications. Decreased vascular supply, whether from injury or preexisting disease, may cause symptoms that both the patient and the physician incorrectly attribute to neurological insult.

Several tests that will help differentiate the etiology of upper extremity sensory abnormalities are available. The following are valuable aids in the evaluation of vascular disorders:

1. *Blood Pressure.* The examiner should take the patient's blood pressure on both the right and the left side. Vascular occlusive disease resulting in altered upper extremity function will typically lower the pressure on the affected side.

2. *Adson's Test.* Adson's test can provide insight into symptoms arising from vascular compression. The test is performed in the following manner: The examiner palpates the patient's radial pulse to establish its rate, force, and amplitude. The patient then rotates his or her head toward the side being tested, raises the chin, and takes a deep breath for a count of 12. The examiner may detect an alteration in the radial pulse as the result of neurovascular compression of the subclavian artery. A positive finding is typically caused by a cervical rib or by the scalenus anticus syndrome (Fig. 2.4*A*). The "reverse Adson's" or Halstead test is demonstrated in Figure 2.4*B*. This variation is performed in conjunction with Adson's test.

3. *Allen's Test.* Allen's test establishes peripheral patency of the vascular system. The patient is instructed to clench his or her fist in order to expel the blood from the area. The examiner then occludes both the radial and the ulnar artery (Fig. 2.5) just proximal to the wrist. The patient is instructed to unclench the fist, and then the examiner releases pressure from the radial artery. The color of the tested side should return to the same color as the opposite extremity within 4 seconds. Failure to return to pretest color within normal time frame indicates occlusion of the collateral circulation. The test is then repeated, and the examiner releases pressure from the ulnar artery to test its patency.

REFLEX EXAMINATION

A reflex is an involuntary motor response to sensory stimuli. Most of the sensory stimuli is directed to either the surface of the skin or to a specific tendon. Initiation of the stretch reflex is typically accomplished by briskly striking either the tendon or the muscle insertion with a rubber hammer. The resulting reflex may be graded from 0 (no response) to 4+ (a clonus response). A 2+ is considered to be normal, and a grade of 1+ or 3+ is considered hypoactive or hyperactive, respectively. The superficial reflex is usually elicited by stroking the skin with the end of the reflex hammer. The abdominal test is a good example of this type of testing.

Significance of Abnormality

Reflex testing is a simple method for evaluating the presence of a complete reflex arc in the patient. The arc extends from the extremity, through the spinal cord, and returns. Conditions such as trauma may damage or totally disrupt the arc and cause a diminishment of the normal reflex. This is a subjective evaluation on the part of the examiner, and therefore, results of reflex testing on one extremity should be compared with results of testing on the opposite extremity.

Types of Reflexes

Reflexes are usually divided into four categories: deep tendon, superficial, visceral and pathological (8). This discussion focuses on the individual areas that most

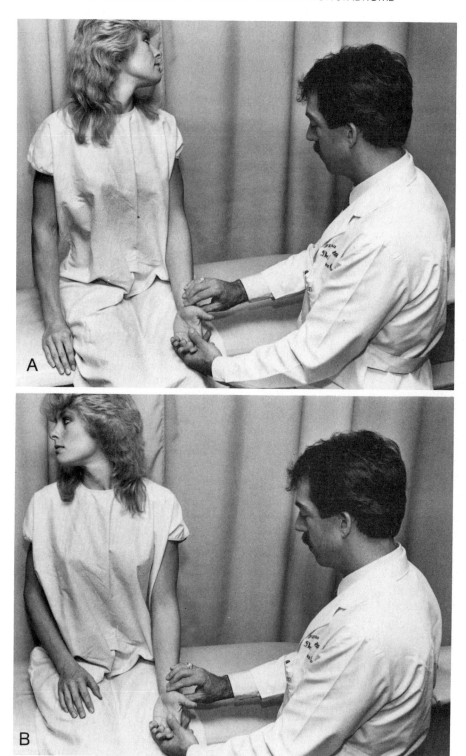

Figure 2.4.   A. Adson's test. The examiner palpates the radial pulse and instructs the patient to rotate the head toward the side being examined. **B.** "Reverse Adson's test"; i.e., Adson's test with the patient's head turned away from the side being examined.

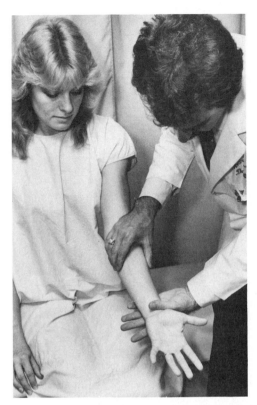

Figure 2.5. Allen's test. The examiner's thumb is positioned to occlude the radial artery.

relate to the examination of the accident victim.

Deep Tendon Reflexes. The deep tendon reflexes may, in theory, be elicited on any muscle in the body. This is obviously impractical and would tend to annoy the patient. Clinical neurologists have identified the following as the important deep reflexes:

1. *Maxillary or Jaw Jerk Reflex.* The maxillary reflex is elicited by lightly striking each half of the patient's mandible while he or she holds it half open. This test measures the reflexes of the masseter and pterygoid muscles on each side. A response is considered normal if the patient's jaw jerks shut. In patients with unilateral frontal lobe lesions, the jaw jerk reflex may be increased only on one side (5). The motor portion of the fifth cranial nerve is being tested in this examination.

2. *Biceps Reflex (C5).* The biceps reflex is elicited by striking the patient's biceps tendon. This action tests the reflex arc of C5-C6 and the musculocutaneous nerve. The response is usually depressed if damage has occurred to the C5 nerve root.

3. *Brachioradialis Reflex (C6).* The brachioradialis reflex also comes from the C5-C6 level, but I consider it primarily for C6. The test is performed by having the patient flex his or her arm while holding the forearm in the neutral position. The tendon located just above the wrist is then struck with the reflex hammer.

4. *Triceps Reflex (C7).* When the triceps tendon just above the elbow is struck with the reflex hammer, a contraction of the triceps muscle should be observed. This test is used to evaluate the radial nerve and the C7 root level.

5. *Patellar or Knee Jerk Reflex (L4).* The patellar reflex test consists of striking the patient's patellar tendon with his or her knee in flexion. The normal response is for the leg to move toward extension. An absence of this reflex is known as Westphal's sign.

6. *Achilles Reflex (S1).* The Achilles reflex is elicited by striking the patient's Achilles tendon with a reflex hammer. The tendon should be slightly stretched by gently dorsiflexing the foot. The foot will normally plantarflex.

Pathological Reflexes. The higher centers of neurological function, the motor cortex and pyramidal tract, will normally inhibit the reactive nature of the contraction and thereby "dampen" the reflexes. An increased reflex (hyperreflexia) or clonus of the muscle indicates a loss of the inhibitory function, and disease (upper motor neuron lesion) may be assumed. The upper motor neuron lesion will allow the neurological unit to return to the primitive defense responses. These responses are created when the lower motor neuron is separated from the rest of the neurological system, and these responses are termed pathological reflexes.

Although there are a wide variety of pathological reflexes that have been identified over the years, there are only a few signs that seem to endure and provide a

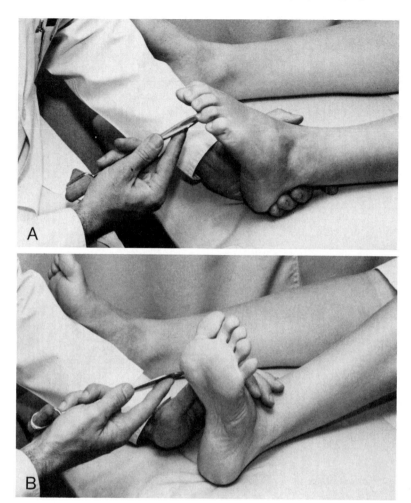

Figure 2.6.   **A.** Plantar flexion of the toes is representative of a normal Babinski reflex. **B.** Fanning of the toes in an abnormal Babinski reflex.

good understanding of the patient's problems. A large majority of patients will present with a wide variety of positive signs because the upper motor neuron lesion will usually not localize into just one sign and not affect the others.

For purposes of this discussion, I separate the pathological reflexes into those of the upper extremities and those of the lower extremities. Many of the names used in these tests are repeated in both extremities, and care must be exercised to avoid confusion. Despite the large number of tests listed in most neurological texts, I include only the most commonly used.

Upper Extremity. The following signs are useful in the evaluation of upper extremity pathology:

1. *Chaddock's Wrist Sign.* The test for Chaddock's wrist sign is performed by stroking the ulnar side of the forearm with the end of the reflex hammer. A positive finding is flexion of the wrist with extension and fanning or separation of the fingers.

2. *Hoffmann's Sign.* The examiner strikes or taps the distal end of the index finger, which produces a clawing movement of the thumb and fingers.

3. *Gordon's Finger Sign.* Have the patient flex or contract his or her fingers and thumb before the test. A positive sign consists of an extension of the fingers when the examiner applies pressure to the pisiform bone.

4. *Trömner's Sign.* Trömner's sign is

similar to Hoffmann's sign. A sharp tap or similar stimulation to the palmer surface, distal ends of the phalanges will produce a reflex contraction of the fingers.

5. *Forced Grasping Sign.*   A return to the primitive reflexes may occur when the patient suffers from an upper motor neuron lesion. The most common example of this is Babinski's reflex. The forced grasping sign is produced when the examiner strokes the palmer surface of the patient's hand. A rapid flexion or grasping motion would constitute a positive finding.

6. *Souques' Sign.*   Souques' sign is useful in evaluating whether or not a patient is exerting a full effort when attempting to raise an injured arm. The patient's fingers will spread out and remain extended while attempting to raise the paralyzed arm.

Lower Extremities. Injuries to the cervical area may also cause long tract signs in the spinal cord and result in pathological reflexes in the lower extremities. The majority of these injuries produce a Babinski

response or initiate a muscular clonus, both of which are indicative of an upper motor neuron lesion. The following signs are usually reliable indicators and should be considered a useful addition to a complete examination:

1. *Babinski Sign.*   The Babinski sign is a well-recognized test for upper motor neuron lesions and reflects a return to the primitive reflex state commonly observed in the infant. Extension of the great toe and a separation of the other toes after the examiner strokes the plantar surface of the patient's foot would be considered a positive sign (Fig. 2.6*A* and *B*). Other activities may stimulate the same pathological action, and each is discussed.

2. *Schäffer's Sign.*   A Babinski reflex is elicited after the examiner squeezes the patient's Achilles tendon.

3. *Oppenheim's Sign.*   A Babinski reflex is elicited after the examiner strokes the patient's tibia firmly.

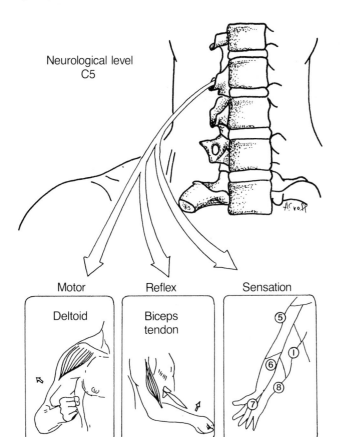

Neurological level
C5

Motor   Reflex   Sensation

Deltoid   Biceps
               tendon

Figure 2.7. Schematic drawing depicting the C5 neurological level. (Adapted from Hoppenfeld S: *Orthopaedic Neurology.* Philadelphia, JB Lippincott, 1977.)

4. *Gordon's Sign.*   A Babinski reflex is elicited when the examiner squeezes the patient's calf muscle.

5. *Rossolimo's Sign.*   Flexion of the patient's toes after the examiner taps the ball of the patient's foot is considered positive.

6. *Gonda Reflex.*   The Gonda reflex consists of extension of the great toe after one of the other toes is bent downward and then quickly released.

7. *Ankle Clonus.*   Clonus is described as a rapid contraction and relaxation of a muscle seen in conjunction with an upper motor neuron lesion. Ankle clonus is produced by forcefully dorsiflexing the patient's foot while supporting the raised leg beneath the patient's knee with the other hand.

8. *Patellar Clonus (Trepidation Sign).*   The patella may reveal clonus by a rapid superoinferior oscillation. The clonus is initiated by quickly depressing the patient's patella while the patient's knee is extended and leg is relaxed.

Measurements

Measurements of the cervical spine are a valuable source of objective evidence. The size of the area is likely to change, and the tape measure is, therefore, the most effective tool for monitoring these changes.

An increase in size of the musculature typically arises from swelling or spasm, and swelling in the cervical area may be observed over an extended time. I have found that swelling in the musculature may last for 6–8 weeks despite physical therapy and immobilization. Another interesting (and surprising) finding is the fluctuation in swelling seen among patients.

My treatment routine includes measurement of the cervical area on each visit. I have observed a similar fluctuation in the amount of swelling and in the report of patient's symptoms and have seen many patients who suddenly complained of pain after several asymptomatic weeks. Swell-

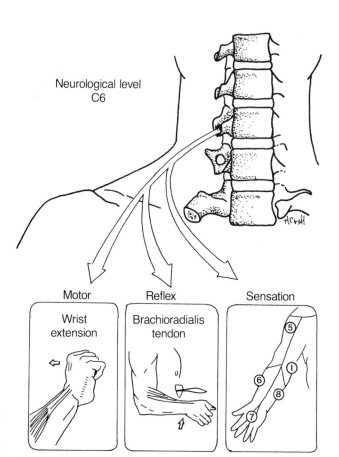

Neurological level
C6

Motor   Reflex   Sensation

Wrist extension   Brachioradialis tendon

Figure 2.8. Schematic drawing depicting the C6 neurological level. (Adapted from Hoppenfeld S: *Orthopaedic Neurology.* Philadelphia, JB Lippincott, 1977.)

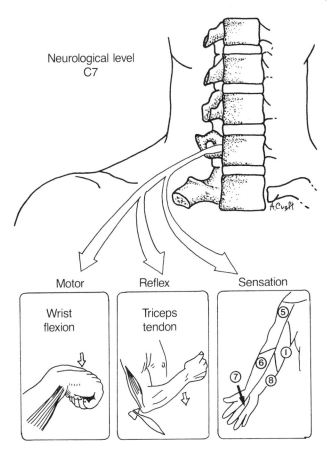

Neurological level
C7

Figure 2.9. Schematic drawing depicting the C7 neurological level. (Adapted from Hoppenfeld S: *Orthopaedic Neurology*. Philadelphia, JB Lippincott, 1977.)

Motor | Reflex | Sensation

Wrist flexion

Triceps tendon

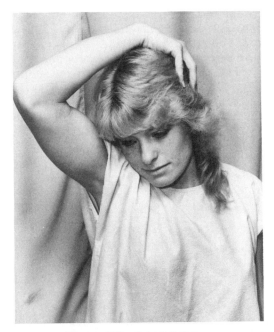

Figure 2.10. Bakody's sign.

ing had been absent during the asymptomatic period, and measurement upon exacerbation showed renewed swelling, almost to the original level. These regularly done measurements have been quite useful when attempting to justify additional treatment or attempting to discover the malingerer.

NEUROLOGICAL LEVEL DIAGNOSTIC GROUPINGS

Alterations in the diagnostic tests previously outlined are of obvious importance in the case of any patient. The findings, however, should be grouped into neurological levels in an attempt to correlate the symptomatic picture with the specifics of the accident and the radiographic picture. Injury of a specific nerve root will often manifest alteration in a variety of functions.

The following diagnostic groups along with appropriate figures and Table 2.2 will

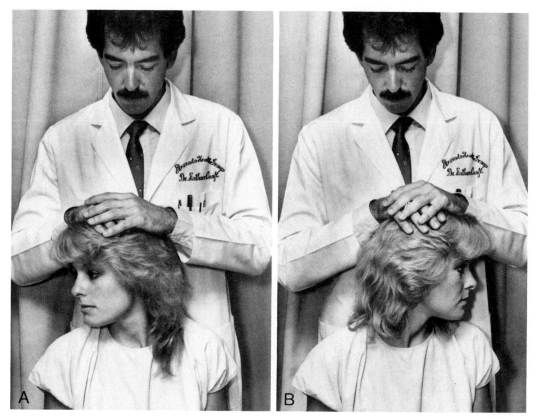

Figure 2.11. **A.** Jackson's compression test. The examiner pushes the patient's head down. **B.** Jackson's compression test on the left side.

be of help to the examiner in correlating structure, function, and diagnosis for each level:

1. *C5 Neurological Level.* The C5 nerve root is the uppermost level of the brachial plexus. It supplies motor innervation to, among others, the deltoid and biceps muscles. The axillary nerve provides sensory innervation to the lateral arm. The biceps reflex is the primary indicator for neurological integrity of the level (Fig. 2.7).

2. *C6 Neurological Level.* The C6 nerve root, along with the C5 nerve root, makes up the upper trunk of the brachial plexus. It supplies motor innervation to the biceps and wrist extensor muscles. The musculocutaneous nerve, which receives some of its supply from C6, supplies sensation to the lateral forearm. The brachioradialis muscle, although it receives sensory innervation from the radial nerve, is largely a function of C6 (Fig. 2.8).

3. *C7 Neurological Level.* The C7 nerve root is the primary supplier of motor innervation to the triceps, finger extensors, and wrist flexor muscles. Branches of the ulnar, radial, and median nerves receive input from C7. The triceps reflex is the primary indicator of C7 neurological function. The third finger on each hand receives its sensory supply from the C7 level (Fig. 2.9).

4. *C8 Neurological Level.* The C8 nerve root arises between the C7 and the T1 vertebra. It supplies sensory innervation to the ring and little finger of the hand and the distal half of the ulnar side of the forearm. The physician must rely on sensory testing and evaluation of the strength of interosseus muscles to establish C8 function. There is no established reflex for C8.

5. *T1 Neurological Level.* The T1 nerve root, like the C8 nerve root, has no known reflex, which forces the examiner to rely on the sensory and the motor function test to establish neurological integrity. The motor

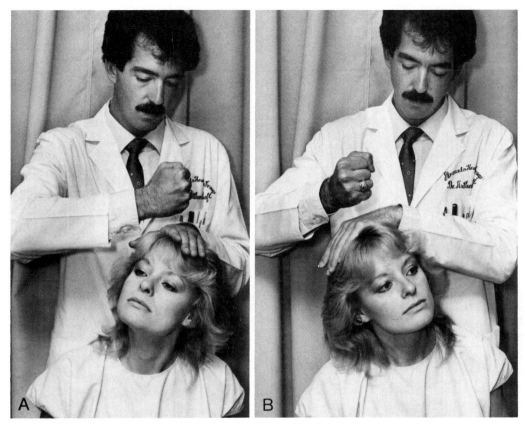

Figure 2.12. **A.** Spurling's test of the left foramina. **B.** Spurling's test of the right foramina.

innervation supplies the interosseus muscles of the hand. The sensory component, provided through the medial brachial cutaneous nerve, supplies the medial side of the arm over the elbow.

ORTHOPAEDIC TESTING

A wide variety of orthopaedic tests have been devised and described over the years. Each test attempts to reproduce the patient's symptoms in order to identify the tissue or structures responsible for the patient's symptomatic picture. The majority of the tests attempt to either increase intrathecal pressure, stretch or compress nerves, or stretch paravertebral muscles.

Nerve Root Compression Tests

The following nerve root compression tests have been found useful in identifying the tissue or structure responsible for the patient's symptoms:

1. *Bakody's Sign.* The patient with a cervical disc herniation or acute radicular pain will often present with the hand of the affected extremity placed on top of the head. This position will usually lessen or eliminate the radicular symptoms (Fig. 2.10).

2. *Jackson's Compression Test.* Jackson describes a test in which the patient is instructed to rotate his or her head first to the right and then to the left. The examiner then exerts downward pressure on the patient's head after each movement. This compresses the nerve root, due to changes in intervertebral foramen size (Fig. 2.11*A* and *B*).

3. *Spurling's Test.* Spurling's test is one of a variety of tests in which the contents of the intervertebral foramen are compressed. The patient is seated on an examination stool and is instructed to rotate and laterally flex the head to either the right or the left. When the head is in maximum rotation and flexion, the examiner delivers a vertical blow to the top of the head (Fig.

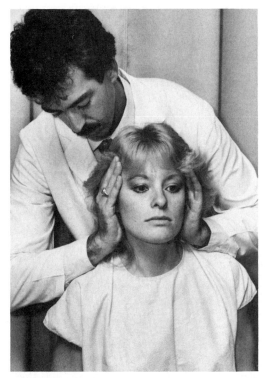

Figure 2.13. Vertical distraction of the cervical spine being applied by the examiner.

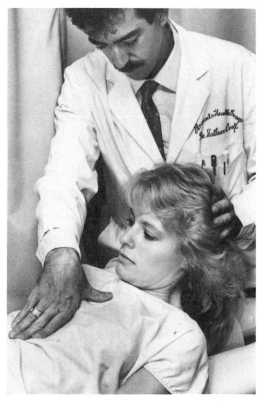

Figure 2.15. Soto-Hall test to traction the spinal cord.

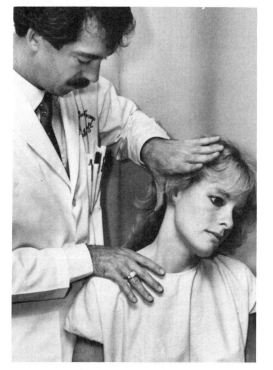

Figure 2.14. Shoulder depression test to stretch the right side.

2.12*A* and *B*). This test should be performed bilaterally.

4. *Maximum Cervical Compression Test.* The maximum cervical compression test is basically the same as Spurling's test but without the vertical blow to the head. The patient first flexes his or her head laterally and then rotates it to the side being tested. This position narrows the intervertebral foramen as much as anatomically possible. It is suggested that this test be performed before Spurling's test.

Muscular Stretch Test

Some orthopaedic tests are designed to stretch the paravertebral muscles and, at the same time, decompress the intervertebral foramen. These tests may cause pain by stretching torn muscles or may relieve symptoms if the nerve root is injured. An examination of the temporomandibular joint should be performed before these tests are carried out, since traction may further irritate the area. These tests include:

1. *Cervical Distraction.* Cervical distraction, as the term implies, consists of a slow, continuous vertical traction being applied to the patient's cervical spine by the examiner. Pain usually indicates muscle injury (Fig. 2.13).

2. *Shoulder Depression.* The shoulder depression test is performed with the patient seated. The head of the patient is laterally flexed away from the side being tested by the examiner who then tractions the shoulder and rotates the patient's face away from the side being tested. This combination of movements may elicite pain either from the muscles or from the adhesions of the dural sleeves around the nerve roots (Fig. 2.14).

OTHER TESTS

A variety of other tests are performed in posttraumatic cases. Some may traction the spinal cord, while others may exert pressure on the neural canal by increasing the intrathecal pressure. Both of the following tests are of help to the examiner in detecting the presence of mass effect lesions that affect the spinal cord:

1. *Valsalva Test.* The Valsalva test or maneuver is designed to increase the intrathecal pressure around the spinal cord. The presence of a space-occupying mass such as a tumor or herniated disc, coupled with an increase in spinal canal pressure, will often result in pain that radiates down the spine or into an extremity.

This test is performed by instructing the patient to take in a deep breath and strain down as if they were going to move the bowels. If pain is elicited, the test is positive.

2. *Soto-Hall Test.* The Soto-Hall test is designed to traction the spinal cord. The spinal cord, when stretched over a mass, will produce a pain that has been described as "electric or lightning like" in quality. The pain usually travels down the spine and often into the legs.

This test is simple to perform and is often modified by a variety of methods. Place the patient in the supine position and instruct the patient to flex his or her neck and touch chin to chest (Fig. 2.15). The test may be modified by helping the patient raise both legs 45–50° and repeat the movement of the cervical spine. The leg position is of help in tractioning the cord from below. The test is positive if pain is elicited.

Summary

1. The physical examination is the foundation upon which all treatment and medical-legal decisions are built. It must be complete and include all items that may be evaluated at the end of the case.

2. The history and physical examination both contain items that are to be used in the prognosis scale.

3. The findings on physical examination should correlate with the history of the accident. Malingering should be suspected if the two do not match.

4. A complete physical examination must include the following areas: osseous, neurological, myofascial, and ligamentous.

References

1. Crellin RQ, MacCabe JJ, Hamilton EBD: Severe subluxation of the cervical spine in rheumatoid arthritis. *J Bone Joint Surg* 5:61, 1962.
2. Foreman SM, Serrins PM: Malignant degeneration of hereditary multiple exostosis: a case history. *J Manipulative Physiol Ther* 7(4): 267–273, 1984.
3. Gilroy J, Meyer JS: *Medical Neurology*, ed 3. New York Macmillan, 1979.
4. Thurber P: *Evaluation of Industrial Disabilities*, ed 2. New York, Oxford University Press, 1960.
5. Chusid JG: *Correlative Neuroanatomy and Functional Neurology*, ed 19. Los Altos, CA, Lange Medical Publications, 1975.
6. DeGowin E: *Bedside Diagnostic Examination*, ed 4. New York, Macmillan, 1981.
7. Guyton AC: *Textbook of Medical Physiology*, ed 7. Philadelphia, WB Saunders, 1986.
8. Baker AB, Baker LH: *Clinical Neurology*. Philadelphia, Harper & Row, 1982.

3

Physical Examination, Part 2

ARTHUR C. CROFT, DC, MS, DABCO

> "To learn how to treat disease, one must learn how to recognize it. The diagnosis is the best trump in the scheme of treatment."
>
> *Jean Martin Charcot (1825–1893)*

Injuries to the cervical spine may present with a myriad of symptoms, depending on the type and severity of damage inflicted. The biomechanics of the head and neck are such that relatively little force is required to produce profound injury. The average head weighs about 10 lb and, mounted on a narrow flexible bony column supported only by muscles and ligaments, makes the cervical spine vulnerable to acceleration/deceleration injury. Severy et al. (1), using anthropomorphic dummies, found that in a 15-mile/hour rear-end collision the head can be accelerated to a force of 10 G. Other factors, such as the relative size and speed of the vehicles involved, road conditions, and position of the head at impact, also greatly influence the outcome of the injury. Chapter 1 provides a detailed description of the biokinetics and

biomechanics involved in how these forces affect the skeleton and soft tissues.

In dealing with cervical spine trauma it is prudent to assume initially that some serious soft tissue, osseous, or nervous system trauma does exist. The clinician should first take a detailed history of the events of the trauma and then make a careful and complete physical examination as is described in Chapter 2.

The importance of the history cannot be overstated and may sometimes contribute more usable information than the physical examination itself, especially when only soft tissue injury is involved. Knowing that the patient as driver had his or her head turned toward the passenger at the time of impact, for example, would allow better understanding of which joints were compressed and which joints were distracted.

As pointed out in Chapter 2, many signs or symptoms of trauma may be occult on initial presentation. One must search carefully for signs of nervous system trauma, soft tissue injury, and occult fracture before proceeding on to treatment. Many times, the patient is in pain at the initial examination, and performance of some tests may not be appropriate or even possible. For example, range of motion tests and certain other orthopaedic tests should not be performed in cases of cervical spine trauma in which fracture or dislocation is possible. If any test is omitted, a note should be added to the patient's chart and this test performed as soon as it can be tolerated or performed safely. Pain can also alter the outcome of certain tests, thereby confusing the clinician, who is wise to assume the worst until proven otherwise. Again, test results that are equivocal should be noted and then the tests repeated as often as necessary until satisfactory results are obtained.

The human body is a dynamic organism, and after injury it may experience several stages of change or reaction. Initially, protective muscle spasm guards and stabilizes damaged structures. Only later may ligamentous instability become apparent. Along with this instability, secondary changes such as nerve root irritation may occur. The patient's condition thus needs to be constantly reassessed during the treatment period.

A potentially serious complication of hyperflexion injuries is *delayed instability* (2, 3). Green et al. (4) reported a 20% incidence of delayed instability in hyperflexion injuries when the posterior ligament complex (ligamentum nuchae, interspinous ligament, ligamentum flavum, and capsular ligament) was disrupted, producing an anterior subluxation of the cervical spine. Even after rigid immobilization of these injuries, severe kyphotic deformity often resulted, sometimes necessitating surgical fusion. Cheshire (5), in an analysis of 257 conservatively treated acute cervical injury patients, found a similar incidence of delayed instability (21%), most commonly seen following initial anterior subluxation (6). Anterior subluxation is considered one of the most unstable of all cervical injuries (5) (Fig. 3.1).

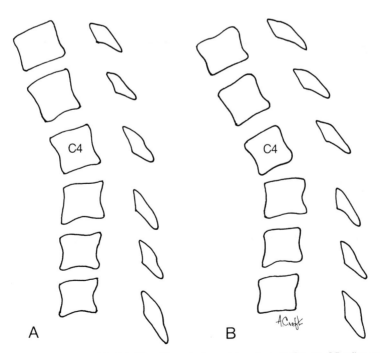

Figure 3.1. Example of delayed instability with anterior subluxation of C4 on C5 after an acceleration/deceleration injury. **A.** Drawing of initial lateral x-ray. **B.** Drawing of neutral lateral x-ray 3 months later, demonstrating delayed instability.

This chapter is divided into six parts: History, Special Neurological Tests, Isokinetic Muscle Testing, Special Radiographic Procedures, Radionuclide Bone Scanning, and Nonirradiating Special Procedures. The topics covered are those generally available tests and procedures that enable the clinician to make an accurate diagnosis and, in turn, provide the most effective treatment available. More detailed information on imaging techniques can be found in Chapters 4 and 5.

History

Certain aspects of the history should alert the clinician to potentially serious underlying pathology. Certainly, when a patient has been thrown about unrestrained inside a vehicle during a violent motor vehicle accident such as a roll-over collision or has been thrown free from the vehicle, the clinician should be highly suspicious for multiple traumas such as rib fractures, fracture-dislocations, musculoligamentous strain/sprains, hematomas, and concussions or contusions to the central nervous system. The examiner should be especially alert to the possibility that a prominent and painful minor injury may mask a quiet but potentially lethal injury.

Loss of consciousness with or without demonstrable head trauma is highly suggestive of concussion. If the patient presents with lacerations to the face or scalp or contusions and ecchymoses over the mastoid area (Battle's sign), for example, a skull fracture should be suspected. Subarachnoid hemorrhage secondary to fracture will usually produce nuchal rigidity. Otorrhagia suggests the possibility of basilar skull fracture, although this injury may also result from traumatic rupture of the tympanic membrane (7). Paralysis, papilledema, fixed dilated pupils, and changes in levels of mentation should also alert the examiner to the possibility of skull fracture. Whenever direct head trauma is significant, skull fracture should be suspected and x-rays should be obtained. Both plain film radiographs and computed tomography (CT) scans should be included. It has been shown that CT is vastly superior to conventional plain film radiography in the investigation of head trauma (8, 9), although a routine skull series is still considered mandatory, as linear fractures may be missed on CT scanning (10,11). Remember that the fracture itself, though most easily visualized, is not the key; the brain damage beneath is.

In general, mild head injuries are characterized by a brief loss of consciousness—perhaps seconds to a few minutes. This is consistent with cerebral concussion. Often, no neurological findings are present, although the patient may have some retrograde amnesia as well as some impairment of memory for a short period of time after the accident (posttraumatic amnesia) (7). A posttraumatic cerebral syndrome (postconcussion syndrome) may occur; it consists of headaches, dizziness, memory loss, inability to concentrate, sleep disorders, irritability, and intolerance to alcohol (7,12–14).

Moderate head injuries are associated with longer periods of unconsciousness;

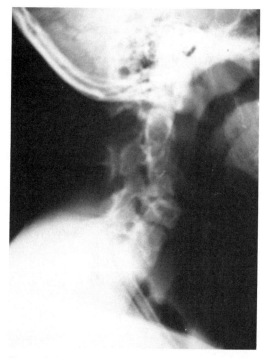

Figure 3.2. Klippel-Feil syndrome. Acceleration/deceleration trauma is concentrated at those levels where motion occurs.

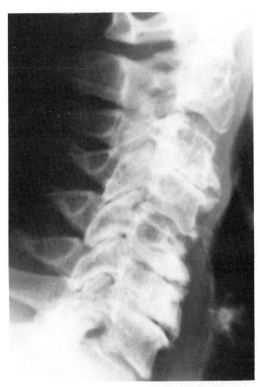

Figure 3.3. Acceleration/deceleration trauma in the presence of advanced degenerative disease.

cerebral edema and contusion may be present. Focal neurological signs are usually present.

Severe head injuries are usually associated with prolonged periods of unconsciousness. Pronounced neurological findings will be present, generally as a result of bleeding into cerebral contusion or laceration.

Examination of the cerebrospinal fluid by lumbar puncture may reveal blood from subarachnoid hemorrhage and a finding of elevated pressure. In the case of concussion or edema alone, the cerebrospinal fluid will usually be normal. Lumbar puncture following head trauma should not be performed in most cases because of the risk of cerebellar herniation.

In all cases of suspected head trauma, the patient should be watched for delayed changes in orientation and alertness, as progressive intracranial hemorrhage may occur. (8). The patient should be observed for 48 hours following such head trauma

and awakened every hour to assess his or her mental status.

Examinations that may be useful diagnostically and prognostically in the head-injured patient include electroencephalography and psychometric testing. CT scanning has, indeed, revolutionized the care of the head trauma patient.

In the presence of certain congenital anomalies or diseases such as Klippel-Feil syndrome, Down's syndrome, ankylosing spondylitis, rheumatoid arthritis, diffuse idiopathic skeletal hyperostosis (DISH) (Forestier's disease), carcinoma, severe osteoporosis, and osteogenesis imperfecta, relatively minor trauma may produce significant damage to the bony and soft tissues.

In Klippel-Feil syndrome (15, 16), the fusion of and the reduction in the number of cervical vertebrae restrict the normal range of motion of the neck and biomechanically reduce the natural resiliency of the spinal column and its supporting structure. Acceleration/deceleration forces then concentrate their energy at the levels where motion occurs (Fig. 3.2). The resulting inability to distribute these forces evenly can greatly amplify the injury. Similar alterations in biomechanics accompany advanced cervical arthrosis and spondylosis (17) (Fig. 3.3), DISH, and anklyosing spondylitis (18, 19).

In Down's syndrome, the underdeveloped or congenitally absent transverse ligament of the atlas predisposes to a traumatic dislocation of the atlas on the axis (20–23), even from trivial trauma. The complications from this type of trauma may be fatal.

Potential atlantoaxial instability is also seen in some cases of rheumatoid arthritis when pannus has destroyed the transverse ligament. After careful physical examination, the initial workup would include lateral stress views taken with great care and under the direct supervision of the clinician to demonstrate changes in the atlantodental interval (ADI) which normally should not exceed 3 mm in adults (24–26). Owing to the ligamentous and capsular laxity seen in infants and children, somewhat greater excursions should be considered normal (27). Because of this difficulty in interpreting the significance of the ADI in children, some have suggested using the adult criteria if the sphenooccipital synchondrosis is complete (28). Locke et al. (29) have reported, however, that in children the ADI is rarely more than 3 mm. Another modality, cineradiography, can also be of help in assessing the integrity of this ligament.

Severe instability at the atlantoaxial joint may produce transient or constant upper motor neuron symptoms and may require surgical fusion (20, 30). Maiman and Cusick (20) found that 21% of these dislocations occurred without a fracture of the odontoid and diagnosis was missed on initial radiological examination in 12% of the cases because of failure to recognize the increased ADI. Subsequent flexion and extension neutral lateral views were needed to make the diagnosis.

DISH, originally described by the French rheumatologist Forestier, causes exuberant osteophytosis to bridge several vertebrae, most often on the anterior surface (31) (Fig. 3.4). Marked limitation of motion from the bony bridging results in a spine that is highly vulnerable to trauma.

Primary or metastatic carcinoma of the spine is occasionally found only after routine radiographic studies are performed following trivial trauma. In Figure 3.5, careful radiographic screening revealed a suspicious lucency of the spinous process at C3. This woman presented at the clinic after a minor rear-end collision that resulted in nagging neck pain. The mass demonstrated on Figure 3.5 was later confirmed to be a metastatic carcinoma.

Lytic vertebrae resulting from carcinoma, infection, or osteopenia are more

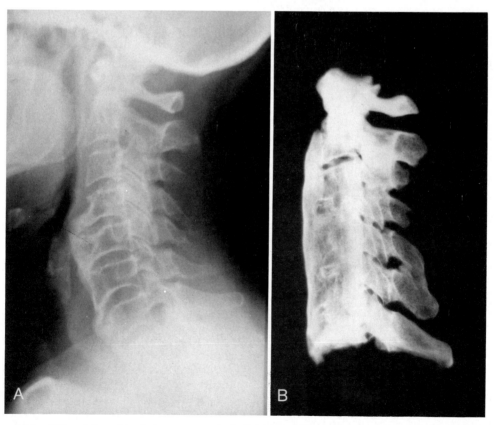

Figure 3.4. Diffuse idiopathic skeletal hyperostosis (Forestier's disease). Forces from acceleration/deceleration trauma concentrate at levels where motion occurs, resulting in greater injury. **A.** Lateral radiograph demonstrating normal disc spacing and exuberant, irregular osteophytes anteriorly. **B.** Dry specimen of Ankylosis.

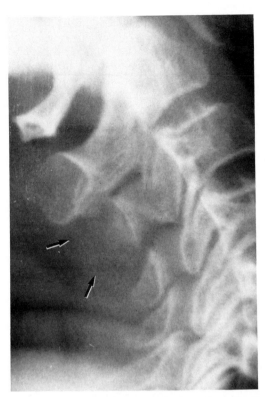

Figure 3.5. This previously asymptomatic patient presented with constant dull pain after a minor motor vehicle accident. The suspicious lucent spinous process at C3 (*arrows*) was later confirmed to be metastatic carcinoma.

susceptible to the forces generated in an acceleration/deceleration injury. Compression fractures are common and, depending upon the integrity of the posterior longitudinal ligament and the spinal canal, may be stable or unstable (Fig. 3.6). CT scanning is useful in assessing the condition of the spinal canal. In some cases, the image should be enhanced with iopamidol or iohexol, a water-soluble contrast medium that is injected into the subarachnoid space (Fig. 3.7).

Another finding that should alert the clinician to a potentially serious condition is dysphagia. Most commonly caused by blood in the retropharyngeal or retrotracheal soft tissues (32–37), vertebral fracture must be excluded at its source. A somewhat less common but potentially fatal cause of dysphagia is esophageal or hypopharyngeal perforation. Soft tissue emphysema, mediastinitis, retropharyngeal abscess, or aspiration pneumonia may ensue

(38–41). This condition has been described in hyperextension injury and is confirmed by barium swallow (42, 43).

Recently, Hann (44) has described retropharyngeal tendinitis of the longus colli muscle in association with secondary calcification, pain, and dysphagia from retropharyngeal soft tissue swelling secondary to hyperextension injury of the neck.

In cases in which dysphagia is present, the clinician should harbor a higher-than-normal index of suspicion for ligamentous disruption, dislocation, subluxation, or fracture and should make careful use of cineradiography, tomography, and CT or bone scanning to uncover the true nature and extent of injuries.

In summary, the importance of the history is often forgotten or underappreciated. Questions that should be asked first and foremost are often omitted because of either absentmindedness or the hurried pace examiners often experience. In practice, it is nearly impossible to remember all of the right questions to ask the patient, and it is far too easy to become sidetracked with other issues. For this reason, I have designed a questionnaire that is given to the patient to fill out at home in a quiet and unhurried setting. This questionnaire should be filled out as soon as possible while conditions are still fresh in the patient's mind.

I have found this form to be invaluable in the workup of patients with soft tissue injuries. It jogs the examiner's memory and helps to prevent critical omissions in the history-taking process. It is not, however, an alternative to the physician-patient consultation and interview.

Special Neurological Tests___

PSYCHOMETRIC TESTING

In the case of head injury, it is important to assess any change in mental functioning. Initially, the clinician will determine the patient's orientation as to person, place, and time. If the patient knows his or her name, where he or she is, and what year, month, day, and time of day it is, the patient is said to be oriented ×3. The patient should be asked to count backward from 100 by 7's. Many organic conditions, such as chronic alcoholism, organic brain syndrome, Alzheimer's disease, and senile dementia, may also affect these simple tests.

If during the initial visit or subsequent visits it becomes apparent that a personality disorder may be producing some functional overlay in relation to the patient's complaints or if a family member alerts you to subtle personality changes, psychometric testing should be performed. One of the most commonly used tests is the Minnesota Multiphasic Personality Inventory (MMPI). In this test, the patient is asked to answer 566 true/false questions. A category of personality profiles results: hypochondriasis, depression, hysteria, psychopathic deviation, masculinity, femininity, paranoia, psychoasthenia, schizophrenia, and hypomania. Recently, Gatchel et al. (45) reported a parallel between levels of back pain and elevations in several parameters of the MMPI. These investigators used also the Millon Behavioral Health Inventory (MBHI), which is a newer test designed and standardized on a medical population, in contrast to the MMPI, which

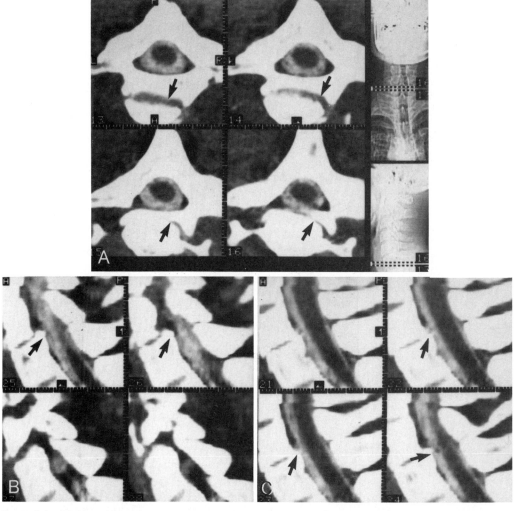

Figure 3.6.   Metrizamide-enhanced study of the cervical spine of a 23-year old man who suffered severe hyperextension/hyperflexion injury from blunt head trauma. Multiple fractures including fracture through the centrum were sustained. Comminuted fragments displace the thecal sac slightly. **A** demonstrates a comminuted fracture of the centrum with minimal vertical compression (*arrows*). **B** demonstrates sagittal reconstructions. **C** demonstrates posterior extrusion of fragments with displacement of the thecal sac (*arrows*). This patient presented with severe temporary neurological deficit but recovered completely.

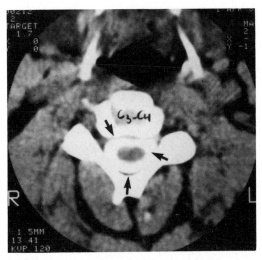

Figure 3.7. Normal axial CT scan of the C3-C4 interspace. The arachnoid space is outlined with contrast media (*arrows*).

Among the advantages of electroencephalography are its noninvasiveness, its relatively low cost, and the fact that the results can be easily reproduced. Among its disadvantages are the frequent occurrence of false positive and false negative results (46). Electroencephalography is performed by a technician trained in the precise placement of electrodes that are attached to standardized positions on the patient's scalp (Fig. 3.8). The patient is seated or placed in a comfortable recumbent position, and a recording lasting at least 20 minutes is taken. The technician will make recordings both with the patient's eyes open and with the patient's eyes closed. Then the patient will be asked to hyperventilate for 3 minutes. This generally causes a change in both the rhythm and the ampli-

was originally designed for a psychiatric population. They believe that in dealing with psychological disturbances associated with physical complaints, the Millon Behavioral Health Inventory would provide more useful information than the MMPI. In both cases, the test results improved (i.e., there was a decrease in the elevation) on several major scales when the patient's physical condition improved with therapy, thereby demonstrating a direct relationship between physical and psychological disorders.

ELECTROENCEPHALOGRAPHY

The electroencephalograph records the electrical activity of the brain, primarily the superficial layer of the cerebral cortex. Many conditions will alter the electroencephalogram (EEG) pattern, including epilepsy (posttraumatic epilepsy as well as the more common forms), brain tumor, brain abscess, meningitis, encephalitis, cerebral vascular accident, congenital defects, cerebral trauma, and subdural hematoma (7). The posttraumatic or postconcussion syndrome is another condition that can often be identified by electroencephalography. Other techniques that have been used to support this diagnosis include brainstem auditory evoked potentials and brain electrical activity mapping (14).

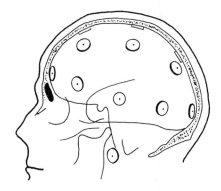

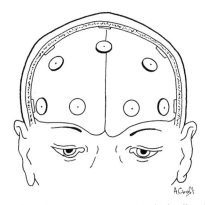

Figure 3.8. Electrode placements in the "ten twenty" system of electroencephalography. (Adapted from Chusid JG: Electroencephalography. In: *Correlative Neuroanatomy and Functional Neurology*, ed 18. Los Altos, CA, Lange Medical Publications, 1982, p 235.)

tude of the EEG waves and may uncover latent abnormalities or accentuate abnormal wave patterns already present. Having the patient stare into a strobe light often enhances epileptogenic foci.

Various forms of waves and rhythms have been described and given different significances. The most important of these rhythms are α, β, θ, and δ. More detailed descriptions of these rhythms can be found in textbooks on electrodiagnostics. As with all of the other electrodiagnostic procedures described in this chapter, the interpretation of the EEG is an art learned only after many years of study and should always be performed by one who is experienced in electrophysiological measurement.

This test is not a definitive tool, and profound lesions may escape the sensitive leads of the electroencephalograph. On the other hand, abnormal findings can occur in normal subjects. Except for the evaluation of seizures, CT scanning has largely supplanted electroencephalography in the evaluation of head trauma.

ELECTROMYOGRAPHY

Electromyography is a method of assessing the integrity of the peripheral nervous system by measuring the electrical activity in skeletal muscles upon insertion of a needle electrode. This test is performed with the patient both at rest and during voluntary muscle contraction.

The principle of electromyography is based upon the motor unit which was first described by Sherrington in the early part of this century. The motor unit consists of the anterior horn cell, its axon, and the muscle fibers innervated by that cell (Fig. 3.9). The proportion of nerve to muscle fibers in a given motor unit is referred to as the innervation ratio, and this ratio varies with the amount of precision required of the muscle. Extraocular motor units have a very low number of muscle fibers, whereas in larger postural muscles such as the quadriceps femoris, one motor neuron may innervate hundreds of fibers. Gradually increasing motor power is the result of an increasing amount of motor unit activation.

The muscle fiber action potential is generated first from the myoneural junction after stimulation by its associated motor neuron. The potential then spreads along the muscle fiber and elicits a contraction.

These electrical potentials can be recorded on an oscillograph and, after being amplified, can be seen on an oscilloscope. There is also an auditory signal that pro-

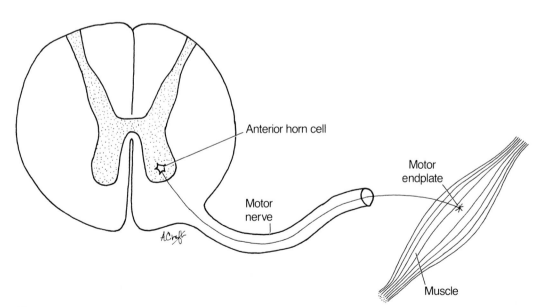

Figure 3.9.   Motor unit. (Adapted from Green L: Electrodiagnostic studies in low back pain. In Finneson BE (ed): *Low Back Pain*, ed 2. Philadelphia, JB Lippincott, 1980.)

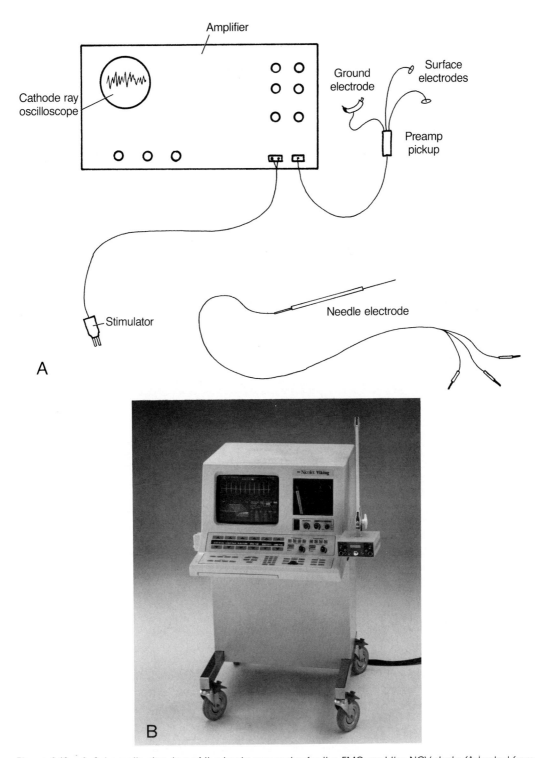

Figure 3.10. **A.** Schematic drawing of the basic apparatus for the EMG and the NCV study. (Adapted from Finneson BE (ed): *Low Back Pain,* ed 2. Philadelphia, JB Lippincott, 1980). **B.** Modern electromyographic unit. (Courtesy of Nicolet Biomedical Instruments.)

duces characteristic patterns with various types of disorders.

The basic apparatus for the electromyogram (EMG) and the nerve conduction velocity (NCV) study consists of an amplifier and cathode ray oscilloscope, a preamp pickup and a ground electrode or reference plate, a stimulator, and a coaxial electrode that is usally a 3–4-cm 24-gauge needle with all but the tip coated with insulating plastic (Fig. 3.10).

Normal muscle at rest shows no action

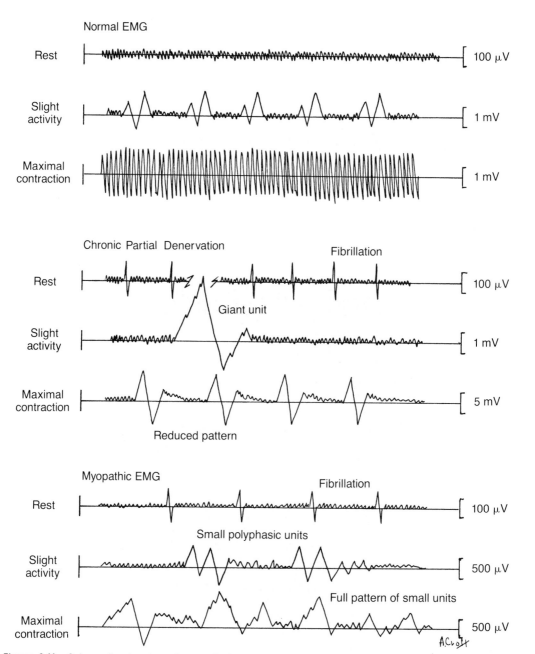

Figure 3.11. Schematic drawing of normal, denervation, and myopathic EMG patterns. (Adapted from Patten J: Peripheral neuropathy and diseases of the lower motor neurone. In: *Neurological Differential Diagnosis.* New York, Springer-Verlag, 1978, p 180.)

potentials, but upon insertion of the needle electrode the clinician may notice "insertion potentials." These may often be given greater importance than they deserve, especially in the absence of any other abnormal findings. Normal compound motor action potentials have an amplitude of 0.5–2 mV and a duration of 3–15 msec and consist of biphasic or triphasic waveforms. Spontaneous muscle activity at rest, such as small fibrillation potentials, is indicative of pathology, as are positive sharp waves. Polyphasic units, i.e., more than 4 phases/waveform, are also indicative of pathology. An increase in amplitude and duration will be seen in cases of chronic partial denervation (Fig. 3.11). Because of the greater overlap of segmental innervation in the cervical spine, fibrillation potentials and positive sharp waves are seen less frequently in the cervical than the lumbosacral region, and their presence along with numerous polyphasic units is an important finding (47, 48).

After the resting potential has been recorded, the patient is asked to gradually increase the force of contraction of the muscle under study. At maximal contraction, the wave pattern becomes quite crowded

Table 3.1.
Electromyographic Testing for Determination of Myotome Level Involvement in the Cervical Spine[a]

C5	Rhomboids
C5, C6	Supraspinatus, infraspinatus, deltoid, biceps brachii
C5–C7	Serratus anterior
C6, C7	Pronator teres, extensor carpi radialis longus
C6–C8	Latissimus dorsi
C7, C8	Triceps brachii, extensor carpi radialis brevis, other wrist and digit extensors, flexor carpi radialis, flexor of the digits
C8-T1	Abductor pollicis brevis, first dorsal interosseus, abductor digiti minimi

[a]Adapted from Eisen A: Electrodiagnosis of radiculopathies. *Neurol Clin* 3(3):495–510, 1985.

in appearance and is characterized by a high-voltage, high-frequency shape. This results from recruitment of additional fibers and is known as an "interference pattern." A reduced or incomplete pattern is typically seen in chronic partial denervation such as occurs in a nerve root compression disorder (Fig. 3.11). Fasciculation potentials and complex repetitive discharges

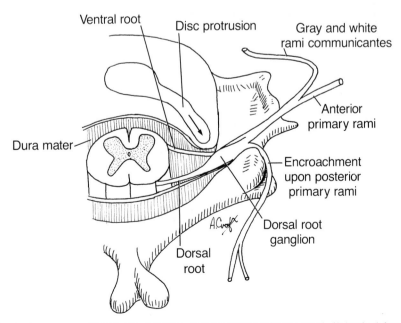

Figure 3.12. Lesions may affect both anterior and posterior primary rami. (Adapted from Warwick R, Williams PL (eds): *Gray's Anatomy*, ed 35. Philadelphia, WB Saunders, 1973.)

are other types of spontaneous activity seen in radiculopathy.

When a nerve is completely severed, denervation fibrillation potentials usually will be noted after 2–3 weeks in all areas supplied by the damaged nerve, although abnormal findings may take up to 6 weeks to appear in distal limb muscles because of the slow progression of axonal degeneration (49). In partial denervations some motor unit potentials can still be elicited, and by careful "mapping" the electromyographer can often locate the nerve root affected and thereby describe the level of compression of the nerve root. When a segmental pattern cannot be demonstrated by this method, however, the diagnosis of nerve root compression becomes less likely. A single root lesion is one involving a specific myotome or dermatome, whereas muscles sharing the same peripheral nerve but different myotomes are spared. Since most muscles receive innervation from more than one spinal root level, weakness from a single root lesion is usually mild (49). Table 3.1 illustrates the muscles usefully tested by electromyography for delineating myotome levels.

In performing needle electromyography, it is important to sample muscles innervated by the posterior primary rami, such as the paraspinal muscles (47, 48). Specificity is most pronounced in the deep layers of these muscles—the multifidi (49–52).

A posteriorly located lesion may not affect the anterior (brachial plexus) divisions, and the results of electromyography may be misleading when only muscles from the anterior divisions are sampled (Fig. 3.12). In the differentiation of root lesions and plexopathies, two features are significant. Radiculopathies may produce fibrillations in the paraspinal muscles, whereas plexopathies, owing to their anterior derivation, will not. And abnormalities of the paraspinal muscles provide clear evidence of a lesion proximal to the dorsal root ganglion. The same can be said of the rhomboids which are innervated directly from the fifth cervical root (49). Fibrillations are not, however, seen with all radiculopathies, and their absence does not confirm a plexus

lesion. Second, sensory nerve action potentials (SNAPs), which are of low amplitude or not detectable, are the rule with axon loss plexopathies. This is in contrast to the radiculopathy in which SNAPs are usually normal even in the presence of profound clinical sensory disturbance. This is due to the lesion being proximal to the dorsal root ganglion, with the peripheral processes of the sensory fibers maintaining continuity with their cells of origin in the dorsal root ganglion (53–55). The abnormal SNAPs could also mean that both preganglionic and postganglionic lesions are present (56); e.g., a nerve root compression may be present with an avulsion injury to the brachial plexus.

NCV STUDY

The NCV study can be a useful tool in differentiating some types of neuropathy and is used in conjunction with electromyography. Nerve conductions can be measured for both sensory and motor nerves, but one of the requirements for this procedure is that the nerve must be available for stimulation at two points along its course. The ulnar and median nerves are the only ones that can be used in the upper extremities, as the radial nerve can be stimulated at only one point.

Motor NCV Study

The technique for the motor NCV study is illustrated in Figure 3.13. First, a suitable muscle is selected (such as the abductor pollicis brevis, in the case of the median nerve, or the first dorsal interosseus muscle, in the case of the ulnar nerve). The time that it takes for an impulse to travel from the proximal stimulus (S1) to the test muscle is known as the "distal latency." The time that it takes for the impulse to travel from a second distally stimulated point (S2) is called the "proximal latency." The NCV is then calculated by application of this information in the equation NCV = D/T, where D equals the distance between S1 and S2, T equals the time between S1 and S2, and the NCV is expressed in meters per second. Normative data are available for both ulnar and median nerves.

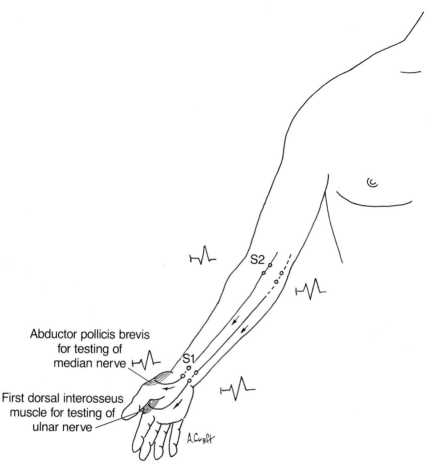

Figure 3.13.   Motor NCV study. Proximal latency equals the time from S2 to the muscle; distal latency equals the time from S1 to the muscle. NCV = D/T (m/sec), where D equals the distance between S1 and S2, and T equals the time between S1 and S2. In this case, the NCV equals 45 m/sec. (Adapted from Patten J: *Neurological Differential Diagnosis*. New York, Springer-Verlag, 1978, p 181.)

Sensory NCV Study

The technique for measuring SNAPs is illustrated in Figure 3.14. Nerve action potentials can be measured both orthodromically (as illustrated) and antidromically. The orthodromic method is usually used. In this case, a sensory nerve is stimulated distally, while pickup electrodes placed proximally record the NCV which is then calculated as previously discussed.

Electromyography verses NCV Study

In general, a nerve root or anterior horn cell disorder would be suspected when the lesion is found to be above the level of the proximal stimulus in a NCV study. NCV is affected much more by a demyelinating disorder than by the axonal lesions seen with nerve root compression. Electromyography, however, is quite sensitive to axonal injury but only after the lesion has had time to produce axonal degeneration. This usually takes 2–3 weeks, although maximal changes may take longer (57). On the other hand, the NCV study will show changes within a week of nerve injury. Therefore, when the EMG is abnormal, demonstrating fibrillation potentials, positive sharp waves, and polyphasic units, and the NCV is normal, a radiculopathy or other condition characterized by axonal degeneration would be suspected. This is especially true when a segmental pattern of denervation can be demonstrated on the EMG. It is important to differentiate between neuropraxia and axonal degeneration because in the latter recovery will be slow and possibly incomplete, whereas in the former it will generally be rapid and complete.

Motor and sensory NCVs in radiculopathies are usually normal. Eisen (49) has stated that the most valuable measurement is the compound motor action potentials. If it is normal 2–3 weeks after the injury, the lesion is neuropraxic in nature. If the amplitude is reduced more than 50%, compared with that of the asymptomatic side, or is less than 2 SD of the normal mean for the muscle being tested, the lesion involves axon loss.

If the NCV and EMG are both abnormal, the diagnosis of nerve root disorder becomes less attractive. This would be especially true if changes in the EMG were not segmental and consistent with specific nerve root levels. Peripheral neuropathy should then be considered as a working diagnosis.

Limitations of Electrodiagnostic Studies

Some of the limitations of these procedures, e.g., latency between onset of the lesion and the time in which the test will be abnormal, have been discussed. Interpretation must be done by an experienced electromyographer and is not as clear-cut and simple as our description has made it sound. Needle insertion is somewhat painful, and some patients may object to this. Localization of nerve root levels is often difficult and can only be confirmed in association with other studies, such as myelography or CT scanning because of the common anatomical variation seen in patients. The brachial plexus may be prefixed or postfixed. When the branch from C4 is large, the branch from T2 is absent, and T1 is decreased in size, the brachial plexus is said to be prefixed. When the branch from C4 is small or absent, C5 is decreased in size, and T1 is larger with T2 present, the brachial plexus is said to be postfixed. Lastly, the precise etiology of a lesion cannot be determined from results of these tests.

Table 3.2.
Electrodiagnostic Findings in Various Disorders

Findings	Suspected Disorder
Normal EMG with or without interference pattern; normal NCV	Upper motor neuron disorder
Abnormal EMG after 2–6 weeks; slow NCV	Entrapment neuropathy
Abnormal EMG with fibrillation potentials, positive sharp waves, large polyphasic units or giant units, and incomplete interference pattern; normal NCV	Anterior horn cell disorder
Abnormal EMG with short-duration, high-frequency polyphasic units, complete low-amplitude interference pattern, and occasional fibrillations; normal NCV	Myopathic muscle
Abnormal EMG in a segmental pattern, with positive sharp waves, fibrillation potential, and incomplete interference pattern; normal NCV	Radiculopathy probable
Abnormal EMG in a nonsegmental pattern with positive sharp waves; normal NCV	Radiculopathy possible, plexopathy possible[a]
Abnormal EMG with slow NCV	Plexopathy possible, peripheral neuropathy, ganglionopathy (e.g., herpes zoster or diabetic radiculopathy), double crush (affects compound sensory nerve action potential)

[a]Standard NCV testing is not adequate to evaluate certain portions of plexuses.

Indications for Electrodiagnosis

Electrodiagnosis has become one of the most important diagnostic tools in neurology. Although the exact nature of the lesion cannot always be identified, the EMG and the NCV study are extremely useful in the differential diagnosis of certain disorders. These tests should not be ordered routinely when a patient presents with neck and arm pain or perhaps numbness in the hands or fingers immediately following a hyperextension/hyperflexion injury. It is quite common for a patient to present with pain or paresthesias along the C8 and T1 dermatomes after this type of injury, and these are often transient (57). If, on the other hand, the clinical picture is suggestive of nerve root compression and if physical findings such as muscle fasciculations, weakness and/or atrophy, and diminished or absent deep tendon reflexes along with corresponding sensory abnormalities are suggestive of a lower motor neuron lesion, the EMG and the NCV study along with other appropriate radiographic studies are certainly indicated (Table 3.2).

Needle electromyography is probably the

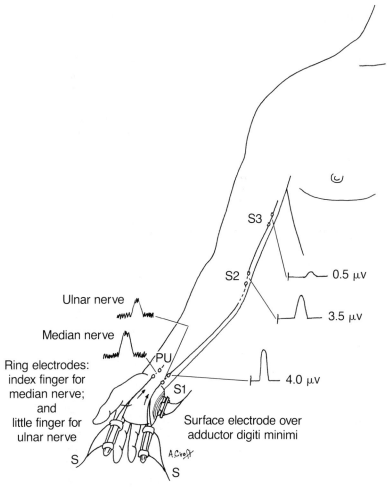

Figure 3.14. Sensory NCV study. Technique for isolating conduction blocks (in this case a block at the olecranon groove). Stimulating S3 produces a small potential. Stimulating S2 produces a slightly larger potential. And stimulating S1 produces the largest potential. *PU*, Pickup electrodes at wrist. (Adapted from Patten J: *Neurological Differential Diagnosis.* New York, Springer-Verlag, 1978, p 181.)

most useful test in a radiculopathy and should therefore precede more invasive radiological testing, such as myelography or CT scanning with contrast, although negative diagnostic testing does not preclude the use of these tests.

Isokinetic Muscle Testing

Over the past decade, a new way of objectively documenting muscle weakness and muscle imbalance has emerged. It utilizes the principles of isokinetics which describes a type of work or exercise performed by muscles or muscle groups such that the harder a particular muscle pushes against a given resistance, the greater the resistance becomes. The test is performed at a speed (in degrees per second) that is preset by the examiner.

In isotonic exercise, a cam system is utilized to produce an even resistance throughout an arc of motion as a way of working a given muscle group more effectively. In exercise with free weights, however, the resistance (weight) remains constant, even though the power of the muscle changes throughout its range of contraction, thereby displaying areas of efficiency and relative inefficiency within the same arc.

Isometric exercise is, of course, familiar to all of us as a way of contracting against a force without changing the length of the muscle. Many Yoga exercises are essentially isometric exercises.

Several companies have refined isokinetics to a very sophisticated level, coupling these machines with a computer system that enables measuring and plotting the torque (in foot-pounds) of a given exercise. Strength and endurance as well as range of motion can also be measured. The

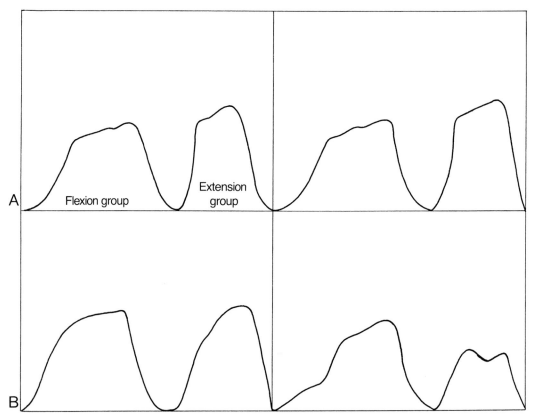

Figure 3.15.   Graph of isokinetic muscle strength tests (torque in ft-lb and subsequent trials. **A.** Normal study with reproducible results. **B.** Abnormal, nonconsistent trial.

primary usefulness of this system has been in the rehabilitation of people with injuries to the peripheral joints, although low-back testing and rehabilitating systems are now in wide use. Normative data continue to accumulate from numerous test centers around the country (58). Another use is in the prevention of injuries. By finding subtle muscle imbalances that could not be detected by other clinical testing, and then by correcting these imbalances (which is done on the same machine), work injuries and sports injuries are theoretically reduced.

With the coupling of the isokinetic unit and the computer, it soon became obvious that a malingerer could not easily fool the machine. (59). Graphs displaying curves of torque and range of motion are generally consistent and homogeneous when the subject sincerely puts forth his or her best effort over three consecutive attempts. If the subject feigns weakness, however, the recording will often be erratic and inconsistent, and in this way the machine along with its computer printout act as a sort of musculoskeletal polygraph capable of snagging most malingerers (Fig. 3.15). This is in contrast to the hand-held dynamometer that merely tests the subject's grip strength. The dynamometer is still the most widely used device, however, and with proper use and interpretation is relatively accurate. There have been many court cases in which isokinetic testing has been accepted as evidence to either prove or dispute the validity of injury and disability claims.

Special Radiographic Procedures

NONCONTRAST RADIOGRAPHY

Foreman and Croft (32) and others (60–64) have pointed to the need for lateral stress views taken in maximal active flexion and extension after hyperflexion or hyperextension injuries to the cervical spine. In spite of the sophisticated laboratory procedures available to the modern clinician, the routine plain film of the cervical spine remains the "gold standard" in the diagnosis and assessment of cervical spine injury and disease. Fractures, dislocations, subluxa-

tions, and various forms of soft tissue injury can be either directly visualized or deduced from these films.

The literature is replete with examples of serious trauma that was missed initially or underappreciated either because the initial trauma seemed relatively trivial, or because no physical signs were initially present to warrant further examination, or because the original x-ray study was incomplete or inadequate. Borovich et al. (8) have described several cases of delayed accumulation of extradural hematoma found only after repeat CT scanning of the skull 24 hours after the first examination. In only one case did neurological deterioration signal the onset of hematoma.

Plain Film Radiography

Plain film radiography is relatively inexpensive, noninvasive, and easy to perform and, with modern high-speed or rare-earth intensifying screens, produces a low dose of ionizing radiation to the patient. I agree with others (60–64) that after serious pathology has been ruled out with anteroposterior (AP) and lateral films, obliques and flexion/extension views should then be obtained if the clinical findings warrant it. Surprisingly, many hospital emergency room physicians do not routinely order stress views in case of acceleration/deceleration trauma.

When plain films are suspicious, or when the trauma has been significant, or when signs of neurological injury are present, further study is indicated. Croft and Foreman (65) recently reported a case in which a normal radiographic abnormality simulated a fracture. After plain films had showed a possible chip fracture of the atlas vertebrae through the lateral mass (Fig. 3.16), linear tomography confirmed the diagnosis (Fig. 3.17). CT scanning, however, ruled out fracture. This case illustrates the logical sequence of radiographic procedure required to rule out serious injury. Plain film radiography remains the first procedure of choice in the evaluation of acute cervical spine trauma.

Three concepts are axiomatic in regards to the investigation of cervical spine trauma:

1. First, do no harm. If a procedure is unlikely to alter the prognosis or the treatment, do not use it. For example, in the case

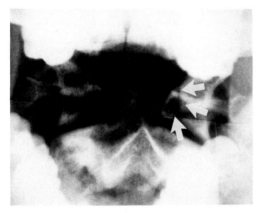

Figure 3.16. AP open mouth view demonstrates suspicious linear radiolucency over the lateral mass of the atlas unilaterally (*arrows*) in a patient suffering from acute upper cervical spine pain following trauma.

of linear fracture of the spinous process of C7 in the absence of neurological findings or other skeletal trauma, other studies are unlikely to yield any further beneficial information and should probably not be performed.

2. Continue to search for a lesion if clinically suspected. In Figure 3.18, a dislocation at C5-C6 was initially missed on routine lateral x-ray because the patient was heavyset and the x-ray beam failed to penetrate the lower cervical spine.

3. Do not accept films of inadequate quality.

Linear Tomography

Linear tomography in addition to plain film radiography is likely to yield even more information with regards to suspected fracture and dislocation. CT scanning provides more detailed evaluation of the cross-sectional soft tissue and bony anatomy of the cervical spinal canal and has been used to define various lesions, including tumor, herniated disc, ossification of the posterior longitudinal ligament, spinal stenosis, facet arthrosis, ligamentous calcification, spondylosis, and fracture. Multiplanar reconstruction (MPR) allows the computer to reconstruct images in planes other than the ones originally recorded.

Cineradiography

Cineradiography (also known as TV-taped radiography or fluorovideo) has a limited but important role in the diagnosis of instability of the cervical spine and, to some extent, in the prognosis of future disability. Macnab (66) has shown that the healing of ligamentous structure is generally incomplete; this instability may result in early and accelerated degenerative changes (67, 68).

Cineradiography are x-rays taken under fluoroscopic control and are recorded on film or, more usually, on videotape. Standard projections of lateral, AP, and oblique cervicals are used, and throughout the examination appropriate spot views are taken. In the lateral views, the patient is instructed to tuck his or her chin and flex the neck all the way forward. Then the patient is instructed to extend all the way back. The same motion should be evaluated in the oblique plane. Other views should include frontal open mouth odontoid views with rotation of the head from right to left and with lateral bending (69). Lateral bending views in the AP direction also should be part of the standard fluoroscopic study. This motion study of the spine may be quite useful in detecting abnormal biomechanics secondary to ligamentous damage that may be unappreciated with plain film radiography.

In a review of 107 cases of cervical spine trauma, with 57 resulting from hyperextension/hyperflexion injury, Buonocore et al. (69) found that 39 cases (68%) of the whip-

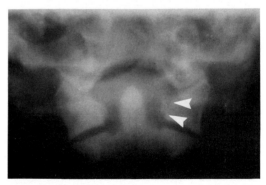

Figure 3.17. Linear tomogram of the same patient as in Figure 3.16 is suggestive of chip fracture of the lateral mass (*arrows*).

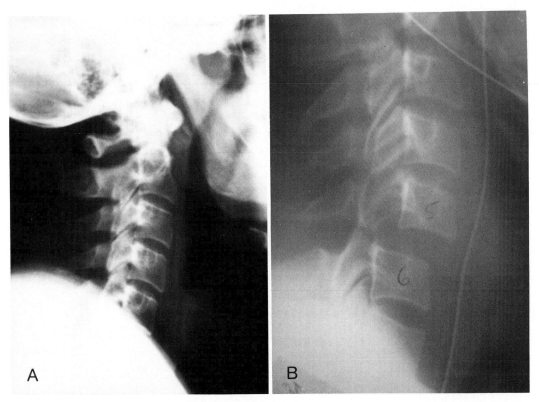

Figure 3.18. Lateral cervical spine film of patient after severe acceleration/deceleration injury. The lower cervical spine was not visualized in **A** because of the lack of penetration. In **B**, complete dislocation at C5-C6 is visualized.

lash injuries studied by cineradiography were interpreted as abnormal. The other 18 were interpreted as normal. In 18 of the 39 cases found to be abnormal, routine x-rays were interpreted as entirely normal. Approximately 25% of these 39 cases underwent operative fusion for stabilization. None of the 18 diagnosed as normal by cineradiography required surgery.

Woesner and Mitts (70) compared plain radiography and cineradiography in 40 cases and found that in 23 cases no abnormalities that were not seen on plain films were detected by cineradiography. In 14 cases of the 40 cases, however, cineradiography did detect abnormal motion not appreciated on plain films. And in 4 cases, the reverse was true—abnormal motion was seen on plain films but not on cineradiography.

The normal biomechanics of the cervical spine as seen on cineradiography have been described by Fielding (71–73), Jones (74–76), Howe (77), and others (61, 78, 79).

Template Analysis

Henderson and Dormon (61) have suggested the use of *intersegmental template analysis* as a sensitive and easy method to obtain information about cervical spine biomechanics in the sagittal plane (64, 80, 81). They constructed acetate overlays on lateral cervical spine films, comparing both extension and neutral lateral views and flexion and neutral lateral views. This was done by placing a transparent acetate over the neutral view and tracing the cortical margins of the occiput to T1. This tracing was then placed over the extension film with the acetate C7 lined up with the film C7. The C6 vertebra was then traced with either a new color or a broken line. Next, the acetate C6 was lined up with the film C6, and C5 was traced. This process was continued

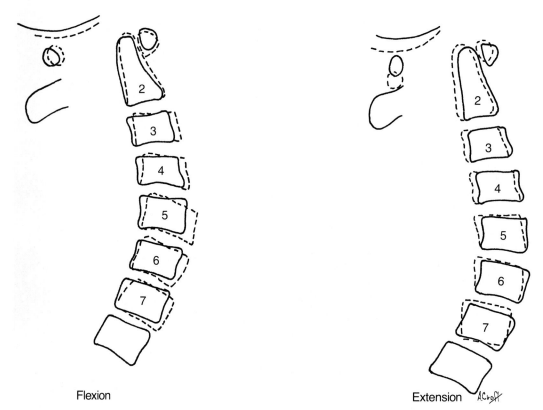

Flexion

Extension

Figure 3.19. Completed template study. *Solid lines* represent neutral position. *Broken lines* represent the extreme flexed or extended position in relation to the vertebra below. (Adapted from Henderson DJ, Dormon TM: Functional roentgenometric evaluation of the cervical spine in the sagittal plane. *J Manipulative Physiol Ther* 8(4):219–227, 1985.)

until all segments had been traced in both flexion and extension. Figure 3.19 represents the completed study. These investigators measured the posterosuperior vertebral body in both neutral and flexion/extension and expressed the sagittal translational movement as a ratio of the translation in millimeters to the body diameter. They called this measurement the "percent sagittal body diameter" (%SBD) (Fig. 3.20). This was effective for segments C3–C7 but was modified for the C2-C3 intersegment by taking the vertical height of the posterior body of C3 (distance *a* in Fig. 3.21) and moving up this distance on the posterior body of C2. The horizontal measurement at level *b* was used in the formula, as described before, to arrive at the %SBD at this level. A different method was used to determine %SBD for occiput-C1 and C1-C2, as is shown in Figure 3.22 in which line *a*, formed by the bisection of a vertical line drawn through the part of the posterior arch of the

atlas with the greatest vertical dimension, forms reference point *b* which then corresponds to reference point *c* on the occiput. The absolute displacement in millimeters between point *c* and C1 is called *d* (it should be noted that this value is subject to magnification). The difference between point *b* and *b1* (*e*) is similarly used to describe motion for C1-C2.

Buetti-Bauml (82) has used a similar technique. His technique was to superimpose the flexion view on the extension view (Fig. 3.23) and, starting from C7, to make the tracings as previously described, resulting in a nomogram (Fig. 3.24). Arlen (83) suggested a possible shortcoming in this technique in that abnormal motion may occur somewhere between full flexion and full extension. He measured the spine and compared measurements in both flexion and extension with that in neutral (Fig. 3.25). Prantl (84), using Arlen's modified technique, studied the spines of 148 symp-

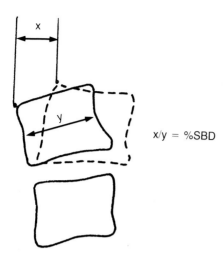

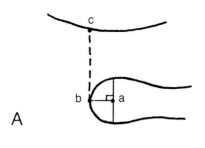

$x/y = \%SBD$

A

Figure 3.20. Schematic drawing demonstrating the ratio of translation of point *x* to sagittal body diameter and given as %SBD. (Adapted from Henderson DJ, Dormon TM: Functional roentgenometric evaluation of the cervical spine in the sagittal plane. *J Manipulative Physiol Ther* 8(4):219–227, 1985.)

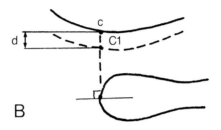

B

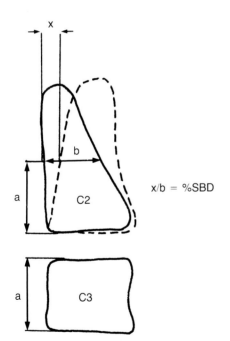

$x/b = \%SBD$

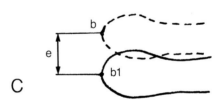

C

Figure 3.22. X-ray analysis of occiput-axis is measured in absolute millimeters and is subject to distortion. **A.** Point *a* is calculated as one half the greatest vertical distance of the posterior arch of the atlas. Bisection of this point corresponds with point *b*. Vertical extension of point *c* on the occiput. **B.** Distance *d* is the measured distance between *c* and *C1* after movement of the occiput. Atlas motion is expressed as distance *e* (*b–b1*). (Adapted from Henderson DJ, Dormon TM: Functional roentgenometric evaluation of the cervical spine in the sagittal plane. *J Manipulative Physiol Ther* 8(4):219–227, 1985.)

Figure 3.21. %SBD at the C2-C3 interspace is calculated by measuring diameter *b* through the C2 body at a distance *a* from the posterior inferior aspect. Distance *a* is the posterior vertical measurement of the C3 body. (Adapted from Henderson DJ, Dormon TM: Functional roentgenometric evaluation of the cervical spine in the sagittal plane. *J Manipulative Physiol Ther* 8(4):219–227, 1985.)

tomatic patients. He compared this technique with the technique of Buetti-Bauml and found Arlen's technique to be significantly more sensitive in detecting biomechanical abnormalities.

The major advantage in using the acetate

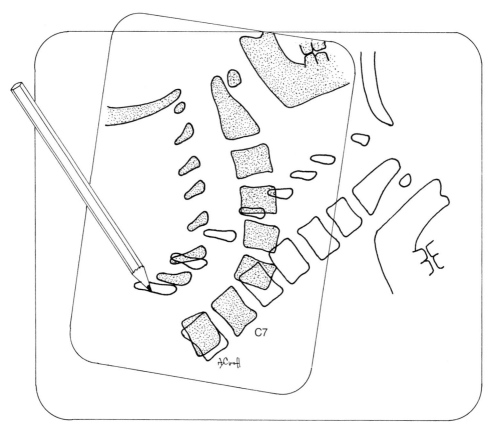

Figure 3.23. Acetate overlay tracing of flexion and extension radiographs. (Adapted from Braakman R, Penning L: *Injuries of the Cervical Spine*. Amsterdam, Excerpta Medica, 1971, p 11.)

overlay method is that it can be accomplished easily and inexpensively and requires only a good set of cervical spine films that includes flexion and extension views. This study can be repeated at a later time for comparison and follow-up evaluation.

CONTRAST RADIOGRAPHY

Myelography

Positive contrast myelography is still used to delineate disc herniation or when nerve root or spinal cord compression is suspected. Usually, surgery is contemplated at this stage, and indications for myelography in disc disease when surgery is not planned are rare (85).

Acute disc herniation partially or completely displaces the intrathecal contrast agent but usually at only one level. This is in contrast to advanced spondylosis in which posterior osteophytes produce transverse bars that may cause multiple level defects in the column of contrast. Incidentally, these bars may not be appreciable on plain films (86, 87).

Nerve root entrapment can be seen on mylographic examination by a defect or lack of filling of the nerve root dural sleeve. Relatively large intraforaminal spurs causing radicular symptoms may not be appreciated on the myelogram, however. When there are questions as to whether myelography is really necessary in cases of disc herniation, it is often useful to use an EMG/NCV study which, if normal, may obviate the need for myelography.

Other indications for myelographic examination include persistent symptoms of nerve root irritation or myelopathy that

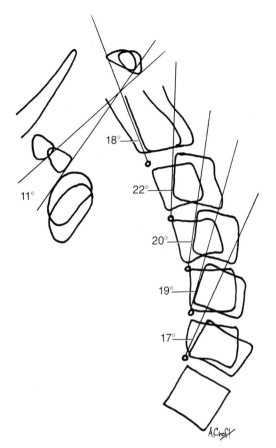

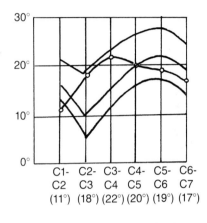

Figure 3.24. Method of acetate tracing described by Buetti-Bauml and the corresponding nomogram. Flexion and extension radiographs are compared. (Adapted from Prantl K: X-ray examination and functional analysis of the cervical spine. *Manual Med* 2:5–15, 1985.)

have proven to be resistant to conservative therapy. There are, however, several pitfalls to the interpretation of these results (86, 88, 89), and since this test is invasive, it may have uncommon but serious complications. Postexamination headaches which may be severe are common. The patient is also exposed to significant amounts of ionizing radiation. Presently, the exposure from myelography is about 20 rads, while that from CT is only about 5 or 6 rads.

Historically, this procedure has not been without risk. The older, oil-soluble contrast agents were associated with several adverse reactions including, most notably, adhesive arachnoiditis (90–92). Metrizamide produced far fewer complications (93–102). The newest nonionic agents, iopamidol and iohexal, are remarkably free from side effects, save for the headaches commonly associated with lumbar puncture.

CT with Contrast

With the advent of MPR, the amount of information available to the physician is staggering. CT without contrast enhancement is painless, noninvasive, and lower in cost than the conventional myelogram ($800 versus $2100). The combination of CT and MPR is rapidly supplanting myelography in the evaluation of trauma, degenerative disease, space-occupying lesions, and most other cases in which myelography had previously been indicated.

In the recent past, it had been suggested by many authors that CT with contrast enhancement myelography alone or in con-

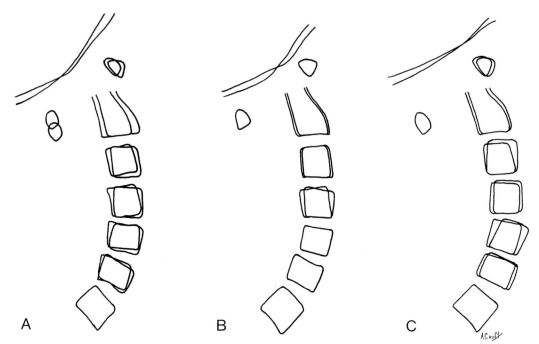

A   B   C

Figure 3.25.   Analysis by acetate overlay methods. **A.** Flexion and extension views are compared according to the method of Buetti-Bauml. **B.** Extension and neutral views are compared according to the technique of Arlen. **C.** Flexion and neutral views are compared by Prantl using Arlen's technique. (Adapted from Prantl K: X-ray examination and functional analysis of the cervical spine. *Manual Med* 2:5–15, 1985.)

junction with standard myelography may be indicated in trauma cases in which acute neurological deficit was present (103). With the recent rapid developments in dedicated spine coils, however, magnetic resonance imaging (MRI) may supplant CT in this type of investigation. Nerve root occlusions and dural tears are found more commonly in the cervical region than in the lumbar region and can be better appreciated radiographically with the use of contrast-enhanced CT than with the use of conventional myelography (104).

Most of the time, CT scanning without contrast and reformatted with MPR will provide all of the information needed to evaluate the patient. The study can always be repeated at a later date with contrast if necessary. When in doubt as to which procedure will yield the most information about a particular condition or differential diagnosis, the clinician should always consult with the neuroradiologist. I prefer to evaluate by plain film first. If the level of the suspected lesion is above the point at which the shoulders begin to obscure detail in the

cervical spine view (usually C4 in a heavy subject), contrast is generally not needed. If, on the other hand, the suspected lesion is below this level, particularly in a patient with a stocky neck, a small amount of contrast agent introduced at the C1-C2 level will go a long way in providing a good diagnostic image while producing very few undesirable side effects.

Discography

Discography consists of injection of a contrast agent into the center of the disc. Under normal conditions, the nucleus pulposus is confined within the surrounding anulus fibrosus. This space is such that under normal conditions only about 0.2–0.3 ml can be injected into it without causing pain. In the case of herniation or disc disease, however, a greater quantity of fluid can be injected—perhaps 0.5 ml or more. When the patient's complaints (i.e., pain) are reproduced, this test is said to be confirmatory at the level of the lesion tested.

Discography is an involved procedure in

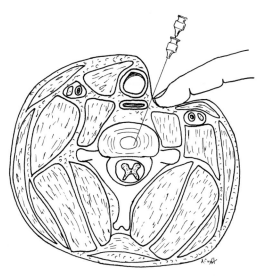

Figure 3.26. Anterolateral approach to the intervertebral disc. (Adapted from Cloward RB: Cervical discography; technique, indications and use in diagnosis of ruptured cervical discs. *Am J Roentgenol* 79:563–574, 1958.)

which meticulous attention to detail must be observed. Several levels are usually tested in hopes of discovering the one level responsible for the patient's symptoms.

After infusion of local anesthetic around the area of the anterior longitudinal ligament (a highly pain-sensitive structure), several needles are passed into the nucleus of each disc by an anterior approach (Fig. 3.26). Once the needles are in place, contrast medium is injected into the disc. X-rays are taken shortly thereafter. With unilateral protrusion, the patient usually feels pain in the neck, shoulder, and arm but rarely as far distally as the elbow. In cases of cord compression, shock-like pain may be experienced in the back and lower extremities (105).

There are several obvious disadvantages to cervical discography, including an increasing incidence of false positive results with advancing age (106, 107). At best, this technique has been used as an adjunct in the diagnosis of disc disease (105). The radiographic appearance of the discogram is considered less significant than the reproduction of the patient's symptoms (108).

Today, this procedure is rarely used (109, 110). With the advent of CT and other new imaging techniques, most believe there is

little if any clinical indication for discography. This issue is, however, hotly debated between supporters and antagonists. There have been several reports in the literature extolling the value of discography under certain conditions (111–115), including a report by Roth (116) who injects local anesthetic into the disc as a means of localizing and treating the offending "painful disc." Many investigators (117–120), however, have found the procedure to be of limited value, and some have strongly condemned it (121). Adverse reactions have included nerve damage and aseptic and infective discitis (118–120).

Angiography

Angiography has some applications in the diagnosis of lesions referable to the cervical spine. This may be true in the case of neurovascular compression syndromes that become symptomatic and persistent after trauma to the cervical spine. Many cases of vertebrobasilar syndrome have resulted from trauma to the vertebral and basilar arteries (see Fig. 7.36). These may require angiography (122).

Angiography, like most other invasive procedures, is associated with several complications. Its use is limited with regard to the majority of conditions discussed in this textbook, and before the clinician considers utilizing a procedure of this type, it is wise to consult with a radiologist and/or vascular surgeon. For more detail on this subject, which is beyond the scope of this textbook, other sources should be reviewed.

Radionuclide Bone Scanning

Bone scanning with various technetium-labeled phosphate compounds is one of the most useful of all the nuclear medicine procedures. In a relatively short amount of time, the entire skeleton can be visualized in a way that not only is easier on the patient and the technician but also is less costly and contributes less radiation exposure to the patient than does conventional x-ray. It is also more sensitive to many conditions of the bone that may not be appreciated by conventional radiography.

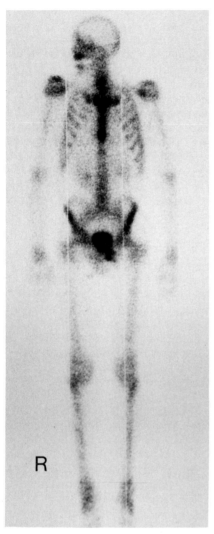

Figure 3.27. Whole-body radionuclide bone scan, anterior view.

The radionuclide substance is adsorbed to the hydroxyapatite portion of the bone matrix in such a way that this adsorption is in direct proportion to the bone's metabolic activity and local blood flow. The final picture allows visualization of metabolically highly active areas of bone. Many conditions, however, may cause an increase in the metabolic activity of bone and show positive on the bone scan, including tumors, fractures, infections, and severe strains that affect the tenoperiosteal junction. Lowered uptake may occur in cases in which blood flow and metabolism are reduced. This may be seen in cases of bone infarct and of early osteomyelitis and in some metastatic deposits.

A large number of findings that may not be related to the skeleton may also be revealed by this type of study. For example, the kidneys and urinary bladder are generally seen as areas of concentration, as they are one of the major clearing organ systems for the radionuclide.

Scans can be confined to a local area such as the legs in cases of suspected tibial stress fracture. Conversely, a technique known as

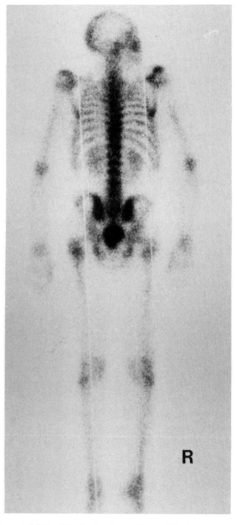

Figure 3.28. Whole-body radionuclide bone scan, posterior view.

whole-body scanning can be done in which the patient is moved on a table past a stationary camera (Figs. 3.27 and 3.28). This application can be of help in evaluating multiple trauma or suspected metastatic disease. In some studies, increased uptake at the site of trauma within several hours has been demonstrated (123). Most authors (124) suggest, however, that within 72 hours most serious bone traumas will show on the radionuclide scan. This technique is also useful in cases of suspected occult fracture.

The test is generally performed approximately 2 hours following injection of a technetium-labeled agent. A radionuclide sensitive scintillation camera picks up a predetermined number of counts over an area and, from this, produces a picture. In general, several areas will normally appear blacker (more active) than the rest of the scan. These include areas of greater bone mass as well as areas of greater overall stress, such as the joints (Figs. 3.27 and 3.28).

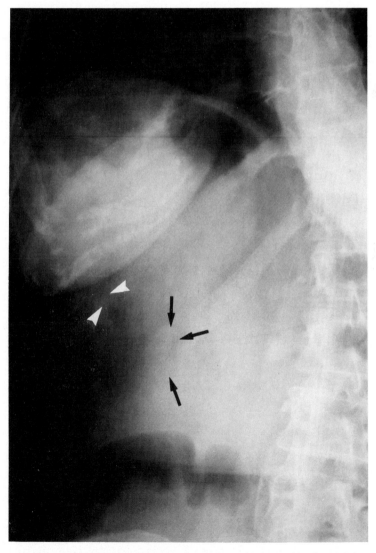

Figure 3.29.   This 60-year-old woman was involved in a motor vehicle accident, sustaining a nondisplaced rib fracture (*arrows*). Above it is an old, ununited rib fracture (*arrowheads*).

After a substantial straining or spraining injury to the neck, a bone scan may show increased activity around the cervical spine. It should not be used as a routine test even in cases of moderate to severe whiplash, and its use strictly for medicolegal substantiation of injury is to be condemned. It is useful as an adjunctive procedure when occult fracture is suspected and plain films, tomograms, or CT scans have been normal or equivocal. When no hard tissue abnormalities have been detected by these methods, however, a strong index of suspicion would be needed to justify further investigation with a bone scan. Certainly, a chronic mild to moderate pain with recurrent headaches would not warrant this degree of suspicion.

Bone scanning may be useful, however, in differentiating a new process from an old one or a fracture from an artifact or congenital anomaly. The activity around a fracture, however, may remain active for several months to as long as 20 years (125). Figures 3.29–3.31 illustrate the usefulness of the radionuclide bone scan in cases of skeletal trauma.

Nonirradiating Special Procedures

MRI

MRI is the newest imaging technique to be used. Introduced in the early 1980's, it is a medical application of nuclear magnetic resonance. MRI, which is also known as "spin imaging" or "spin mapping," produces no ionizing radiation hazard. The resonance is produced by placing the body in a magnetic field and then subjecting it to phased radiofrequency waves. The nucleus of hydrogen, a single proton, is most sensitive to this resonance.

MRI can produce coronal, sagittal, or axial images similar to CT scans. The test takes 20–40 minutes, depending upon the series chosen (Figs. 3.32–3.35). In some areas of the body, MRI is more sensitive than

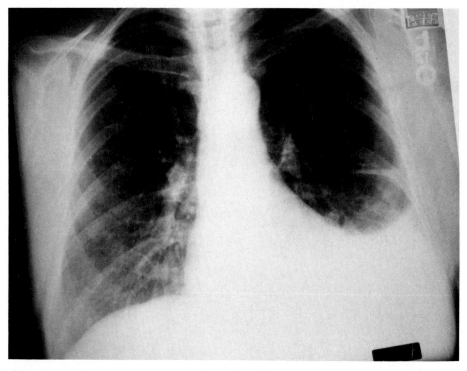

Figure 3.30. X-ray of the same patient as in Figure 3.29. This patient had been released to bed rest but had developed dyspnea later that night. This film was taken the following day. Four hundred ml of fresh blood was removed from the left lung at thoracentesis.

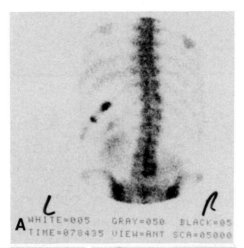

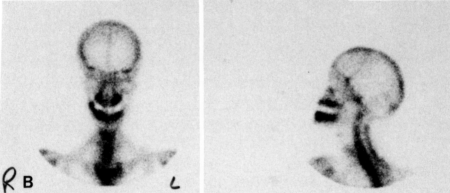

Figure 3.31. **A.** Radionuclide bone scan of same patient as in Figures 3.29 and 3.30 shows areas of increased uptake in the left lower posterior rib cage at the areas of fracture. Both were fresh, but only one was visible on the plain films. **B.** Increased uptake was also present in both maxilla and mandible. The patient had recently undergone extensive periodontal surgery.

CT scanning because it is able to differentiate between various tissues on the basis of their relative concentrations of water. For example, gray and white matter in the brain contain, respectively, 84 and 71% water (126), allowing for discrimination between the two.

At present, however, both the purchase (between $1.2 and $2.2 million) (127) and the maintenance (126) of MRI scanners are quite expensive. Hence, the cost to patients and insurance companies is likewise very high. A cervical spine series at my hospital in 1986 cost more than $800—significantly more than a CT scan. New applications for MRI, such as spectroscopic analysis, may become clinically useful. Many authors have declared MRI to be superior to CT and conventional plain film and myelographic techniques in the diagnosis of many cervical spine lesions, such as degenerative changes, spinal stenosis, trauma, disc herniation or degeneration, tumor, infection, syringomyelia, and Chiari malformation (128–130). Certainly, at this time, two statements can be made: (*a*) the indications for MRI versus CT are in flux, and specific applications should be discussed with the radiologist or neuroradiologist, and (*b*) the final chapter has not been written in this issue. I prefer to use MRI in cases of suspected myelopathy and CT in cases of suspected radiculopathy. Chapter 5 provides a more detailed discussion of this subject.

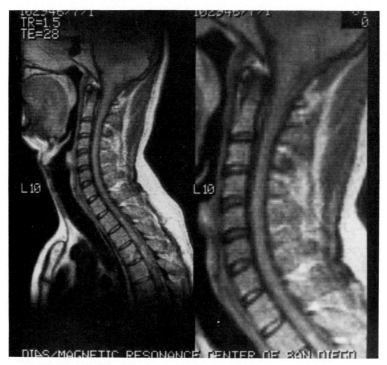

Figure 3.32. Magnetic resonance image of the cervical and upper thoracic spine. Sagittal view with close-up of cervical spine.

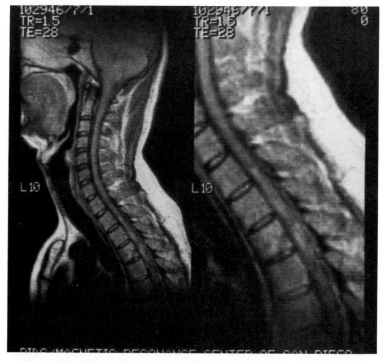

Figure 3.33. Magnetic resonance image of the cervical and upper thoracic spine (same patient as in Figure 3.32). Sagittal view with close-up of upper thoracic spine.

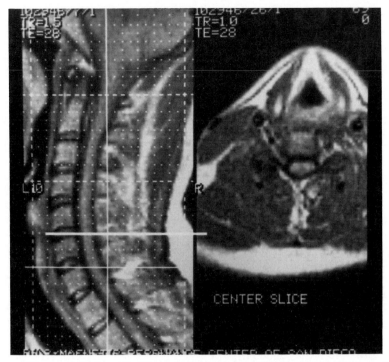

Figure 3.34. Magnetic resonance image of the cervical spine (same patient in Figures 3.32 and 3.33). Axial view.

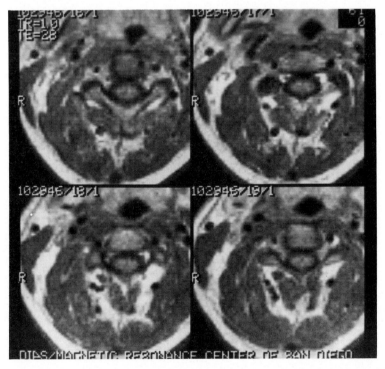

Figure 3.35. Magnetic resonance image of the cervical spine (same patient as in Figures 3.32–3.34). Axial views.

THERMOGRAPHY

Thermography is a method of measuring the heat patterns of the human body. Interest in measuring these patterns is not new, however. About 2000 years ago, Hippocrates spread a very thin layer of mud on his patients and observed the irregular drying pattern of the mud as it caked.

Infrared light waves were discovered by Sir William Herschel in 1800. Several years later, his son, Sir John Herschel, created the first thermogram. Infrared light waves, which are invisible to the naked eye, are of a longer wavelength and lower frequency than red light, hence the term infrared.

To understand what some of the clinical applications of thermography might be, the physiology that influences this process needs to be understood. Under normal conditions, the core temperature of the body is kept at a a steady 37° Celsius. This is, of course, affected both endogenously and exogenously. A greatly increased metabolism or strenuous muscular activity produces endogenous heat. Exogenous heat is heat from any outside source.

The body attempts to maintain its desired core temperature by perspiration (evaporation), conduction to air (convection) and, lastly, radiation. In the latter case, peripheral circulation opens, allowing core blood to pass to the skin which directly radiates infrared to the outside, thereby dissipating heat. This accounts for about 60% of our normal heat loss, depending on ambient temperature and the type of clothing worn (130). Surface vasodilation and vasoconstriction are controlled primarily by the sympathetic nervous system, although other minor factors are involved (131).

It had been argued that processes that produce increased local heat, such as tumors or muscle spasm, are responsible for changes in the thermographic (infrared) pattern seen on the skin surface. Love (132) has shown that aerobic metabolism in normal muscle tissue could not increase local tissue temperature by even 0.2° Celsius. And Nilsson et al. (133) have stated that the current methods of thermography were not sensitive enough to detect heat from, for example, a source such as a tumor or a muscle in spasm. Others (134) have held that motor root fiber irritation producing mus-

cle spasm and increased muscle metabolism in the paraspinal area (135) will account for the heat patterns seen with this modality. Christianson (136), however, has stated that there is little evidence supporting these views. He has also said that any local metabolism could not account for a significant rise in temperature because the increased blood flow that would be required for the active muscle tissue would also serve to dissipate any increased local heat. He noted that these paraspinal heat patterns rarely define any known myotome and that paraspinal hot spots are frequently quite small and often linear—a pattern more suggestive of a nerve or blood vessel than a muscle group (Fig. 3.36). Spinal thermography is generally accepted as detecting irritation of sensory fibers of the dorsal root, not ventral root motor fibers.

Christianson (136) has proposed that the most likely explanation for the various heat patterns typically seen in thermography is the phenomenon of antidromic stimulation of sensory fibers from local cutaneous regions. The distal terminals of C-fibers, which primarily carry pain impulses, contains a very powerful pain-producing sub-

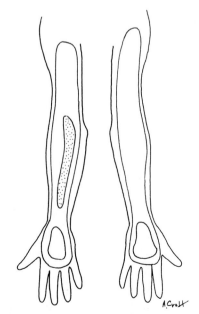

Figure 3.36.   Schematic drawing of a thermogram of the ventral aspects of the arms, forearms, and hands, demonstrating a linear hot spot (*stippled area*).

stance that also acts as a vasodilator. This is known as substance P. It is released upon antidromic stimulation of dorsal root ganglia (137–139). The effects of substance P release may be seen as a warm area or narrow stripe. It is postulated that in addition to vasodilation, local heat production, and pain, muscle spasm may be associated with substance P release—hence the association between muscle spasm and the abnormal thermogram.

The issue again becomes clouded when investigators try to explain the dermatomal pattern of dorsal root irritation, which often is seen as a cooler area rather than a warmer area (135). Wexler (140) has postulated that through a series of central nervous system reflexes, local vasoconstriction mediated by the sympathetic nervous system is responsible for the colder patterns commonly seen in thermography and that, in general, an acute injury will produce a warm derma-

tome, whereas a chronic condition will present with a cool dermatome.

Christianson (136) has offered an alternate hypothesis based upon the release of substance P. According to his hypothesis, chronic irritation may produce an eventual depletion of substance P, which would then account for chronic vasoconstriction. More research is needed to verify these models.

Presently, there are two forms of thermography equipment available—liquid crystal and infrared electronic. Wexler (141) claims that liquid crystal equipment gives about the same results as the more sophisticated electronic infrared equipment. Liquid crystal equipment is composed of boxes with flexible latex covers that are coated with heat-sensitive crystals and stretched over one end. These crystals emit colors that vary according to the temperature. These boxes are inflated with air, and the latex ends are placed against the patient. After a given

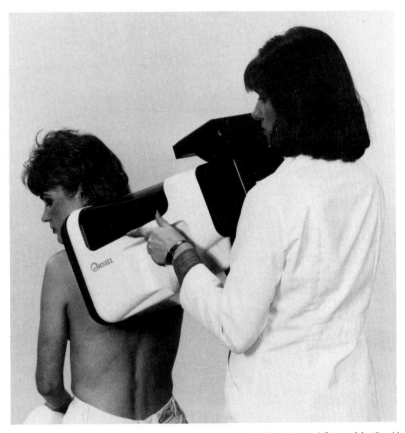

Figure 3.37.   Liquid crystal thermographic equipment. (Courtesy of Qmax Medical Inc.)

period of time, when the crystals have registered a color "heat picture," a 35-mm photograph is taken of this heat pattern, and the examination proceeds to the next test area. The major advantage of this form of thermography equipment is cost—usually under $6000 (Fig. 3.37). The disadvantages are that much more time is needed to scan large or multiple areas of the body and there is no way of controlling the sensitivity or color variance between temperature increments. Another disadvantage is that some third party payers will not reimburse for the use of liquid crystal thermography equipment.

Electronic infrared thermography is technologically superior to liquid crystal thermography, but purchase of electronic infrared thermography is vastly more expensive. Most units on the market today cost more than $35,000 (Fig. 3.38). There are several advantages to using this system, however. The operator can control subtle variances in temperature with different color sequences, thereby enhancing any asymmetry found. The images obtained are in real time and can be stored on floppy disc for future recall and photographing. Computer cathode ray tube displays provide typical curser movements to allow the operator to focus in on specific areas (Fig. 3.39). One of the biggest advantages of electronic infrared thermography equipment is that the procedure is much faster than that with use of liquid crystal equipment.

Microwave thermography is the newest form of heat-sensing technology. With this type of thermography, antenna or microwave scanners are placed next to the skin. Its major advantage will be to detect deep-seated abnormalities not detectable with

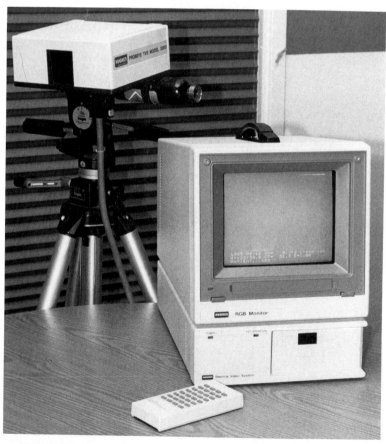

Figure 3.38.   Infrared thermographic equipment and computer. (Courtesy of Hughes Aircraft Co.)

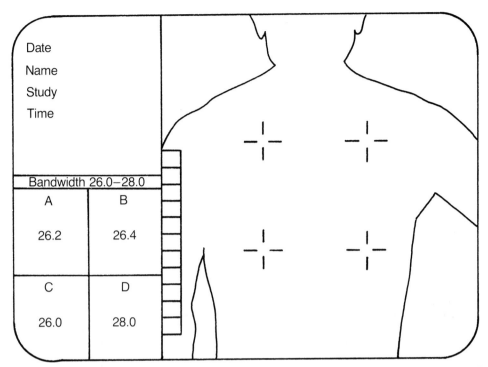

Figure 3.39. Schematic drawing of the computer cathode ray tube display used in electronic infrared thermography equipment.

infrared thermography. The images are reproduced as in electronic infrared but currently have a lower resolution than that provided by infrared thermography equipment.

The protocol for thermographic testing must be rigidly followed in order to ensure accuracy and reproducibility. The patient is disrobed and allowed to equilibrate to ambient temperature for 15–20 minutes. Prior to this test, the patient should not bathe, take medications, sunbathe, have any form of physiotherapy, drink hot or cold beverages, smoke, or use ointments (142). The test room must be draft free and temperature stable, in the range of 66–75° Fahrenheit. After the first test is performed, the patient is then escorted back to the equilibration room to reequilibrate for another 15–20 minutes, and the test is then repeated. In total, three separate tests are performed to ensure accuracy. Wexler (141) has reported no false negative results when this protocol has been followed.

Feldman and Nickoloff (143), using liquid crystal equipment, thermographed the neck, shoulders, and upper extremities of 100 asymptomatic actively employed factory workers and found symmetry in the overwhelming majority. They have recommended that when asymmetry is found an organic basis for it should be sought.

It is claimed that thermography and electromyography together will yield a 94% accuracy result (144). The sensitivity of thermography is claimed by some (141) to be roughly equivalent to that of myelography in the detection of nerve root irritation. If Wexler's claim of no false negatives is true and generally reproducible, a negative or normal thermogram would certainly seem to obviate the need for more invasive and hazardous testing, such as myelography. The cost of thermography is significantly less than that of myelography.

Conclusion

It has been said many times that the history is often the single most important part of the physical examination. An understanding of the complex biomechanics and kinematics of the cervical spine and related soft tissue during the acceleration/deceleration trauma is fundamental to the understanding of the effects of specific aspects of a particular type of injury. For example, what position the head was in at the time of impact in the acceleration/deceleration trauma. This most valuable information can only be gleaned from a careful and unhurried history.

Beyond the history and standard physical examination, the clinician must decide what further testing, if any, is indicated. This decision should be based first and foremost on the urgency of the moment. Evidence of fracture, dislocation, hemorrhage, or gross neurological deficit require immediate action. Most often, however, the injury is less than critical in nature, and the clinician must temper his or her desire to identify, quantify, and document organic lesions, through the use of sophisticated, invasive, perhaps potentially harmful (and usually expensive) diagnostic procedures, with a consideration for the basic tenet, "first, do no harm." If the results of a test are unlikely to change the form of treatment rendered, that test can often be deferred or avoided completely. For example, some have argued that thermography should be used routinely at the beginning of the case and then again at the end of treatment. Although this procedure is noninvasive and in no way harmful to the patient, it is expensive, and in this author's opinion, its use at the beginning of treatment offers no real advantage in the management of most soft tissue injuries. Very often the patient will recover with little or no residual disability or pain, and thermography serves no purpose other than to document that the patient was, at least initially, in pain. In general, it serves its greatest function in the evaluation of a chronic or perhaps permanent condition.

At the other end of the spectrum, however, we as clinicians must not become lackadaisical or routine in our management of these cases. Time is a great teacher, and with a thorough understanding of the anatomy, neurology, biomechanics, and physiology of the soft tissue injury as well as an understanding of the uses and limitations of the wide variety of diagnostic procedures available, coupled with the day-to-day experience of the physician-patient interaction, we can easily manage a case from beginning to end, rationally and prudently.

It is well known that seemingly minor trauma can produce significant injury. The symptoms may be late in appearance, however. Omission of proper diagnostic steps may result in misdiagnosis of an underlying lesion that, if left untreated, could become chronic and highly resistant to treatment later. In the worst of all possible scenarios, this misdiagnosis could result in death.

Summary

1. The history should be as complete as possible and should include a careful description of the biomechanical forces to which the patient was subjected.

2. Psychometric testing may be indicated in the overall evaluation of patients who have sustained appreciable trauma. This type of evaluation may be indicated in (a) patients who have suffered concussion or other head injury, (b) patients who seem to react inappropriately to their condition or in whom some form of functional overlay is suspected, and (c) patients with a history of some form of personality disorder.

3. Electroencephalography (EEG) may be useful in demonstrating certain posttraumatic conditions. Postconcussion syndromes can be produced from acceleration/deceleration trauma in the absence of blunt head trauma.

4. Electromyography (EMG) and the NCV study should be employed in suspected cases of radiculopathy or lower motor neuron lesion. Pathological changes, however, may not be demonstrable for 3 weeks or more.

5. Isokinetic testing may be useful in evaluating and documenting muscle weakness.

6. The importance of plain films in the evaluation of trauma cannot be overstated. In hyperextension/hyperflexion injuries to the cervical spine, flexion and extension views should be added to the standard five-view

cervical spine series for evaluating interseg-mental instability. In cases of protracted pain and disability in which delayed instability may be a factor, these flexion/extension views should be repeated at later dates.

7. Cineradiography or fluorovideo radiogra-phy plays an important role in the diagnosis of aberrant spinal biomechanics that may be secondary to chronic muscle contracture, scar tissue formation, or ligamentous instability.

8. Intersegmental template analysis is another method of demonstrating altered spinal biomechanics. In this technique, an acetate overlay is placed on lateral cervical spine films taken with the patient in flexion, neutral, and extension. Several techniques are described.

9. Most cases of disc protrusion or herniation can be demonstrated with CT scanning. This technique is, in many ways, superior to mye-lography, in that it is painless, is noninvasive, delivers less radiation, is less expensive and, with MPR, provides more information than does standard myelography. In some cases, contrast-enhanced myelography with CT may be indicated. The newer nonionic com-pounds iopamidol and iohexol are remark-ably free from side effects.

10. Discography, once used to diagnose disc disease, has been largely abandoned.

11. Angiography, like most other invasive pro-cedures, is associated with several compli-cations. With regard to the majority of conditions discussed in this textbook, its use is limited.

12. Technetium bone scanning is useful in detecting metabolic bone disease, tumor, infection, occult fracture, and severe strains that affect tenoperiosteal junctions. It may be useful in differentiating a new process from an old one or a fracture from an arti-fact or anomaly.

13. MRI is the newest imaging technique. It can provide information in multiple planes simi-lar to CT with MPR. It is produced not with ion-izing radiation but with phased radiofrequency waves. Perhaps its major advantage over CT is its ability to discrimi-nate between different types of soft tissue—an achievement that is largely dependent upon the specific hydrogen ion concentra-tion of tissues.

At present, however, certain areas of the spine, notably the neuroforamina are not as easily visualized on MRI as they are on CT with MPR. Cortical bone is nearly devoid of signal. Therefore, both CT and MRI have applica-tions in the evaluation of the cervical spine and, in many cases, may be complemen-tary to one another.

14. Thermography, a way of establishing asym-metrical heat emission patterns on the body surface, has been shown to be effective in evincing soft tissue injuries. Careful protocol must be followed, however, and results must be reproducible in order that they stand up to scientific scrutiny. Several theories as to the exact mechanism or mechanisms involved in production of these dermal heat pattern changes have been proposed, and cer-tainly more research is needed in this area.

References

1. Severy DM, Mathewson JH, Bechtol CP: Controlled automobile rear-end collisions, an investigation of related engineering and medical phenomena. *Can Serv Med J* ll:727, 1955.

2. Jackson R: *The Cervical Syndrome*, ed 4. Springfield, IL, Charles C Thomas, 1977, pp 62–64.

3. Pennecot GF, Leonard P, Peyrot Des Gachons S, Hardy JR, Puliequen JC: Traumatic ligamentous instability of the cervical spine in children. *J Pediatr Orthop* 4(3):339–345, 1984.

4. Green JD, Harle TS, Harris JH: Anterior subluxation of the cervical spine: hyperflexion sprain. *AJNR* 2:243–250, 1981.

5. Cheshire DJE: The stability of the cervical spine follow-ing conservative treatment of fractures and disloca-tions. *Int Paraplegia* 7:193–203, 1970.

6. White AA, Johnson RM, Panjabi MM, Southwick WO: Biomechanical analysis of clinical stability in the cervi-cal spine. *Clin Orthop* 109:85–95, 1975.

7. Chusid JG: Trauma to the central nervous system. In Chusid JG (ed): *Correlative Neuroanatomy and Functional Neurology*, ed 18. Los Altos, CA, Lange Medical Publi-cations, 1982, p 340.

8. Borovich B, Braun J, Guilburd JN, Zaaroor M, Michich M, Levy L, Lamberger A, Grushkiewicz I, Feinsod M, Schachter I: Delayed onset of traumatic extradural hematoma. *J Neurosurg* 63(1):30–24, 1985.

9. Vicario S, Danzl D, Thomas DM: Emergency presen-tation of subdural hematoma: a review of 85 cases diag-nosed by computerized tomography. *Ann Emerg Med* 11(9):475–477, 1982.

10. Sugiura M, Mori N, Yokosuka R, Jamamoto M, Iman-aga H, Sugimori T, Jimbo M, Kitamura K, Kono H: Head injury in children—with special reference to CT find-ings (author's translation). *No Shinkei Geka* 9(6):697–704, 1981.

11. Cohen RA, Kaufman RA, Meyers PA, Towbin RB: Cra-nial computed tomography in the abused child with head injury. *AJR* 146(1):97–102, 1986.

12. Thurber P, Thurber P Jr: *Claims Medical Manual*,ed 3. Palo Alto, CA, Pacific Books, 1960, pp 74–76.

13. Ford JS: Posttraumatic headache. *Headache* 4(1):3–11, 1985.

14. Jacome DE, Risko M: EEG features in post-traumatic syndrome. *Clin Electroencephalogr* 15(4):214–221, 1984.

15. Scher AT: Cervical spine fusion and the effects of injury. *S Afr Med J* 56:525–527, 1979.

16. Edstein NE, Epstein JA, Zilkha A: Traumatic myelopathy in a seventeen-year-old child with cervical spinal stenosis (without fracture or dislocation) and a C2-C3 Klippel-Feil fusion: a case report. *Spine* 9(4):344–347, 1984.

17. Turek SL: The cervical spine. In Turek SL (ed): *Orthopaedics: Principles and Their Applications,* ed 3. Philadelphia, JB Lippincott, 1977, p 766.

18. Foo D, Bignami A, Rossier AB: Two spinal cord lesions in a patient with ankylosing spondylitis and cervical spine injury. *Neurology* 33:245–249, 1983.

19. Murray GC, Persellin RH: Cervical fracture complicating ankylosing spondylitis: a report of eight cases and review of the literature. *Am J Med* 70:1033–1041, 1981

20. Maiman DJ, Cusick JF: Traumatic atlanto-axial dislocation. *Surg Neurol* 18(5):388–392, 1982.

21. Greenberg AD: Atlanto-axial dislocation. *Brain* 91:655–684, 1968.

22. Mouradian WH, Fietti VG, Cochran GV, Fielding JW, Young T: Fractures of the odontoid: a laboratory and clinical study of mechanisms. *Orthop Clin North Am* 9:985–1001, 1978.

23. Wachenheim A: *Roentgen Diagnosis of the Craniovertebral Region.* New York, Springer-Verlag, 1974, pp 360–364.

24. Gehweiler JA, Osborne RL, Beecher RF: *Radiology of Vertebral Trauma.* Philadelphia, WB Saunders, 1980, pp134–138.

25. Steel HH: Anatomical and mechanical considerations of the atlanto-axial articulation. *J Bone Joint Surg* 50A:1481–1482, 1968.

26. White AA, Panjabi MM: Clinical biomechanics of the occipito-atlanto-axial complex. *Orthop Clin North Am* 9:867–878, 1978.

27. Harris JH Jr: *The Radiology of Acute Cervical Spine Trauma.* Baltimore, Williams & Wilkins, 1981, p 2.

28. Wachenheim A: *Roentgen Diagnosis of the Craniovertebral Region.* New York, Springer-Verlag, 1974, pp 94–95.

29. Locke GR, Gardner JE, Van Epps EF: Atlas-dens interval (ADI) in children. *Am J Roentgenol Radium Ther Nucl Med* 97:135, 1966.

30. Alexander E, Forsyth HF, Davis CH, Hashold BS: Dislocation of the atlas on the axis. The value of early fusion of C1, C2 and C3. *J Neurosurg* 15:353–371, 1958.

31. Rothman RH, Simeone FA (eds): *The Spine,* ed 2. Philadelphia, WB Saunders, 1982, vol 2, p 992.

32. Foreman SM, Croft AC: Diagnosis of whiplash injuries. *Calif Chiro Assoc J* 11(4):26–27, 1986.

33. Penning L: Prevertebral hematoma in cervical spine injury: incidence and etiologic significance. *AJR* 136:553–561, 1981.

34. Schneider RC, Livingston KE, Cave AJE, Hamilton G: "Hangman's fracture" of the cervical spine. *J Neurosurg* 22:141–154, 1965.

35. Elliot JM, Roger LF, Wissinger JP, Lee JF: The hangman's fracture. Fractures of the neural arch of the atlas. *Radiology* 104:303–307, 1972.

36. Hyperextension injury of the cervical spine with rupture of the esophagus. *J Bone Joint Surg* 42B:356–357, 1960.

37. Scher AT: The value of retropharyngeal swelling in the diagnosis of fracture of the atlas. *S Afr Med J* 58:451–452, 1980.

38. Stringer WL, Kelly DL Jr, Johnston FR, Holliday RH: Hyperextension injury to the cervical spine with esophageal perforation. Case report. *J Neurosurg* 53:541–543, 1980.

39. Spenler CW, Benfield JR: Esophageal disruption from blunt and penetrating external trauma. *Arch Surg* 111:663–667, 1976.

40. Mengoli LR, Klassen KP: Conservative management of esophagus perforation. *Arch Surg* 91:238–240, 1965.

41. Faroog PA, Raji MR: Esophageal perforation with fracture dislocation of cervical spine due to hyperextension injury. *Br J Radiol* 55:369–372, 1982.

42. Stringer WL, Kelly DL, Johnson FR, Holliday RH: Hyperextension injury of the cervical spine with esophageal perforation. *J Neurosurg* 53:541–543, 1980.

43. Pollock RA, Apple DF, Purvis JM, Murray HH: Esophageal and hypopharyngeal injuries in patients with cervical spine trauma. *Ann Otol* 90:323–327, 1981.

44. Hann CL: Retropharyngeal-tendinitis. *AJR* 130:1137–1140, 1978.

45. Gatchel RJ, Mayer TG, Capra P, Diamond P, Barnett J: Quantification of lumbar function. Part 6: the use of psychological measures in guiding physical functional restoration. *Spine* 11(1):36–42, 1986.

46. Patten J: *Neurological Differential Diagnosis.* New York, Springer-Verlag, 1978, p 266.

47. Hoover BB, Caldwell JW, Krusen EM, et al: Value of polyphasic potentials in diagnosis of lumbar root lesions. *Arch Phys Med Rehabil* 51:546–548, 1970.

48. Waylonis GW: Electromyographic findings in chronic cervical radicular syndromes. *Arch Phys Med Rehabil* 49:407–412, 1968.

49. Eisen A: Electrodiagnosis of radiculopathies. *Neurol Clin* 3(3):495–510, 1985.

50. Gough JG, Koepke GH: Electromyographic determination of motor root levels in erector spinae muscles. *Arch Phys Med Rehabil* 47:9–11, 1966.

51. Johnson B: Morphology, innervation, and elecromyographic study of the erector spinae. *Arch Phys Med Rehabil* 50:638–641, 1969.

52. Penderson HE, Blunck CJF, Gardner E: The anatomy of lumbosacral posterior rami and meningeal branches of spinal nerves (sinuvertebral nerves). *J Bone Joint Surg* 38A:377–391, 1956.

53. Bonney G, Gilliatt RW: Sensory nerve conduction after traction lesions of the brachial plexus. *Proc R Soc Med* 51:365–367, 1958.

54. Kimura J: *Electrodiagnosis in Diseases or Nerves and Muscles: Principles and Practices.* Philadelphia, FA Davis, 1983.

55. Stanwood JE, Kraft GH: Diagnosis and management of brachial plexus injuries. *Arch Phys Med Rehabil* 52:52–61, 1971.

56. Narakas A: Traumatic brachial plexus injuries. In Dyck PJ, Thomas RK, Lambert EH (eds): *Peripheral Neuropathy,* ed 2. Philadelphia, WB Saunders, 1984.

57. Wilbourn AJ: Electrodiagnosis of plexopathies. *Neurol Clin* 3(3):511–529, 1985.

58. Mayer TG, Smith SS, Keeley J, Mooney V: Quantification of lumbar function. Part 2: sagittal plane trunk strength in chronic low-back pain patients. *Spine* 10(8):765–771, 1985.

59. Tessler SR: Sports device may solve whys of "bad back" *Detroit News* pp 10–20, August 16, 1984.

60. Jackson R: *The Cervical Syndrome,* ed 4. Springfield, IL, Charles C Thomas, 1977, pp 212–215.

61. Henderson DJ, Dormon TM: Functional roentgenometric evaluation of the cervical spine in the sagittal plane. *J Manipulative Physiol Ther* 8(4):219–227, 1985.

62. Hviid H: Functional radiography of the cervical spine. *Ann Swiss Chiro Assoc* 3:37–65, 1963.

63. Howe JW: Cineradiographic evaluation of normal and abnormal cervical spinal function. *J Clin Chiro Arch* 2: Winter, 1972.

64. Henderson DJ: Kinetic roentgenometric analysis of the cervical spine in the sagittal plane: a preliminary study. *Int Rev Chiro* 35:2, 1981.

65. Croft AC, Foreman SM: Unilateral pseudonotch of the atlas vertebra simulating fracture. *ACA J Chiro* 23(12):44–50, 1986.

66. Macnab I: Acceleration injuries of the cervical spine. *J Bone Joint Surg* 46A:1797–1799, 1964.

67. Ehni G: *Cervical Arthrosis: Diseases of the Cervical Motion Segments.* Chicago, Year Book, 1984, pp 54–55.

68. Turek SL: *Orthopaedics: Principles and Their Applications,* ed 3. Philadelphia, JB Lippincott, 1977, p 742.

69. Buonocore E, Hartman JT, Nelson CL: Cineradiograms of the cervical spine in diagnosis of soft-tissue injuries. *JAMA* 198(1):143–147, 1966.

70. Woesner ME, Mitts MG: The evaluation of cervical spine motion below C2: a comparison of cineroentgenographic and conventional radiographic methods. *Am J Roentgenol Radium Ther Nucl Med* 115(1):148–154, 1972.

71. Fielding JW: Cineradiography. *J Bone Joint Surg* 45A:1543, 1957.

72. Fielding JW: Cineradiography of normal cervical spine. *J Bone Joint Surg* 39A:1280–1288, 1957.

73. Fielding JW: Normal and selected abnormal motion of cervical spine from second cervical vertebra to seventh cervical vertebra based on cineradiography. *J Bone Joint Surg* 46A:1779–1781, 1964.

74. Jones MD: Cervical spine cineradiography after traffic accidents. *AMA Arch Surg* 85:974–981, 1962.

75. Jones MD: Cineroentgenographic studies of patients with cervical spine fusion. *Am J Roentgenol Radium Ther Nucl Med* 87:1054–1057, 1962.

76. Jones MD: Cineradiographic studies of collar immobilized cervical spine. *J Neurosurg* 17:633–637, 1960.

77. Howe JW: Observations from cineroentgenological studies of the spinal column. *ACA J Chiro* 7(10):65–70, 1970.

78. Lane GR: Cervical spine: its movement and symptomatology. *J Clin Chiro* 1(1):128–145, 1971.

79. Whitehead LC, Moon C: The cineradiographic evaluation of normal and aberrant flexion motion in the cervical spine. *Int Rev Chiro* 35:2, 1981.

80. Grice AS: Preliminary evaluation of 50 sagittal cervical motion radiographic examinations. *J Can Chiro Assoc* March, 1977.

81. Conley TN: Stress evaluation of cervical mechanics. *J Clin Chiro* 1(3):45–62, 1974.

82. Buetti-Bauml C: *Funktionelle Rontgendiagnostik der Halswirbelsäule.* Stuttgart, Thieme, 1959.

83. Arlen A: *Biometrische Rontgenfunktionsdiagnostic der Halswirbelsäule.* Heidelberg, Fischer (Schriflenreihe Mannelle Medizin, Bd 5).

84. Prantl K: X-ray examination and functional analysis of the cervical spine. *Manual Med* 2:5–15, 1985.

85. Hitselberger WE, Witten R: Abnormal myelograms in asymptomatic patients. *J Neurosurg* 28:204–206, 1968.

86. Rothman RH, Simeone FA (eds): *The Spine,* ed 2. Philadelphia, WB Saunders, 1982, vol 1, p 461.

87. Ehni G: Extradural spinal cord and nerve root compression from benign lesions of the cervical area. In Youmans J (ed): *Neurological Surgery.* Philadelphia, WB Saunders, 1982, pp 25–94.

88. Jackson R: *The Cervical Syndrome,* ed 4. Springfield, IL, Charles C Thomas, 1977, p 236.

89. Ehni G: *Cervical Arthrosis: Disease of the Cervical Motion Segments.* Chicago, Year Book, 1984, p 146.

90. Erlacher PR: Nucleography. *J Bone Joint Surg* 34B:204, 1952.

91. Finney LA, Gargano FP, Buermann A: Intraosseous vertebral neurography in the diagnosis of lumbar disc disease. *Am J Roentgenol* 92:1282–1292, 1964.

92. Finneson BE: *Low Back Pain.* Philadelphia, JB Lippincott, 1980, p 160.

93. Hansen EB, Fahrenkrug A, Praestholm J: Late meningeal effects of myelographic contrast media with special reference to metrizamide. *Br J Radiol* 51(605):321–327, 1978.

94. Haughton VM, Ho KC, Larsen SJ, et al: Comparison of arachnoiditis produced by meglumide locarmate and metrizamide myelography in an animal model. *Am J Roentgenol* 131:129–132, 1978.

95. Praestholm J: Experimental evaluation of water soluble contrast media for myelography. *Neuroradiology* 13:25–35, 1977.

96. Wray AR, Templeton J, Laird JD: Seizure following lumbar myelography with metrizamide. *Br Med J* 23–30, 1978.

97. McCormick CC, ApSimon HT, Chakera TM: Myelography with metrizamide—an analysis of the complications encountered in cervical, thoracic and lumbar myelography. *Aust NZ J Med* 11(6):645–650, 1981.

98. Skalpe IO: Adhesive arachnoiditis following lumbar myelography. *Spine* 3(1):61–64, 1978.

99. Skalpe IO: Adhesive arachnoiditis following lumbar radiculography with water-soluble contrast agents. A clinical report with special reference to metrizamide. *Radiology* 121(3):647–651, 1976.

100. Haughton VM, Ho KC, Larson SJ, Unger GF, Correa, Paz F: Experimental production of arachnoiditis with water-soluble myelographic media. *Radiology* 123(3):681–685, 1977.

101. Kelley RE, Daroff RB, Sheremata WA, McCormick JR: Unusual effects of metrizamide lumbar myelography. Constellation of aseptic meningitis, arachnoiditis, communicating hydrocephalus, and Guillain-Barré syndrome. *Arch Neurol* 37(9):588–589, 1980.

102. Hopkins RM, Adams MD, Lau DH, Creighton JM, Hoey GB: Ioglucomide: a new nonionic myelographic agent. Preclinical studies. *Radiology* 140(3):713–717, 1981.

103. Rothman SLG, Glenn WV Jr: *Multiplanar CT of the Spine.* Baltimore, University Park Press, 1985, p 375.

104. Rothman SLG, Glenn WV Jr: *Multiplanar CT of the Spine.* Baltimore, University Park Press, 1985, p 376.

105. Turek SL: *Orthopaedics: Principles and Their Applications,* ed 3. Philadelphia, JB Lippincott, 1977, p 759.

106. Fernstrom U: A diskographical study of ruptured lumbar intevetrebral disks. *Acta Chir Scand [Suppl]* 258, 1960.

107. Holt EP: The fallacy of cervical diskography: report of 50 cases in normal subjects. *JAMA* 188:799–801, 1964.

108. Rothman SCG, Glenn WV Jr: *Multiplanar CT of the Spine.* Baltimore, University Park Press, 1985, p 659.

109. Ehni G: *Cervical Arthritis: Diseases of the Cervical Motion Segments.* Chicago, Year Book, 1984, p 46.

110. Jackson R: *The Cervical Syndrome,* ed 4. Springfield, IL, Charles C Thomas, 1977, pp 190–191.

111. Brenner A, Roosen K, Hartjes H, Buch A, Ruhnan K: Diskographic—myelographic. *Neurochirurgia* 27(1):8–11, 1984.

112. Kikuchi S, Macnab I, Moreau P: Localization of the level of symptomatic cervical disc degeneration. *J Bone Joint Surg* 63B(2):272–277, 1981.

113. Distelmier P, Lins E: Technik und aussagekraft der diskographic bei der diagnostik zervikaler syndrome. *Rontgenblatter* 29(4):178–183, 1976.

114. Simmons EH, Segil CM: An evaluation of discography in the localization of symptomatic levels in discogenic disease of the spine. *Clin Orthop* 108:57–69, 1975.

115. Collins HR: An evaluation of cervical and lumbar discography. *Clin Orthop* 107:133–138, 1975.

116. Roth DA: Cervical analgesic discography: a new test for the definitive diagnosis of the painful-disk syndrome. *JAMA* 235(16):1713–1714, 1976.

117. Merriam WF, Stockdale HR: Is cervical discography of any value? *Eur J Radiol* 3(2):128–141, 1983.

118. Laun A, Lorenz R, Agnoli AL: Complications of cervical discography. *J Neurosurg Sci* 25(1):17–20, 1981.

119. Agnoli AL, Laun A: Komplikationen bei ossovenographie und diskographie im halsbereich. *Rontgenblatter* 30(12):616–620, 1977.

120. Roosen K, Bettag W, Fiebach O: Komplikationen der

zervikalen diskographie. *Fortschr Geb Rontgenstr Nuklearmed* 122(6):520–527, 1975.

121. Holt EP Jr: Further reflections on cervical discography. *JAMA* 231(6):613–614, 1975.

122. Louis R: Traumatismes du raekis cervical.l. Entorses et hernies discales. *Nouv Presse Med* 8(22):1843–1849, 1979.

123. Rosenthall L, Hill RO, Chuang S: Observation on use of ^{99m} Tc-phosphate imaging in peripheral bone trauma. *Radiology* 119:637, 1976.

124. Martin P: The appearance of bone scans following fractures, including immediate and long term studies. *J Nucl Med* 20:1227, 1979.

125. Alazraki N: Bone imaging by radionuclide techniques. In Resnick D, Niwayama G (eds): *Diagnosis of Bone and Joint Disorders.* Philadelphia, WB Saunders, 1981, vol 1, p 660.

126. Coyle BA: MRI: a revolutionary new tool. *Calif Chiro Assoc J* 13–15, July 1985.

127. Hendee WR, Morgan CJ: Magnetic resonance imaging part II—clinical applications. *West J Med* 141(5):638–648, 1984.

128. Hyman RA, Edwards JH, Vacirca SJ, Stein HL: 0.6T MR imaging of the cervical spine: multislice and multislice and multiecho techniques. *AJNR* 6(2):229–236, 1985.

129. Modic MT, Weinstein MA, Pavlicek W, Boumphrey F, Starnes D, Duchesnean PM: Magnetic resonance imaging of the cervical spine: technical and clinical observations. *AJR* 141(6):1129–1136, 1983.

130. Guyton AC: *Textbook of Medical Physiology,* ed 5. Philadelphia, WB Saunders, 1976, p 956.

131. Gautherie M: Temperature and blood flow patterns in breast cancer during natural evolution and following radiotherapy. In Gautherie M, Albert E (eds): *Biomedical Thermology.* New York, Alan R Liss, 1982.

132. Love TJ: Thermography as an indicator of blood perfusion. *Ann NY Acad Sci* 335:429–437, 1980.

133. Nilsson SK, Gustafsson SF, Torell IM: Skin temperature over a heat source: experimental studies and theoretical calculations. *Ann NY Acad Sci* 335:416–428, 1980.

134. Pochaczevsky R, Wexler CE, Meyers DH, Epstein JA, Marc JA: Thermographic study of extremity dermatomes in the diagnosis of spinal root compression syndromes. In Gautherie M, Albert E (eds): *Biomedical Thermology.* New York, Alan R Liss, 1982.

135. Wexler CE: Thermography. In: *Neuromusculoskeletal Disorders Symposium,* Glen Cove, NY, January 22–23, 1983.

136. Christianson J: Thermographic physiology. In Rein H (ed): *The primer on Thermography.* Orlando, FL, Harry Rein, 1983, pp 4–6.

137. Holton P: Further observations on substance P in degenerating nerves. *J Physiol (Lond)* 149:35, 1959.

138. Nicoll RA, Shenker C, Leeman SE: Substance P as a transmitter candidate. *Ann Rev Neurosci* 3:227–268, 1980.

139. Olgart L, Gazelius B, Brodin E, Nilsson G: Release of substance P-like immunoreactivity from the dental pulp. *Acta Physiol Scand* 101:510–512, 1977.

140. Wexler CE: Lumbar, thoracic and cervical thermography. In Gautherie M, Albert A (eds): *Biomedical Thermology.* New York, Alan R Liss, 1982.

141. Wexler CE: Thermography finds multitude of applications. *JAMA* 247(24): 3296–3302, 1982.

142. Rein H: *The Primer on Thermography.* Orlando, FL, Harry Rein, 1983, pp 20–21.

143. Feldman F, Nickoloff ED: Normal thermographic standards for the cervical and upper extremities. *Skeletal Radiol* 124:235–249, 1984.

144. Rein H: *The Primer on Thermography.* Orlando, FL, Harry Rein, 1983, pp 13–14.

4

Clinical Radiographic Examination

STEPHEN M. FOREMAN, DC, DABCO

The radiographic examination is an objective, essential part of the physical examination process. Some physicians argue that those patients who will require a radiographic examination will be detected by a complete physical examination and, therefore, that widespread utilization of radiographic procedures is unjustified. Jacobs and Schwartz (1) reviewed the cases of 233 consecutive patients who had suffered a cervical spine injury and on whom an attempt was made to predict the incidence of radiographic evidence of trauma. They found that emergency room physicians were able to successfully predict the presence of radiographic changes with only a 50% accuracy. This finding certainly appears to refute the view that widespread use of radiographic procedure is unjustified.

The treating physician will benefit from a radiographic examination, as it can be used to detect the presence of both fractures and dislocations that would preclude the performance of a standard orthopaedic examination. A second area of benefit comes from the medicolegal standpoint. The radiographic report creates an objective record of the patient's osseous and ligamentous integrity immediately after the accident. Some patients who may appear to be "normal" on initial examination and, therefore, are not given a radiographic examination may have delayed instability and later develop a serious anterior flexion deformity (2). From a legal standpoint, such a patient would have been better served had the physician ordered x-rays during the initial examination.

The order in which the films are taken is often arranged in a fashion that allows the radiologist to discover fractures or instability that would preclude the flexion and

137

extension views. The neutral lateral view, usually consisting of a cross-table lateral view, is typically the first film obtained in posttraumatic cases. A large number of fractures may be visualized on the neutral lateral view, and it is quite effective for structural assessment. Some fractures, particularly those of the atlantoaxial junction, may be difficult to appreciate on the neutral lateral view. The superimposition of the lateral masses of the atlas and the odontoid process obliterates the detail necessary to establish the presence of small, nondisplaced fractures. An anteroposterior (AP) open mouth view should be used to supplement the neutral lateral view, as it clearly delineates the structes that were superimposed on the lateral view. Shaffer and Doris (3) found the two views used in combination would increase the diagnostic yield to 100% in those patients with questionable lateral views.

Lines of Measurement_____

As previously mentioned, the neutral lateral view serves as the initial source of information regarding the structural integrity of the neural canal. It has been established that certain lines that can be mentally visualized on the radiograph can be

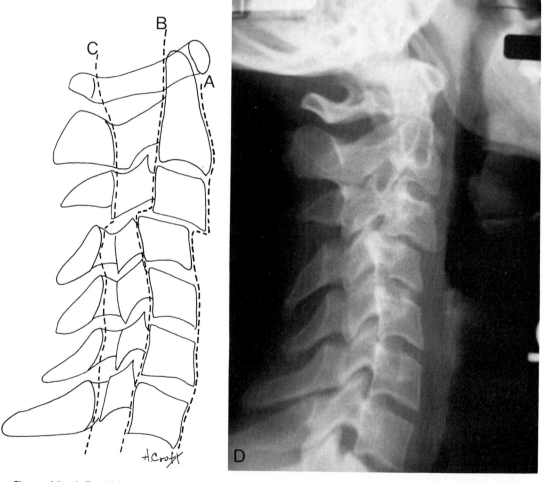

Figure 4.1. **A.** The AVL extends from the anterior arch, inferiorly, to C7. There should not be any alteration of this smooth line. **B.** The PVL should be smooth and unbroken and extend from the posterior aspect of C1 down to C7. **C.** The PCL should be drawn directly over the spinolaminal line and represents the posterior wall of the spinal canal. **D.** Radiograph provided for comparison.

used to assist the physician in determining the degree of potential instability. In the normal patient, these lines are smooth and symmetrical. Damage to or disruption of the longitudinal ligaments, ligamentum nuchae, or capsular ligaments will usually result in sufficient instability between the vertebral segments to cause a disruption of one or more of these lines. These lines are the anterior vertebral, the posterior vertebral, and the posterior canal and should be visualized mentally with each set of radiographs.

ANTERIOR VERTEBRAL LINE

The anterior vertebral line (AVL) should be visualized as a smooth, unbroken arc extending from C2 to C7 along the anterior border of the vertebral bodies (Fig. 4.1A). Patients who present with either a straight or a kyphotic curve should also have a smooth line, and any disruption of this line should be noted.

A disruption of the AVL may be caused by a variety of conditions including compression fractures and bilateral and unilat-

eral facet dislocations. Small nondisplaced avulsion fractures may not alter the line.

POSTERIOR VERTEBRAL LINE

The posterior vertebral line (PVL), also known as George's line, like its anterior counterpart, should also be visualized in a smooth, unbroken manner extending from C2 to C7 along the posterior border of the vertebral bodies (Fig. 4.1B). This line delineates the anterior wall of the spinal canal, and its disruption may localize the source of a neurological deficit.

A change in the PVL is not always seen with an alteration of the AVL. For example, a bilateral facet dislocation will interrupt both lines, compared to a vertebral body fracture which may only present with a change in the AVL.

In addition to the possible shift of the PVL, the examiner should inspect the relative height of the posterior border of the intervertebral discs. The height of an area that is suspect should be compared with the height of the other intervertebral discs. Fractures of the posterior elements or severe hyperflexion injuries may allow tearing of the posterior longitudinal ligament which may be revealed by the increase in disc height (Fig. 4.2).

POSTERIOR CANAL LINE

The posterior canal line (PCL) is visualized directly over the spinolaminal line from levels C1 to C7. The spinolaminal line is the short cortex line produced by union of the right and the left lamina to the spinous process. The absence of the spinolaminal line, usually seen at the level of the atlas, indicates a failure of fusion (Figs. 4.3 and 4.4A and B).

The PCL delineates the posterior border of the spinal canal (Fig. 4.1C). The physician may observe an alteration of this line even when the other two are within normal limits.

Posttraumatic Series

Since a hyperextension/hyperflexion injury is a phenomenon of motion, the static radiographic examination should attempt

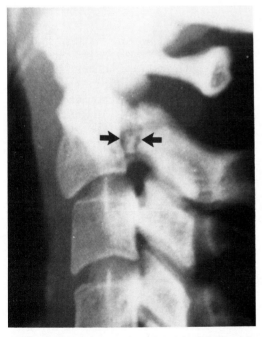

Figure 4.2. Lateral cervical view of a hangman's fracture at C2 reveals a separation in the neural arch (*arrows*). The posterior intervertebral disc height is increased.

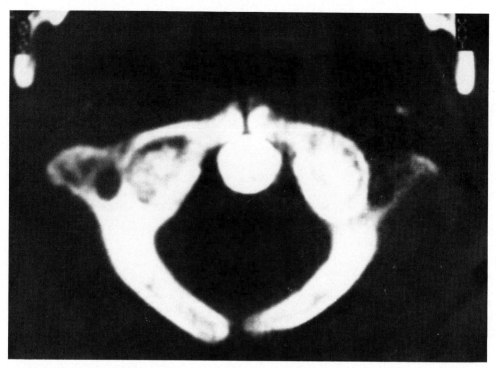

Figure 4.3.   Axial view of the atlas reveals an absence of union in both the anterior and the posterior arch.

to reproduce the extremes of the cervical movement. The other, nonmovement views are designed to delineate areas that are suspect and recognized as high risk for trauma. A complete posttraumatic series should include the neutral lateral, flexion and extension laterals, right and left obliques, AP open mouth, AP lower cervical, and right and left pillar views. Each view is required for a complete osseous and ligamentous evaluation. These various positions are discussed and reviewed in this chapter with regard to their specific function.

LATERAL VIEWS

The neutral lateral view, particularly the cross-table lateral view in cases involving moderate to severe trauma, is used for the rapid assessment of the structural integrity of the spinal canal. The AVL, PVL, and PCL are used to localize both subtle and gross changes in the shape and stability of the neural canal.

Other areas must also be included when the lateral view is reviewed. The vertebrae may have been fractured. Gross changes are usually quite apparent, but subtle fractures that are either small, nondisplaced, or both may be more difficult to appreciate. Small avulsions and ligamentous tears may be suspected by changes in the paraspinal soft tissue areas. The soft tissue areas that must be observed for change include the retropharyngeal and retrotracheal spaces, the atlantodental interval (ADI), and the interspinous spaces.

Retropharyngeal Space

The retropharyngeal space is a radiographic landmark located between the anterior border of the cervical vertebrae and the posterior border of the pharyngeal air shadow (Fig. 4.5). This area is a potential space composed of loose tissue and may be infiltrated by either blood or air or both. The space extends from the anterior arch of the atlas inferiorly to the level of either the third or the fourth cervical segment.

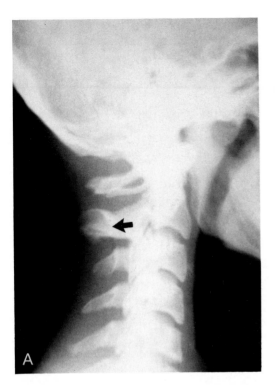

colli tendon and is composed of either calcium pyrophosphate or hydroxyapatite crystals, and this condition is termed retropharyngeal tendonitis (4).

This area, when evaluated on a neutral lateral projection taken at 72 inches, will vary 3–7 mm in width. Harris (5) has reported that this area, when measured anterior to C3, should not exceed 4 mm in width in an adult. Other authors believe that its maximum width is in the range of 2.0–5.0 mm (6–9).

Retrotracheal Space

The retrotracheal space is composed of a continuation of the same prevertebral loose tissue found in the retropharyngeal space, is located anterior to C4, and extends inferiorly to C7. This area is significantly larger than that of the retropharyngeal space and should not exceed 22 mm in width (10).

The retropharyngeal and retrotracheal spaces are significant because they may be

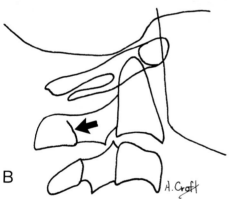

Figure 4.4. **A.** Lateral view of the cervical spine reveals an absence of the spinolaminal line. A normal spinolaminal line (*arrow*) is shown at C2. **B.** Line drawing of **A.**

The retropharyngeal space anterior to the odontoid process may contain a calcific deposit. This mass will be amorphic in nature and will usually produce a variety of upper cervical symptoms. The patient with this mass will typically complain of pain upon extension, cervical rotation, and swallowing. The deposit is located in the longus

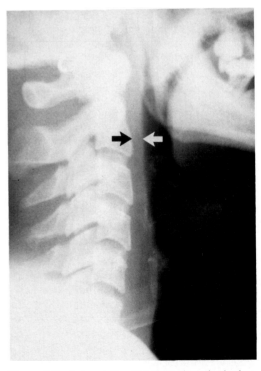

Figure 4.5. Lateral view of a normal cervical spine. The retropharyngeal space (between the *arrows*) should not exceed 4 mm.

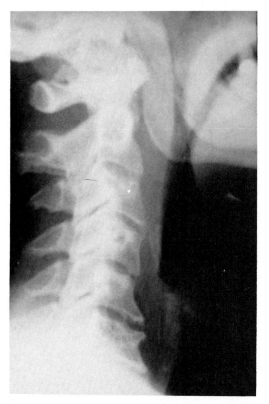

Figure 4.6. Lateral cervical view reveals broad widening of the retropharyngeal space. Note that offending fracture is not visualized.

is seen. Other processes, such as an abscess or goiter, may increase the size of this space (Fig. 4.8). One other abnormality that may be seen in either the retrotracheal or the retropharyngeal space is air. The presence of air typically arises from tearing of either the trachea or the esophagus and is recognized by long, thin radiolucent streaks within the spaces (Fig. 4.9A and B). The width of the space may or may not be altered.

Posttraumatic esophageal perforation is a potentially serious injury. Bacteria may exit the esophagus through the tear and cause moderate to severe complications, such as mediastinitis, retropharyngeal abscess, cervical abscess, aspiration pneumonia, and death (10, 12). This serious condition is also seen in nontraumatic situations. Hunter et al. (13) have reported several cases in which the patient suffered deep laceration in the esophagus after eating a taco, hence the term "taco tear." It

the only areas to demonstrate a radiographic change when the patient has suffered a nondisplaced fracture. The retropharyngeal space is usually only altered in upper cervical fractures. The resultant vascular insult causes a slow accumulation of blood that will cause either a localized widening or a small, semicircular impression on the posterior aspect of the pharyngeal shadow (Fig. 4.6).

Penning (11) reviewed the cases of 30 consecutive cervical spine injury patients and found that in 18 a widening of the retropharyngeal space as previously described had been demonstrated. The hematomas found were localized almost exclusively at the C1–C4 levels. Smaller hematomas were associated with types I, II, and III odontoid fractures (Fig. 4.7).

Retrotracheal hematomas and subsequent changes in the retrotracheal space are not as common. The wider space allows more blood to accumulate before a change

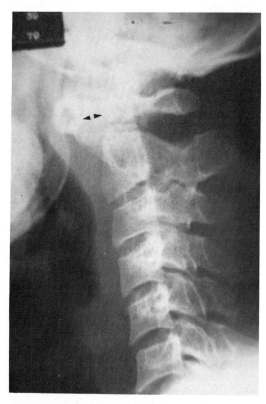

Figure 4.7. Lateral cervical view reveals type II fracture and anterior dislocation of the atlas. A large displacement (*arrows*) due to a combination of the fracture and the dislocation is shown.

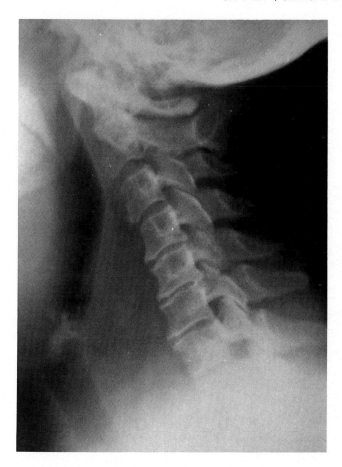

Figure 4.8. A huge increase in the retrotracheal space can be seen. This enlargement was seen in a posttrauma patient, but the cause turned out to be a goiter.

should be pointed out that the presence of either a nasogastric or an endotracheal tube will invalidate the measurements of the previously mentioned spaces (6).

ADI

The ADI is the space located between the posterior surface of the anterior arch of the atlas and the anterior surface of the odontoid process (Fig.4.10). This space is lined with a synovial membrane and is maintained by the transverse atlantal ligament.

Various authors have argued over the size of the ADI as visualized on the neutral lateral view. It is generally acknowledged that the ADI should not exceed 3 mm in adults (14, 15). Some authors (14) believe that the ADI can be as large as 5 mm in children. Locke et al. (7) studied 200 children and found that the ADI did not exceed 3 mm.

Widening of the ADI is the result of either an absence or a rupture of the transatlantal ligament, which allows the atlas to shift anteriorly in relation to the odontoid. The neutral lateral view may not reveal the increase in size. The ADI should be measured on the lateral view, and its size should be compared with that on the flexion view.

Some congenital and acquired conditions may affect the ADI without trauma. These conditions often predispose the individual to severe damage after only mild trauma. Some arthritides, such a rheumatoid, juvenile rheumatoid, psoriatic, and that resulting from *Yersenia* infection, may damage the transatlantal ligament by synovial hyperplasia. The hyperplasia or pannus formation that so adversely affects the transatlantal ligament may also cause severe erosions of the odontoid process (Fig. 4.11*A* and *B*). Congenital conditions such as Down's syndrome (16) can present with an absence of the transatlantal ligament.

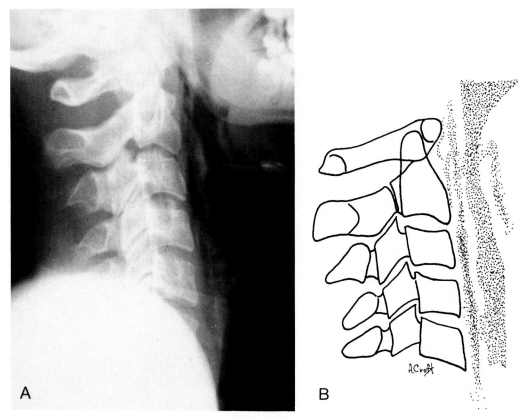

Figure 4.9. **A.** Long, thin radiolucent lines of air in the retropharyngeal and retrotracheal space are demonstrated. A small fracture can be seen on the superior surface of the lamina at C2. **B.** Line drawing of **A.**

Treatment of these patients usually consists of posterior fusion through the spinous processes of the atlas and axis.

Interspinous Space

The spaces between the spinous processes are maintained by the ligamentum nuchae and the interspinous ligament. These ligaments allow for movement of the cervical spine and limit the flexion of the area. Hyperflexion injuries, which combine both stretching and shearing forces, may partially tear, stretch, or totally disrupt these posterior structures.

Radiographic changes consisting of an asymmetrical widening between the spinous processes (Fig. 4.12) may be apparent on the neutral lateral view. The radiographic changes are dependent upon the degree of ligamentous damage and the presence of spasm. Muscle spasm may restrict the shifting between the vertebral segments and disguise ligamentous instability.

The tearing and change in strength of an interspinous ligament will cause an asymmetrical widening of the affected level. The spinous processes are said to have a "fanning" appearance. The damage may also cause an alteration in the cervical curve. An abrupt change in vertebral alignment at a single spinal level is usually due to ligament damage and is to be expected. Changes in the cervical curve that are a result of myospasm tend to cause fanning over an area of four to five segments (Fig. 4.13).

Other changes that may be seen with posterior element injury include malalignment of the posterior facet, narrowing of the anterior disc space, and possible wid-

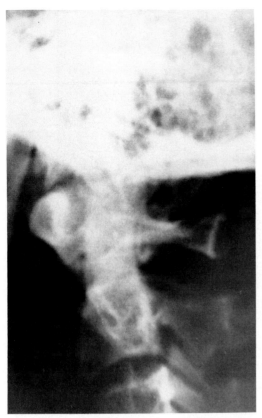

Figure 4.10.   Lateral view demonstrates a widening of the ADI. This measured 6 mm on the original film. Compare this interval with that on Figure 4.6.

of the head may shift the atlas forward and reveal the changes that were not apparent on the neutral lateral view. If the ADI increases to 5 mm or more, it should be assumed that the transverse ligament has ruptured. This area should be considered extremely unstable, and a neurosurgical consultant should be sought.

Repeat examinations with the flexion lateral view may need to be conducted after the paravertebral muscle spasm has been reduced. Pain upon flexion may indicate excessive movement of an articular facet secondary to ligament damage not discovered on the initial series. In cases of delayed instability alluded to earlier, pain may also arise upon flexion. The initial lateral flexion view may reveal an acute angulation at one specific vertebral level. An anterior angulation of 11° or less should be considered within normal limits (2). Fielding and Hawkins (17) defined instability as "weakness of intervertebral bonds that render them unable to withstand trauma tolerable to the normal spine and allows actual or potential abnormal excursion of one segment or another, implying a potential or actual compromise of neural elements." This weakening and subsequent increase in acute angulation occurs in about 20% of patients with anterior subluxation (2).

ening of the posterior disc space. An increase in the distance between the anterior-inferior corner of the articular facet and posterior-superior corner of the vertebra below may be seen. This distance should not exceed 1–2 mm in the normal patient. All of these changes would take place at the level of ligamentous injury.

FLEXION LATERAL VIEWS

The lateral view taken with the cervical spine in flexion incorporates (a) the radiographic information found on the neutral lateral view and (b) the changes demonstrated through motion. This view is designed to allow inspection of the articular facets and the integrity of the posterior ligament complex.

When this view is being studied, the ADI deserves special attention, since the weight

EXTENSION VIEW

The extension lateral view, like its flexion counterpart, allows visualization of the extreme limit of cervical movement and, with this motion, evaluation of the posterior-inferior sliding of the articular facets. This sliding should be smooth and allow the spinous processes to approximate. The atlas, in relation to the occiput, does not follow this pattern and usually has a paradoxic movement pattern. When the patient extends his or her head, the posterior arch should approach the occiput. A failure of this movement may indicate fixation or fusion of the occipitoatlas junction.

Other changes, particularly along the anterior aspect of the vertebral bodies, may be observed on the extension lateral view. The hyperextension movement places the anterior longitudinal ligament under a

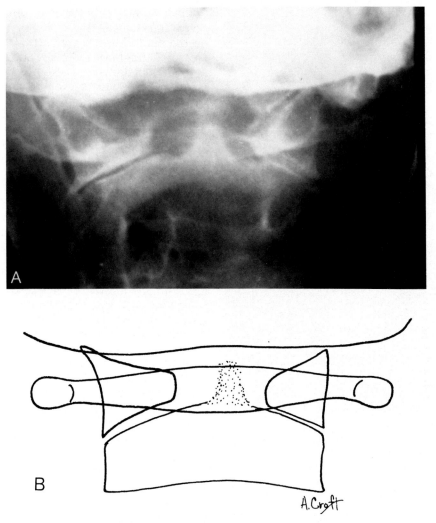

Figure 4.11.   **A.** AP open mouth view of the axis reveals severe bony erosions of the odontoid process. This process is referred to as "whittling" of the dens. **B.** Line drawing of **A.**

great, sudden vertical traction, resulting in either osseous or ligamentous damage. In addition to the clinical findings of swollen anterior cervical musculature, radiographic changes in the intervertebral discs may be seen. The sudden vertical traction may damage the anterior longitudinal ligament and cause an increased anterior disc height. The other posttraumatic change that may be observed is the presence of small pockets of gas in the anterior edge of the disc. This gas is usually seen as a thin radiolucent shadow and is referred to as a vacuum defect or lucent cleft [18]. The defect is produced by trauma and should not be confused with the vacuum phenomenon pro-

duced by degeneration and associated with conditions such as intervertebral osteochondrosis [19]. The location of the gaseous defect is the primary diagnostic feature by which these two entities may be differentiated. The degenerative vacuum phenomenon is linear and located horizontally in the center of the disc (Fig. 4.14). The lucent clefts produced by trauma are located anteriorly and are often adjacent to the vertebrae. The presence of these clefts may be apparent within hours, and although they may resolve within a few months, they may last as long as 5 years [20].

The more severe examples of hyperex-

The oblique views are a valuable tool and should be used to assess the patency of the foramen. Preexisting degenerative changes of the facets, uncinate processes, and the height of the cervical discs will affect the size and symmetry of the foramen. The hypertrophic changes seen in the facets and uncinate processes often result in an encroachment into the foramen. This degenerative change has been described as having an hourglass appearance. These changes are common in patients over 50 years of age and are typically found at the C5–C7 levels.

Structural abnormalities and disease processes may alter the symmetry and patency of the IVF. Enlargement of the IVF may be caused by benign processes such as neurofibromatosis. Structural changes of the IVF may occur in conditions that disturb vertebral segmentation, such as Klippel-Feil syndrome (Fig. 4.16).

The normal apposition of the posterior articulating surfaces is easily inspected on an oblique view. The superior facet should

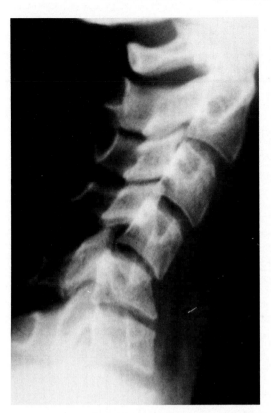

Figure 4.12. Lateral cervical spine view demonstrates a sudden widening of the spinous processes between C5 and C6.

tension may produce an avulsion fracture on the anterior-inferior corner of either C2 or C3 (Fig. 4.15). Other levels may be involved, but the upper cervical spine is most commonly affected. Holdsworth (18) depicted this fracture and classified it as an extension teardrop fracture. The avulsion may be minimally displaced, and the first observation may be a localized increase in the retropharyngeal space. Hyperextension-dislocation will, in contrast to the small avulsion, produce a diffuse prevertebral soft tissue hematoma that extends from the nasopharynx to the clivus (21).

OBLIQUE VIEWS

Oblique views, when properly taken, allow the examiner an unobstructed view of the intervertebral foramen (IVF). Proper exposure and positioning allow examination of the lamina, pedicles, and interfacet joints.

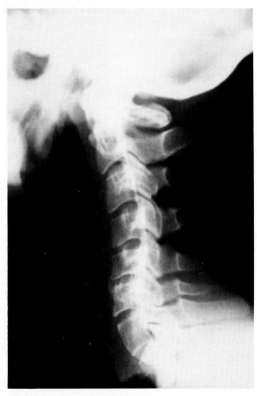

Figure 4.13. Multiple-level (C3–C5) spinous process fanning is seen.

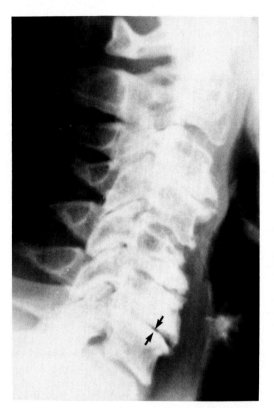

Figure 4.14.   Lateral view of the cervical spine shows a typical linear radiolucent gas accumulation, the so-called vacuum phenomenon, at C6-C7 disc level (*arrows*).

be oriented posteriorly in relation to the inferior facet. If the patient is suffering from a unilateral facet dislocation, the superior facet will be positioned anterior to the inferior facet (Fig. 4.17*A–C*). Other changes associated with a unilateral facet dislocation will be an anterior vertebral body shift in relation to the inferior segment and an increase in the height of the posterior aspect of the intervertebral disc at the affected level.

Unilateral facet dislocation may be accompanied by a fracture of the articular pillar. A disruption of the smooth flowing cortex line caused by a superimposition of the articular masses is indicative of this problem (Fig. 4.18).

AP OPEN MOUTH VIEW

The AP open mouth view is valuable because it reveals the alignment and struc-

tural integrity of the atlas, dens, occiput, and axis. The normal view (Fig. 4.19) reveals the atlas sitting directly upon the axis and the lateral borders of each structure perfectly aligned. The atlantoaxial joint spaces should be equal and symmetrical. The bifid spinous process of the axis should be found in the midline.

The dens is subject to fracturing. Anderson and D'Alonzo (22) classified the odontoid fractures into three types. These three types (I, II, and III) are differentiated by their location and prognosis. A complete discussion of these three fractures and their clinical significance is found in Chapter 6.

Two congenital malformations are occasionally mistaken for odontoid fractures: the os odontoideum and ossiculum terminale. The os odontoideum is a failure of fusion of the dens with the body of the axis (Fig. 4.20*A* and *B*). A gap between the structures is usually present. Differentia-

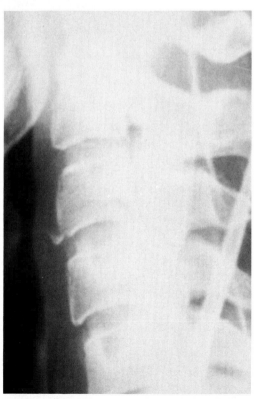

Figure 4.15.   A small avulsion fracture is seen at the inferior corner of C3. Also note the small semicircular impression on the pharyngeal air shadow, which is indicative of a retropharyngeal hematoma.

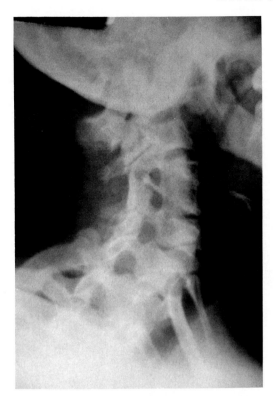

Figure 4.16. Oblique view of the cervical spine demonstrates segmentation abnormalities at C4-C5. An alteration of the IVF is also noted.

tion of the os odontoideum and a type II fracture should follow two lines of reasoning. First, the os odontoideum will demonstrate as smooth borders between the segments. A sclerotic border or cortex line may be visualized. Second, a type II fracture of the odontoid will usually be accompanied by a prevertebral soft tissue hematoma and a widening of the retropharyngeal space. This widening should be considered a significant diagnostic sign, and this finding justifies further imaging studies. With type II fracture, there will be an irregular border and no sclerosis on the edges.

Agenesis of the odontoid process may also be noted. This is a congenital anomaly that may cause instability in the upper cervical spine complex. The absence of an anchor post for the atlas may allow for excessive movement (Figs. 4.21*A–D* and 4.22*A* and *B*). The patient seen in Figure 4.21 was

asymptomatic even with the 1.5-cm movement of the atlas.

The odontoid is supplied by a limited number of blood vessels. Fractures of the dens, particularly the type II fracture, may cause a non-union and signs of ischemic necrosis distal to the injury (Fig. 4.23). Sclerosis, deformity, and softening of the odontoid are likely complications. This area may be compared to the avascular necrosis seen in fractures of the scaphoid.

The second developmental variation is the ossiculum terminale. This entity is found normally in children as a primary ossification center at the superior end of the odontoid. This may be visualized in children as old as 11 years. In adults, the presence of the center represents a non-union or persistent epiphysis and is sometimes mistaken for a type I fracture. The differential diagnosis should follow the same lines of reasoning as described for the os odontoideum.

Other conditions or anatomical structures may simulate fractures in the atlantoaxial area. Keats (23) has described a vertical lucency over the odontoid process that is caused by the airspace between the front incisors and that may be mistaken for an odontoid fracture.

The Jefferson or "burst" fracture of the atlas disrupts the neural arch and is often recognized on the AP open mouth view by the lateral edges of the articular masses seen extending over the outer margins of the axis (Fig. 4.24). A complete discussion of the mechanics of this injury and its clinical significance can be found in Chapter 6.

At times, the AP open mouth view will reveal a lateral displacement or subluxation of the atlas on the axis. The shift is observed by comparing the spaces between the lateral border of the odontoid and the medial border of the lateral mass of the atlas. This alteration from the normal position may be the result of torn alar ligaments or secondary to a rotation of the atlas. Differentiation of the two etiologies is accomplished by observing the motion of the atlas during lateral flexion.

Two supplemental AP open mouth views taken with the patient in right and left lateral flexion may be employed when a differentiation is required. The lateral flexion views are designed to delineate the

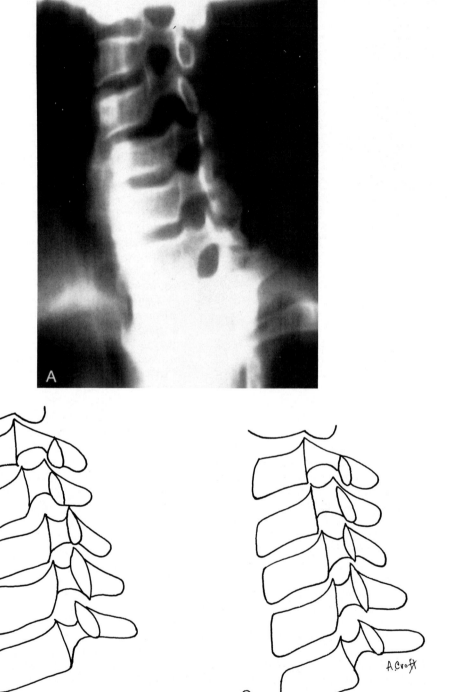

Figure 4.17. **A.** Oblique tomogram of the cervical spine shows a unilateral facet dislocation of C5 on C6. **B.** Line drawing of **A. C.** Line drawing of the normal orientation of the facets in the oblique position.

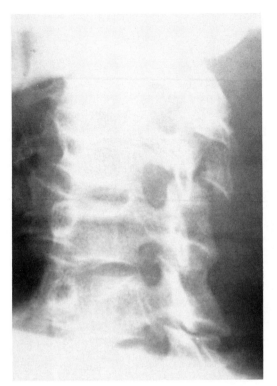

Figure 4.18. Oblique view demonstrates an articular facet fracture. The fragment has moved laterally and disrupts the normal flowing margin.

amount of aberrant movement present in the atlas. The method of examination may be either plain film radiography or fluoroscopic procedures. Damage to the alar ligaments must be considered if the right and left lateral flexion films reveal aberrant movement of the atlas. Excessive lateral movement is atypical, as the function of the atlas is to facilitate the rotation rather than lateral movement of the head. The lateral flexion views of the upper cervical spine area are not part of the usual posttraumatic series and should be incorporated if the atlas is laterally displaced or alar ligament damage is suspected.

AP LOWER CERVICAL VIEW

The AP lower cervical view is used to review the alignment and structural integrity of the lower five cervical vertebrae. The atlas and axis are usually not visualized because of the superimposition of the mandible. Some radiographic views, such as those provided by the Ottonello method (24), rely on rapid movement of the mandible in the hope that the movement may obliterate the structure and allow visualization of the entire cervical spine. I have

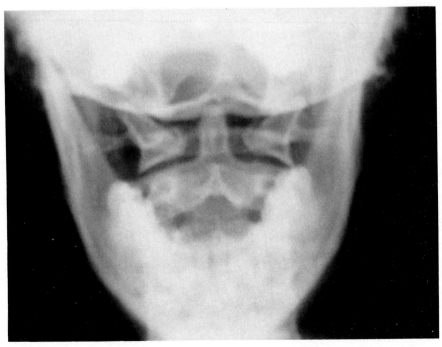

Figure 4.19. Normal AP open mouth view.

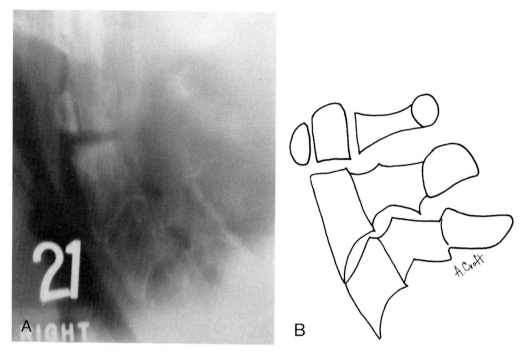

Figure 4.20.   **A.** Lateral tomogram of the atlantoaxial complex reveals a smooth radiolucent line through the base of the odontoid process. The smooth sclerotic border and absence of trauma support the diagnosis of an os odontoideum. **B.** Line drawing of **A.**

found the method ineffective, and the risk of missed pathology does not justify the utilization of this or similar techniques.

The AP lower cervical view allows inspection of the uncinate processes, the joints of Luschka, the superior and inferior endplates, and the intervertebral disc spaces. These structures are not always easily seen, as the cervical spine is a curved structure and the result is radiographic dis-

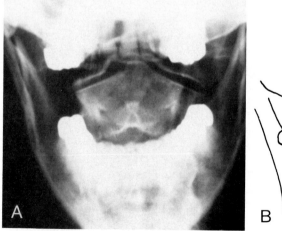

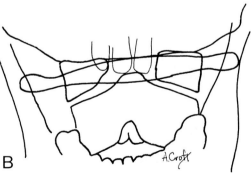

Figure 4.21.   **A.** AP open mouth view shows agenesis of the odontoid process. The remnant is insufficient to maintain stability. **B.** Line drawing of **A.** **C.** Lateral flexion view of the same patient shows the anterior arch of the atlas in a relatively normal position. **D.** Line drawing of **C.**

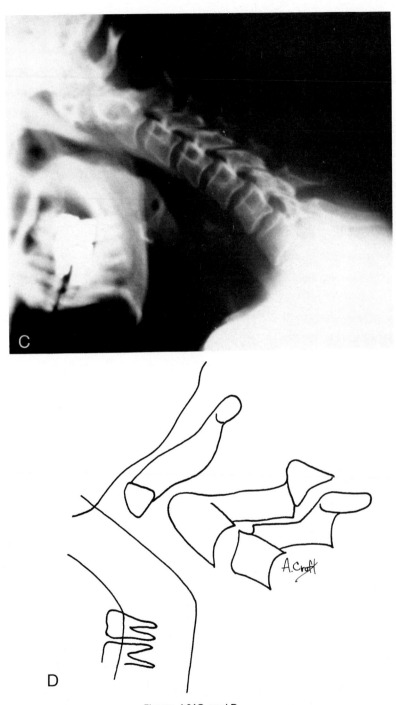

Figure 4.21C and D.

tortion. The majority of this distortion is eliminated if the tube is angled 15° cephalad. This angle has been found to produce the best results.

The lateral masses, even with tube angulation, are superimposed and create one long, flowing cortex line on each side of the cervical spine. A sharp disruption in this

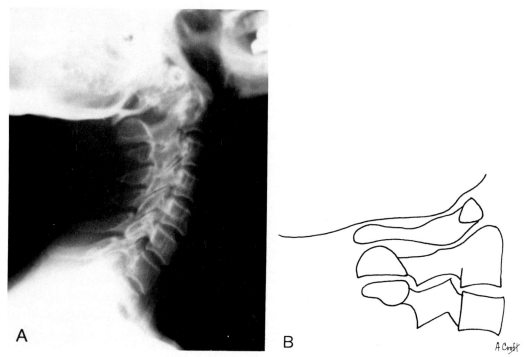

Figure 4.22. **A.** Extension view of the same patient as in Figure 4.21 demonstrates a marked posterior movement of the atlas. **B.** Line drawing of **A.**

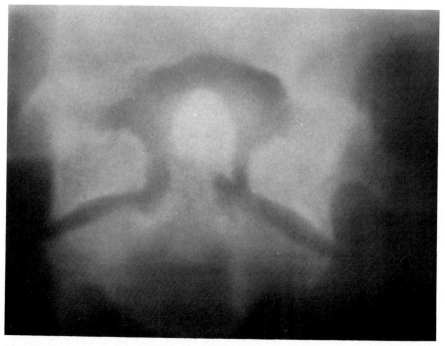

Figure 4.23. AP open mouth tomogram demonstrates a type II fracture of the dens. The upper portion of the dens shows an increased density which was attributed to ischemic necrosis.

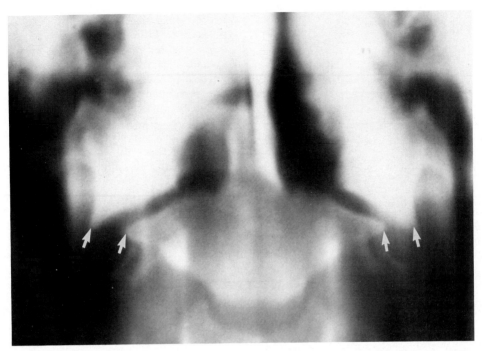

Figure 4.24. AP open mouth tomogram reveals a marked displacement of the lateral masses of the atlas compared with the axis (*arrows*).

line is usually the result of a fracture. Posterior facet arthrosis may cause exuberant calcification and irregularity of the line.

The tracheal air shadow, also seen on the AP lower cervical view, should be midline and should taper in a superior direction. Space-occupying lesions such as hematomas and goiters may displace it laterally in the cervical area. Tracheal deviations in the upper thoracic area are usually the result of mediastinal masses, pulmonary collapse, or aberrant tissue growths such as intrathoracic goiter.

The spinous processes should be midline and equally spaced. Each spinous process should be located and be either "teardrop" or bifid in shape. An abnormal distance between the two spinous processes is a typical finding when there has been a tearing of the interspinous ligament. With a clay shoveler's fracture, a "double" spinous process may be seen. This radiologic appearance is produced by the original spinous process and the "new" spinous process that, in actuality, is the proximal edge of the fractured process. These two structures are not superimposed and, due to the

superior-inferior orientation of the spinous processes in that area, create two images.

Hyperflexion injuries are notorious for causing compression fractures. These compressions typically occur at the C5-C7 level and are readily apparent on lateral views. The AP lower cervical view shows the fracture as a change in the height between the superior and the inferior endplate (Fig. 4.25). Rotation of the patient's head during the accident may have caused an uneven collapse which compresses one side of the vertebral body to a greater degree.

Rotation of the patient's head may also cause a great deal of stress on the uncinate processes. Fractures of these structures are usually minimally displaced and may cause only slight retrotracheal swelling. The AP lower cervical view may be the only standard view that affords the examiner an unobstructed view.

The joints of Luschka, also known as the uncovertebral joints, are subject to degenerative changes. These structures will demonstrate as an increased sclerotic margin, a decreased joint space, and a rounded, ir-

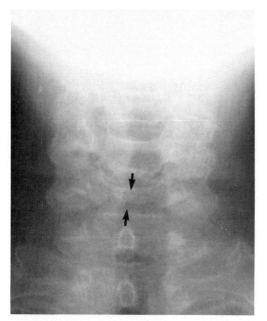

Figure 4.25. AP lower cervical view reveals a decreased vertebral height at the C6 level (*arrows*). This finding is typical of compression fractures.

regular superior surface. The degenerative changes seen in these osseous or intervertebral disc structures are significant in that they may change the direction of therapy, and this information is utilized in the patient's prognosis. A complete discussion of the significance of degenerative changes may be found in Chapter 11.

The last area of interest on the AP lower cervical view is the apices of the lungs. This area is usually seen on the inferior edge of the film, and the presence of apical thickening is of obvious significance. The superior sulcus is a common sight for neoplastic change, such as a Pancoast tumor. In this area a neoplastic condition could produce cervical symptoms that may be incorrectly attributed to a recent automobile accident. A full discussion of Horner's syndrome can be found in Chapter 9.

PILLAR VIEWS

The pillar view described by Weir (25) is often overlooked and is not utilized in many practices. It is designed to afford the examiner a close, unobstructed view of the lateral masses in the coronal plane. This view is important to the posttraumatic series because on the other projections the

lateral masses remain obscured. The fractures of the lateral masses are typically secondary to lateral flexion of the head, and visualization of this area is particularly important in that the articular pillars may be the sites most frequently affected by relatively minor trauma without bone abnormality (26, 27). Fractures may affect either one or both sides of the articular pillars. These fractures are typically compressive in nature and classified as either unilateral or bilateral.

Unilateral compressive articular fractures present as a difference of more than 2 mm in vertical height compared with that of the opposite side. A bilateral compressive fracture presents as a difference of more than 2 mm in vertical height between the medial and the lateral border of an articular pillar. This change would be found on both the right and the left articular pillar. Vines (26) in his study found that the most common location for the articular compression is the sixth cervical vertebra.

Interpretation remains difficult despite the specialized views used to visualize the pillars. Simple asymmetry and variations in pillar height are insufficient for the definitive diagnosis of a fracture. Free osseous fragments or signs of reparative changes occurring after the injury are required before a definitive diagnosis may be made (27). Imaging techniques that may allow better visualization of the articular structures are discussed more fully in Chapter 5.

COMPARATIVE STUDIES

Comparative studies of the spine after several weeks of treatment can be controversial. Some physicians routinely re-x-ray their patients despite the lack of a sound clinical indication. Despite the question of overutilization and other ethical questions, there are several occasions when a second or even a third examination may be of benefit to both the patient and the examiner. The indications for reexamination include suspected fractures, known fractures, ligament damage, and a loss of biomechanical integrity.

Suspected Fractures

A patient who on the initial films is suspected of suffering a fracture should be reexamined 2 or 3 weeks later in an attempt to visualize the calcium infiltrated hematoma at the site of the injury. The views that demonstrate this area are usually the only ones that are repeated.

Alternative methods for the detection of nondisplaced fractures would include scintigraphy, also known as a bone scan, and computerized tomography. Scintigraphy would be the examination of choice, as the area of interest can be quickly localized in a cost-effective manner. Further discussion of these imaging procedures is found in Chapter 5.

Known Fractures

A fracture visualized on the initial series should be examined during the healing process if there is a question concerning either the rate or the extent of healing. Follow-up is especially important if the fracture is located in an area of questionable vascularity. Type II odontoid fractures, for example, are highly susceptible to ischemic necrosis and delayed union.

Ligament Damage

Subtle ligament damage is not always apparent on an initial series. Posttraumatic myospasm may have been sufficient to prevent subtle shifts in vertebral alignment. Studies done in the absence of spasm may reveal the ligament damage.

Biomechanical Integrity

Some disciplines place a great deal of importance on the biomechanics of the spine. A loss of the normal lordotic curve of the cervical spine, as viewed on the neutral projection, should be reevaluated at the end of treatment. Permanent loss of the cervical curve is often a precursor to future degenerative joint disease and will affect the patient's final prognosis.

Conclusion

Despite the variety of views in this post-traumatic series, certain areas of interest are often obscured and overlooked. Small, nondisplaced fractures may only be inferred by soft tissue alterations. In these cases, further examination with utilization of sophisticated imaging techniques is required. The indications and clinical benefits derived from these techniques are discussed in Chapter 5.

Summary

1. Physical examination and history after trauma are insufficient. Radiographic examination is mandatory in the evaluation of these cases.

2. Visualization of biomechanical lines and the use of soft tissue measurements are essential to radiographic interpretation.

3. A minimum of seven views are essential to inspect each of the areas for osseous trauma.

Supplemental views or studies may be employed if positive findings are detected.

4. Comparative studies are warranted to look for suspected fractures, ligament damage, and biomechanical integrity. Comparative studies are also used to follow the healing progress of known fractures.

References

1. Jacobs LM, Schwartz R: Prospective analysis of acute cervical spine in injury; a methodology to predict injury. *Ann Emerg Med* 15:45–49, 1986.
2. Gree JD, Harles TS, Harris JH: Anterior subluxation of the cervical spine: hyperflexion sprain. *AJNR* 2:243–250, 1981.
3. Shaffer M, Doris P: Limitation of the cross table lateral view in detecting cervical spine injuries: retrospective analysis. *Ann Emerg Med* 10(10):508–512, 1981.
4. Hann CL: Retropharyngeal tendinitis. *AJR* 130:1137–1140, 1978.
5. Harris JH: *The Radiology of Acute Cervical Spine Trauma.* Baltimore, Williams & Wilkins, 1978.
6. Jackson H: The diagnosis of minimal atlanto-axial subluxation. *Br J Radiol* 23:672, 1950.
7. Locke GR, Gardner JE, Van Epps EF: Atlanto-dens interval (ADI) in children. *Am J Roentgenol Radium Ther Nucl Med* 97:135, 1966.
8. Cattell HS, Filtzer DL: Pseudosubluxation and other normal variations of the cervical spine in children. *J Bone Joint Surg* 47A:1295, 1965.
9. Clark WM, Gehweiler JA, Laib R: Twelve significant signs of cervical trauma. *Skeletal Radiol* 3:201–205, 1979.
10. Tomazek D, Rosner M: Occult esophageal perforation

associated with cervical spine fracture. *Neurosurgery* 14(4):492–494, 1984.

11. Penning L: Prevertebral hematoma in cervical spine injury: incidence and etiological significance. *AJR* 136(3):553–561, 1981.

12. Shinger WL, Kelley DL, Johnston FR, Holliday RH: Hyperextension injury of the cervical spine with esophageal perforation. *J Neurosurg* 53:541–543, 1980.

13. Hunter TB, Proteil RL, Horsley WW: Food laceration of the esophagus. *AJR* 140:505–506, 1983.

14. Fielding JW, Cochran B, Lawsing JF III, Hohl M: Tears of the tranverse ligament of the atlas. *J Bone Joint Surg* 56(A):1683, 1974.

15. Hinck VC, Hopkins CE: Measurements of the atlanto-dental interval in the adult. *Radiology* 84:945, 1964.

16. Peuschel SM, Scola FH, Perry CD, Pezzullo JC: Atlanto-axial instability in children with Down's syndrome. *Pediatr Radiol* 10(3):129–132, 1981.

17. Fielding JW, Hawkins RJ: Roentgenographic diagnosis of the injured neck. In: *Instructional Course Lectures*, American Academy of Orthopaedic Surgeons. St Louis, CV Mosby, 1976, vol 25, pp 149–170.

18. Holdsworth F: Fractures, dislocations and fracture-dislocations of the spine. *J Bone Joint Surg* 52A:1534, 1970.

19. Foreman SM: Radiographic differential diagnosis of common spinal degenerative disorders. *J Manipulative Physiol Ther* 8(1):23–27, 1985.

20. Reymond R, Wheeler P, Perovic M, Block B: The lucent clefts. *Clin Radiol* 23:188–192, 1972.

21. Edeiken-Monroe B, Wagner LK, Harris JH: Hyperextension dislocation of the cervical spine. *AJR* 146:803–808, 1986.

22. Anderson LD, D'Alonzo RT: Fractures of the odontoid process of the axis. *J Bone Joint Surg* 56A:1663, 1974.

23. Keats TF: *Atlas of Normal Roentgen Varients That May Simulate Disease*, ed 3. Chicago, Year Book, 1984.

24. Merril V: *Atlas of Roentgenographic Positions and Standard Radiologic Procedures*, ed 4. St Louis, CV Mosby, 1975.

25. Weir DC: Roentgenographic signs of cervical injury. *Clin Orthop* 1975.

26. Vines FS: The significance of occult fractures of the cervical spine. *Am J Roentgenol* 107(3):493–504, 1969.

27. Abel MS: Clinical and roentgenological aspects of occult fractures of smaller elements of cervical vertebrae. *Am J Surg* 97:530 542, 1959.

5

State-of-the-Art Cervical Magnetic Resonance/ Computed Tomography Imaging

WILLIAM V. GLENN, JR., MD

Introduction

OVERVIEW: THE GOOD NEWS AND THE BAD NEWS

The primary goal of this chapter is to provide referring physicians, who are confronted with cervical acceleration/deceleration trauma, with a "snapshot" regarding imaging capabilities of surface coil magnetic resonance (MR) and high-resolution computed tomography (CT). In its depiction of the current state of the art, this snapshot must be both challenging and careful. *Challenging* because the following pages illustrate how accurate these imaging systems can be when properly utilized. This contrasts, however, with how imperfectly realized and underutilized these state-of-the-art imaging capabilities really are in day-to-day practice. *Careful* because CT and MR have developed so quickly that any definitive statements of their comparative worth may not apply 5 years hence. Although the technological advances in CT have now leveled off, the developments in MR continue to reflect rapid progress. It is difficult to predict the ultimate role of either modality.

Both modalities have already shown their value in many types of clinical imaging problems. Therefore, to the extent that cervical fractures, dislocations, disc bulges and/or herniations, degenerative ridges, nerve root canal (NRC) spurs, facet joint abnormalities, and spinal cord injury and/or encroachment all come into play in the evaluation of cervical acceleration/deceleration trauma, the combined imaging modalities of CT and MR have much to offer.

The *good news* is that both modalities have the virtue of demonstrating soft tissue *and* bony changes in tomographic layers in multiple perspectives. Examples include axial, sagittal, coronal, and even oblique planes. More recently, the added advantages of creating curved planes, three-dimensional surface-shaded views, and even stereoscopic presentations provide for more viewing flexibility and, in many cases, easier understanding of complex anatomic relationships.

The *bad news*, however, is that both imaging modalities are static. Neither has the ability to provide "fluoro" tomography in order to assess how one segment moves in relation to another. And because both MR and CT require 20–40-minute scan times, patients are required to hold as perfectly still as possible. That typically means a comfortable position that minimizes whatever neck or arm pain resulted in the patient's visit in the first place. And both scanners have horizontal couches, meaning that the spine is imaged with both pain and gravitational loading minimized.

THE CHANGING X-RAY "GOLD STANDARD" IN EXAMINING THE SPINE

During the two decades from 1960 to 1980, myelography was the imaging "gold standard" by which spine surgeons confirmed their clinical diagnoses and then proceeded to a treatment plan. About 1980, articles began to announce the computerized imaging era that has now evolved into surface coil *m*agnetic *r*esonance *i*maging (MRI or MR) and x-ray *h*igh-*r*esolution *c*omputed *t*omography (HRCT) (1–3). Each physician has had to adjust to these changes. Radiologists are currently in the throes of optimizing diagnostic imaging workups, and referring physicians are modifying their prior complete dependence on plain films and myelography in order to take advantage of whatever is better about the mutiplanar sectional imaging capabilities of MR and CT. None of us, however, move at the same speed with regard to new technology.

CARDINAL RULE: MULTIPLE VIEWS

Historically, radiologists have endorsed the idea that one single x-ray view of something, especially something complicated, is not always representative. What is abnormal about a particular structure may not be readily apparent in the first x-ray view obtained. It may actually take a combination of visual perspectives to thoroughly cover an area of interest, particularly if it happens to be anatomically complex. A thorough review of present CT capabilities, technically and diagnostically, will clearly show that multiplanar CT and MR (axials plus sagittals and perhaps coronals) are available from virtually every high-resolution scanner.

RADIOLOGIST'S AND REFERRING PHYSICIAN'S OBLIGATIONS

The *radiologist* must perform, organize, and interpret the images produced by MR and CT. Specific clinical problems may occur as isolated abnormalities producing the signs and symptoms of neck pain or cervical radiculopathy. Since the clinical management for each of these potential sources of pain may be different, and because it may be impossible to differentiate the precise cause of symptoms, it is incumbent upon the radiologist to provide a precise MR or CT analysis of the various anatomical components at each vertebral segment (i.e., a segmental road map). In the process he or she may describe significant anatomic changes that appear subjectively abnormal but, in fact, may be clinically silent. To not be able to describe such changes due to an incomplete examination would be irresponsible. To ascribe undue clinical significance to each and every (clinically silent) anatomical aberration, however, would likewise be irresponsible.

The *referring physician* has an obligation to understand the results of the expensive imaging test he or she has ordered. This means understanding both the written consultation report and the image sequences. He or she is the last arbiter of what the imaging results mean in terms of patient management decisions. He or she must be able to take the radiologist's detailed mapping of the anatomic changes and sort out what is contributory and what is noncontributory for each particular clinical situation. He or she must be sufficiently comfortable in his or her own review of the image sequences to be able to disagree with the radiologist's opinion and, thereby, engage that radiologist in a discussion to resolve any different opinions. Both will benefit, and more importantly, so will the patient.

The first (and crucial) step is an organized presentation of the anatomic facts and a set of images to substantiate those facts.

Because there are typically lots of pictures, it is important to have an easily understood recipe for the organization of the filmed images. This may, at first, seem to be a macro issue of concern only to radiologists reading the films. Not so. The referring physician must be able to understand (and read) the spine imaging films. He or she has to decide how everything fits together and to what extent the imaging examination explains the patient's complaint or comes up substantially short of helping in that task. Carefully organized teaching materials designed specifically for referring physicians must be available (5–16) so that the diagnostic images from CT or MR can effectively play their very crucial role. If there is confusion regarding image organization on film, however, there will be corresponding reluctance to feel confident about what the images mean. Too often the latter situation prevails. Generally, this confusion is due to too many film format

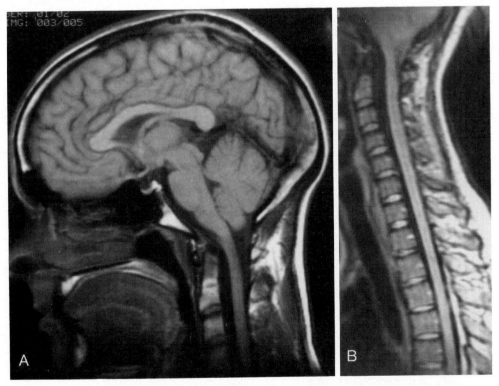

Figure 5.1. Normal cervical cord (MR). The cervical lordotic curvature is normal. Disc spaces show normal height and normal high MR signal intensity. The central canal is widely patent. The cord is visualized from the posterior fossa to approximately T4-T5. There is no focal cord enlargement, cavitation, or areas of increased signal intensity (as might be seen in either a demyelinating process or compressive gliosis).

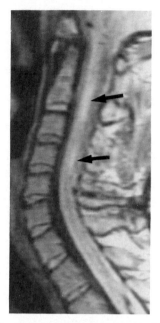

Figure 5.2. Cervical multiple sclerosis (MR). The focal area of increased signal intensity (*arrows*) very likely represents a focal demyelinating plaque in a young female patient with symptoms and periventricular deep white matter foci of increased MR signal intensity (Brain images not shown) consistent with multiple sclerosis.

variations. The subject is addressed in detail in a recent monograph (7) that visually illustrates the many different (and, therefore, confusing) approaches to CT film formatting.

If a referring physician completely understands how the image sequences are placed on the films, he or she will not have any trouble keeping track of just which interspace, which foramen, etc., any single image might represent. It is part of his or her obligation (to the patient) to know. It is the radiologist's responsibility to provide the organization, the films, the report, and the necessary educational materials to make all these elements properly mesh together.

CURRENT CLINICAL SITUATIONS JUSTIFYING MR, CT, OR BOTH

When should an examination (and what type) be ordered? This is an interesting and very practical question for which there currently is no definitive answer. Some leading academic radiologists believe that MR will completely replace CT within 5–10 years. Those of us actually reading the im-

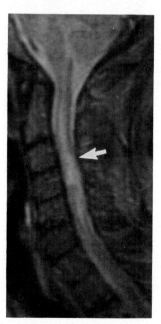

Figure 5.3. Cervical cord tumor (MR). Focal enlargement of the cord (*arrow*) strongly suggests expansile tumor.

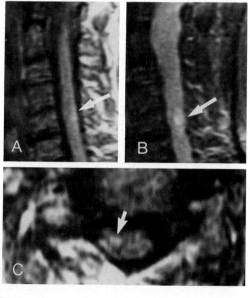

Figure 5.4. Cervical cord hemorrhage (MR). An area of increased signal intensity on both first (**A**) and second (**B**) echo images is shown (*arrows*) in a patient with clinical presentation highly consistent with cord hemorrhage and confusion. **C.** Axial view.

aging studies produced by the best of both modalities available have come to the following tentative conclusions which certainly can apply for the next 2–3 years.

In the lumbar spine, MR and CT are basically of equal value in diagnosing disc abnormalities. Those who tout MR as superior to CT in the diagnosis and characterization of disc herniations are usually the same people who do not usually perform CT in a complete multiplanar fashion. When *complete* high-detail sagittal CT image sequences are routinely available, the advantage of sagittal MR sequences is minimized. Only MR is capable of detecting the physiological degenerative change of the nucleus pulposus, by alterations in disc space MR signal intensity. Both MR and CT can detect more advanced degenerative changes which are reflected by loss of disc space height (provided sagittal CT reformations are done). Because of the closer image spacing and superior bone detail provided by CT, the lumbar spine evaluations for stenotic change or degenerative facet joint abnormalities are clearly better done with CT than with MR. As a general statement, complete multiplanar CT and surface coil sagittal and axial MR are basically quite equivalent in imaging the lumbar spine.

In cervical spine imaging, there are more distinct differences. For patients considered to have cervical myelopathy, with the primary emphasis in the diagnostic imaging examination being to evaluate the cord, MR is the clear choice. It involves no invasive intrathecal instillation of contrast material, as would be the case with CT. Moreover, MR is capable of intrinsically evaluating the cord for focal enlargements, which CT can also do, but MR can diagnose cord cavitation and increased signal intensity, such as occurs with multiple sclerosis plaque formation or gliosis, which CT cannot do. Examples of MR use are in imaging normal cord (Fig. 5.1), multiple sclerosis plaque (Fig. 5.2), cord tumor (Fig. 5.3), cord hemorrhage (Fig. 5.4), cord gliosis from compression (Fig. 5.5), cord atrophy and syrinx (Fig. 5.6), and congenital abnormalities (Fig. 5.7).

Evaluation of disc abnormalities in the cervical regions is also very well done with MR. Multiplanar reformatted CT is very good, but MR has the added advantage of demonstrating any internal physiological degenerative changes of the disc space, per se, as manifest by loss of normal high MR disc space signal intensity at one or more cervical interspace levels. Examples of cervical disc imaging by MR (Fig. 5.8) and CT (Fig. 5.9) are provided.

Cervical MR can show central spondylitic ridging, but it does not show it as well as does complete multiplanar reformatted CT, particularly with the closely spaced sagittal images. For definition of small bone detail or any soft tissue pathology that can only be demonstrated with ultrathin sections, CT would have a significant potential advantage, since CT is capable of generating multiplanar image sequences with spacings of 1–2 mm, whereas MR on a routine basis can only accommodate 3-mm-thick slice sections with usually 1.5-mm interslice gaps. Contiguous MR 3-mm sections can be obtained by doubling the scan time.

For evaluation of cervical radiculopathy off the midline, there is a shift in the optimum imaging modality. The key situations for evaluation are entrapment of cervical nerve roots as they traverse from medial to lateral from within the spinal canal to outside the spinal canal. Their course is much more oblique than in the lumbar spine. The osseous-ligamentous tunnels or NRCs through which these nerve roots pass are correspondingly much smaller with considerably smaller margins for error allowed. Moreover, the ganglia are located much more strategically with regard to endplate ridges (after Rauschning's anatomy work) than is the case in the lumbar spine. This places a particular premium on the ability to evaluate, in very thin sections at oblique orientations, the potential for NRC encroachment by joint of Luschka osteophytes as well as by endplate osteoarthritic ridges. In the case of NRC stenosis evaluated by surface coil MR imaging, the stenotic foramina are often simply not visualized. This, by default, implies neural entrapment but falls short in terms of demonstrating precisely where and why. It is the strong preference of our clinical practice to recommend CT rather than MR for

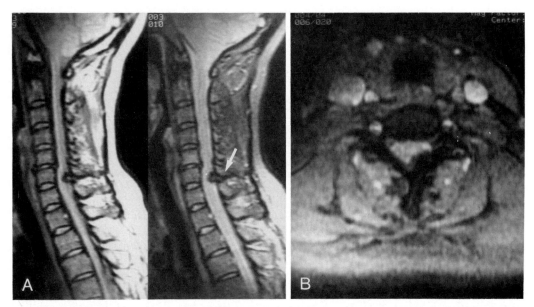

Figure 5.5.   Central canal encroachment with probable cord compression (MR). A fractured left C6 lamina was suspected from this MR study and later proven with a radionuclide bone scan and confirmatory CT scan. Note the more dramatic sagittal appearance of encroachment (**A**) than what is observed on the axial image (**B**).

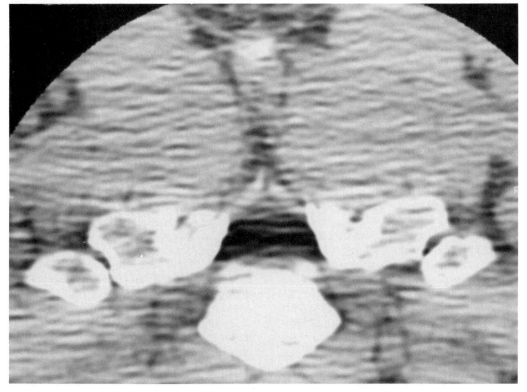

Figure 5.6.   Cord atrophy and syrinx (MR).

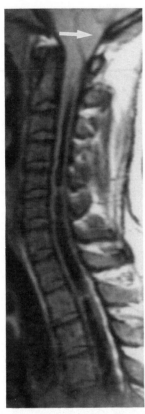

Figure 5.7. Arnold-Chiari malformation (MR). Cerebellar tonsils (*arrow*) are very low lying, actually protruding inferior to a large foramen magnum. This patient also has an extensive cervical and upper thoracic syrinx with the appropriate clinical symptoms.

Clinical situations justifying both MR and CT examinations are definitely more prevalent in the cervical region than in other levels of the spinal column. As discussed previously, these two modalities offer some similarities in their ability to demonstrate central canal stenosis, central discs, and spondylolytic ridging. There are, however, distinct differences in their abilities to make intrinsic evaluations of the cord and of potential bony encroachments of the small and obliquely oriented cervical NRC.

Any situation in which one examination has been performed and fails to explain adequately a significant cervical spine problem should immediately raise the possibility of using the other examination, for correlation. The diagnostic process is furthered if the second examination simply verifies the first. There is also benefit if they do not agree. If the first was negative and the second was positive, the gain is a potential explanation for the patient's clinical presentation. Suppose the first examination was positive but not in accord with the clinical presentation and then the second examination was negative. This places more burden on the presumptive clinical diagnosis, assuming it is a condition that one or both of the imaging tests should be capable of demonstrating. If both examinations were to be positive and for the same reasons, the clinical diagnosis is strongly supported. If both examinations were positive but for different reasons, the referring physician must then decide which findings from which examination best support his clinical diagnosis. More information is never bad.

As a general rule, an older patient with clinical symptoms that potentially represent a combination of myelopathy (cord compression?) and radiculopathy (root entrapment) should probably have both MR and CT ordered outright. Both examinations should absolutely precede any consideration for cervical myelography. CT will show the spondylolytic endplate ridges, NRC reductions, and any significant central canal stenosis due to ridges or subluxations. MR will pick up several different types of intrinsic cord abnormalities. MR will also provide more vertical coverage by demonstrating a portion of the posterior

evaluation of cervical radiculopathy. These are usually older patients for whom degenerative disc changes as would be manifest by loss of disc space signal intensity on MR could be accurately presumed. CT clearly defines the central canal dimensions or encroachments thereto. If the referring physician is comfortable that the primary diagnostic problem is very likely *not* a cervical cord problem, complete multiplanar CT is the procedure of choice. Examples of the use of these modalities are in imaging the relationship of exiting neural elements to endplates laterally (Fig. 5.10), presumed cervical NRC stenosis by MR (Fig. 5.11), definite cervical NRC stenosis by CT (Fig. 5.12), and oblique sagittal thin slice NRC imaging by CT (Fig. 5.13).

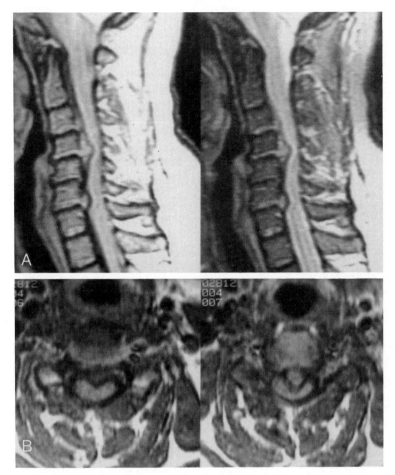

Figure 5.8.   Central cervical disc herniations (MR). At C4-C5, there is a massive disc herniation, and at C6-C7, a moderate disc herniation. The axial images **(B)** correspond to C4-5, showing this disc abnormality to be maximum centrally. Both levels would reflect significant myelographic abnormalities if a myelogram were performed (not necessary in view of clear MR findings).

fossa as well as several upper thoracic interspaces, neither of which are usually included in the CT/multiplanar reconstruction examination that concentrates on four interspaces and simply surveys one or two other levels.

Imaging Concept, Recommendations for Scanning Technique, and Case Organization on Film

Who should be responsible for scanner function, the scanning technique, and the case organization on film? The equipment

manufacturers, x-ray technologists, and radiologists have the combined role of making sure the equipment performs state-of-the-art imaging examinations. The variables at issue are: minimizing scan time, maximizing image resolution (slice thickness, slice intervals, use of surface coils), and complete coverage of the specific area of interest (multiple sequences: axials, sagittals, obliques). These are only part of the challenge, however.

Delivering the results (to the requesting physician) in terms of smooth image sequences and written consultation reports is also highly important. To optimize these steps in the imaging process, it is necessary to ask the referring physicians how they

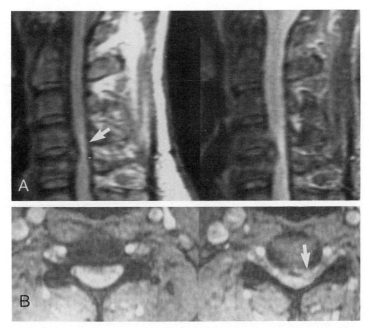

Figure 5.9.   Central cervical disc herniation (MR). The C5-C6 disc has herniated (*arrow*), causing cord compression anteriorly as manifest by a high signal area which is most likely gliosis.

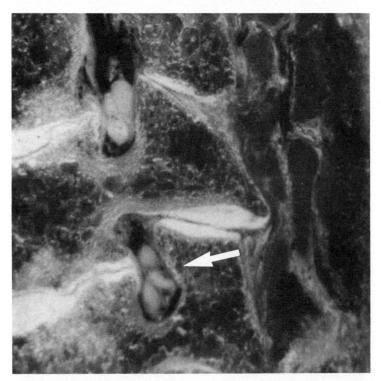

Figure 5.10.   Detailed cryosectioned anatomy of cervical NRC. The strategic relationship between the exiting neural elements and the lateral margins of the cervical endplates is demonstrated. Note that the roots and ganglia are immediately adjacent to the endplates and, therefore, very vulnerable to osteophytes and ridges protruding from the endplates. (Courtesy of Wolfgang Rauschning, Uppsula, Sweden, and of the Foundation for Advanced Medical Display Technology, Los Angeles.)

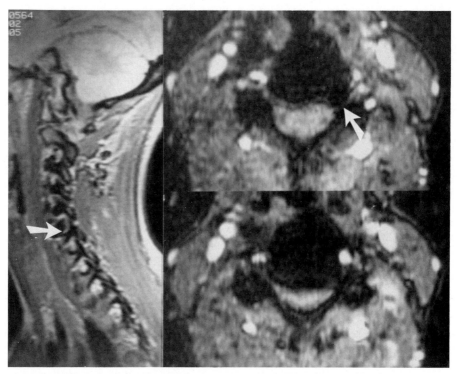

Figure 5.11.   NRC stenosis (MR). The left C5-6 NRC has a lage lateral spur (*arrow*) causing severe NRC or foraminal stenosis.

best understand (and want) the results conveyed. It is *not* appropriate for radiologists to decide that (*a*) referring physicians do not need to receive the films, (*b*) axial images are sufficient and sagittals are superfluous, (*c*) teaching referring physicians how to read the films is inappropriate, and (*d*) presenting image sequence results should conform to what radiologists prefer rather than to what referring physicians might prefer (or really need). The radiologist *must realize his or her role as a facilitator, advise manufacturers* what pulsing sequences, what surface coils, and what image presentation software are needed, and *ask referring physicians what* presentation and educational capabilities *they need* to maximize the use of the imaging tests

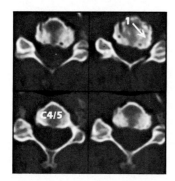

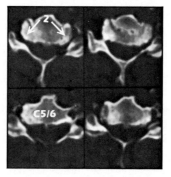

Figure 5.12.   Cervical NRC stenosis (CT). These contiguous 1.5-mm axial images show endplate ridging and joint of Luschka osteophytes and hypertrophy that severely encroaches on NRC dimensions on the left at C4-C5 (*arrow at 1*) and bilaterally at C5-C6 (*arrow at 2*).

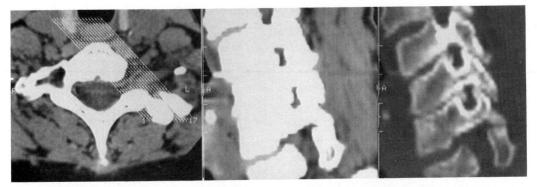

Figure 5.13. Oblique thin slice CT imaging of cervical NRC. Reformatted sagittals (*center* and *right*) demonstrate one of the soft tissue and bone images represented by the oblique reference lines on the reference axial image (*left*). Oblique sagittal images show four cervical interspaces, with the middle two NRCs or foramina being stenotic from endplate ridging extending laterally.

being ordered. Ultimately, the referring physician will determine the role of both CT and MR. The more referring physicians know, the better the advice they can offer. And as that advice is utilized, the more imaging examinations will be ordered. It is both appropriate and self-serving for radiologists to listen carefully.

In the next several sections, brief explanations on how the CT and MR scanners work and how they are best operated for cervical spine diagnosis are provided, with references given for more detailed explanations. Case organizational strategies (regarding the patient's films) that have evolved with the help of many referring physicians are presented as examples of the sort of interactive communication process that makes for better examinations and better results. The lesson to be learned is that the next good suggestion can come from anyone, regardless of his or her imaging experience. This combination has kept me and my colleagues very much on the leading edge, far ahead of many leading academic centers, and the subject of considerable mimicry by CT and MR equipment manufacturers for add-on features in scanning, filming, case presentation, etc.

CT

Imaging Concept

CT is a sectional imaging device in which a rotating gantry containing an x-ray tube and an arc of detectors rotates about the body. Patients lie horizontally on a couch that is incrementally advanced into the thin, highly collimated x-ray scanning beam. The x-ray beam is turned on only when the gantry is taking data in order to produce a picture. Current high-resolution CT scanners obtain data for a "slice" or axial image section in scan times of 1–10 seconds, compared with a scan time of longer than 6 minutes required for the very first CT scanners introduced in 1973. Each image section or slice ranges in thickness from 1.5 to 10 mm. Successive images are stored in the scanner's computer for later viewing and for photographing. Because the images can be obtained parallel to each other, in perfect registration, the sequence of axial images can be further processed or reformatted into alternative planes of view (i.e., sagittal, coronal, obliques, etc.) without the need for further scanning. The possibilities are discussed further under "Future Developments."

Recommendations for Scanning Technique

Slice Thickness and Scanning Intervals. The imaging examination should obtain sufficient data to routinely provide whatever images (even after the fact) are deemed important. I recommend routinely obtaining a closely spaced, continuous, parallel sequence of nongantry tilted axial images. In the cervical spine, the image interval should be 1.5–2 mm, with 1.5-,

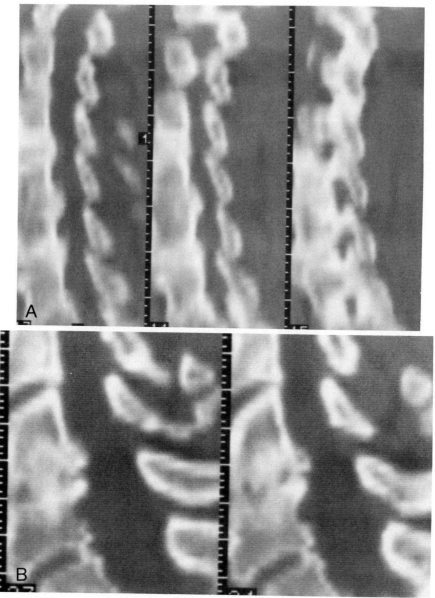

Figure 5.14. Scanning protocols and cervical reformatted image quality. A lumbar scanning protocol adapted for cervical work and a high-resolution cervical scanning protocol that limits the range of coverage but maximizes reformatted image detail are compared. **A.** Sagittal images of more than six cervical segments are from 37 5-mm-thick axial images taken every 2.5 mm. **B.** Much more high bone resolution (crucial in cervical work) is shown in reformatted images derived from 37 1.5-mm-thick axial images taken every 1.5 mm. The latter protocol is what I routinely use in my practice. (From Rothman SLG, Glenn WV Jr: *Multiplanar CT of the Spine*. Rockville, MD, Aspen Systems, 1985, p 395.)

2-, or 3-mm slice thicknesses utilized; best results are obtained with 1.5-mm scan intervals and a 1.5-mm slice thickness.

Arriving at this scanning protocol was a lesson I and my colleagues had to learn the hard way. One of the common pitfalls was

protocols, which are rigid and highly structured, have to be significantly modified for proper cervical work. Our initial attempts took the standard 5-mm-thick lumbar CT slice and spaced successive slices at 2.5 mm (50% overlap) rather than at the standard

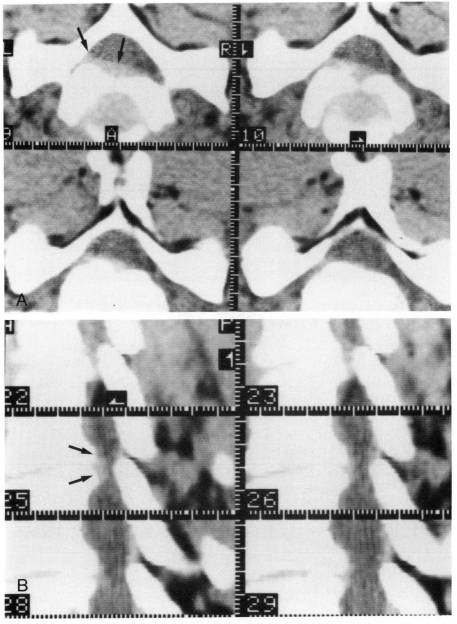

Figure 5.15. Star athlete's cervical disc (scanning diagnosis originally missed). The difference between surgery and no surgery was the difference between the first and second examinations on this patient. The coarser cervical CT technique used to obtain the image in Figure 5.14A did not show the soft disc component but was sufficient to demonstrate the left-sided endplate ridge (not something that occurred acutely, in a professional athlete with acute onset of new symptoms). The second study (shown here) represents the turning point in cervical CT scanning protocols. There is clearly a soft disc component (*arrows*) that is separate from the endplate ridging. (From Rothman SLG, Glenn WV Jr: *Multiplanar CT of the Spine*. Rockville, MD, Aspen Systems, 1985, p 430.)

3-mm spacing for lumbar imaging. A cervical study was targeted to cover five to six interspace levels with reformatted image quality as depicted in Figure 5.14A. We were readily able to identify gross abnormalities, e.g., severe central canal stenosis,

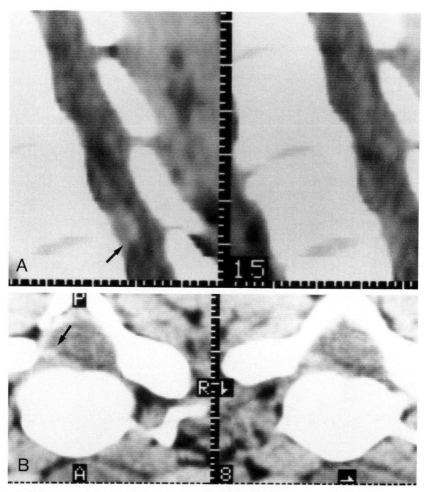

Figure 5.16.   Lateral herniated cervical disc with calcification. Sagittal (**A**) and axial (**B**) views show a lateral disc herniation with a small peripheral calcification (*arrows*). This is the sort of very fine detail that would not be possible to detect with the coarser cervical scanning technique used to obtain the image in Figure 5.14A. (From Rothman SLG, Glenn WV Jr: *Multiplanar CT of the Spine.* Rockville, MD, Aspen Systems, 1985, p 431.)

rotatory scoliosis, subluxations, or large discs. Subtle but important abnormalities such as strategically located foraminal spurs and small lateral discs were not routinely detected. From the standpoint of diagnostic accuracy, these deficiencies and the somewhat crude reformatted imagery, as depicted in Figure 5.14A, led to frustration on the part of the radiologist as well as a distinctly underwhelming response (a drop in clinical utilization) from referring physicians. This experience was by no means unique. Radiologists at many facilities who had developed confidence and expertise in lumbar CT had also met with considerable disappointment when attempting to ex-

tend their imaging capabilities to the cervical spine.

The solution to these problems was two-part. First, the protocols had to be changed so that the differences in gross sizes of anatomic structures between lumbar and cervical spines were taken into account. Larger lumbar structures can be imaged with thicker 5-mm slices, and coarser structures can be imaged with 3-mm scanning intervals. Second, there needed to be considerably more flexible image manipulation and display options for optimum cervical studies than for lumbar studies. By paying more attention to a categorization of cervical spine disorders I and my colleagues were able to better tailor the type of scanning and filming protocols. For those very common circumstances in which degenerative diseases of the disc and the vertebral joint are of primary clinical interest, a thin slice scanning protocol is absolutely essential. This means 1.5-mm-thick axial slices obtained every 1.5 mm with equal close spacing in the reformatted sagittal and coronal sequences. In Figure 5.14*B* is demonstrated the significant resolution difference in terms of sagittal reformatted image bone detail that could be obtained from 37 thin section axial slices covering not six but only three vertebral segments. Note that the lumbar-like scanning protocol underlying the coarser sagittal reformatted image bone detail demonstrated in Figure 5.14*A* was also obtained from 37 axial slices.

Soft tissue disc detail is illustrated in Figure 5.15 in which the horizontal and verti-cal CT resolution is sufficient to distinguish between both spondylitic ridging and soft tissue disc component. This same case (of a well-known baseball pitcher) was imaged in accordance with the protocols used for Figure 5.14*A*, and the soft disc component was missed! Two weeks later, he was rescanned with thin sections; demonstration of the soft disc herniation in addition to the ridge meant surgery for him and a change in cervical scanning protocols for me and my colleagues. That was the case that did it. A similar case (Fig. 5.16) is that of a lateral herniated disc that would have been picked up on a coarser scanning protocol but that had not been shown with the same level of detail as demonstrated with the high-resolution thin section technique.

The need for more flexibility in terms of imaging manipulation and display options can be illustrated by the rather common

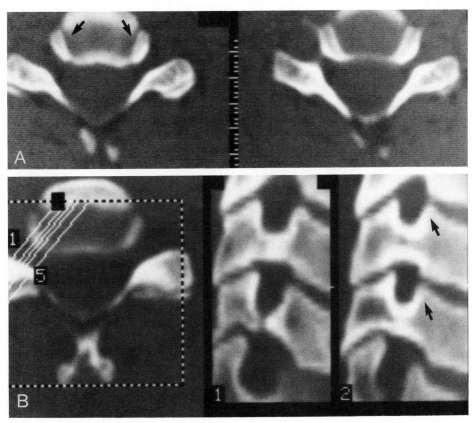

Figure 5.17. Carefully angled oblique sagittals. Normal uncinate processes are shown in both axial (**A** and **B**, *left*) and oblique (**B**, *right*) bone window images. Normally, there is 1–2 mm of cartilage between the uncinate process and the inferior endplate of the upper vertebra. (From Rothman SLG, Glenn WV Jr: *Multiplanar CT of the Spine*. Rockville, MD, Aspen Systems, 1985, p 433.)

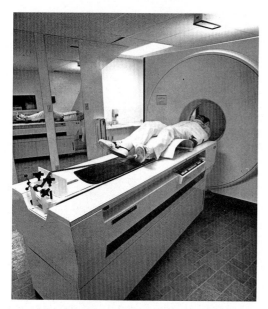

Figure 5.18. Traction device and patient positioning. The patient's head is gently restrained in a plastic head holder. Arms are pulled down passively. The traction device (Cat-Trac cervical traction device from CT Innovations, 536 East First Avenue, La Habra, CA 90631) is positioned below the patient's body, thus reducing shoulder pain. (From Rothman SLG, Glenn WV Jr: *Multiplanar CT of the Spine*. Rockville, MD, Aspen Systems, 1985, p 396.)

cervical and upper thoracic levels have a much wider scan field requirement to accommodate the shoulders. The shoulders' bulk, particularly that of the humeral heads, causes typical shoulder streaking artifacts. To minimize such artifacts, the shoulders need to be passively pulled down to remove, wherever possible, humeral heads from the scanning field. This is best accomplished by placing soft, broad armbands, on the forearms and attaching these bands to a device that allows gentle but constant traction as shown in Figure 5.18. The patient is not told to pull down on the rope because this nearly always produces motion artifact, owing to minor twitches. Another difference from lumbar scanning is that breathing during the scanner rotations (when raw data are being obtained) can cause motion artifacts as shown in Figure 5.19. Patients must be instructed to take slow but steady shallow breaths. Motion artifacts from swallowing can be avoided in almost all cases if patients are encouraged to swallow between scans rather than during the data acquisition phase when the scanner gantry is rotating. Many imaging centers advocate the use of water-soluble intrathecal contrast material (i.e., iohexol and iopamidol) as essential in the proper performance of cervical CT examinations. I

requirement to generate oblique sagittal reformatted views as closely spaced as in Figure 5.17. This does not supplant the need for obtaining orthogonal sagittal and coronal or curved coronal images. More often these oblique foraminal reformatted views, necessary on both sides, are obtained in addition to the other image sequences. Furthermore, they require (*a*) more user interaction to appropriately angle the oblique images and (*b*) a separate operation for left-sided cervical NRCs and their right-sided counterparts. The scanning technologist's job is, therefore, more tedious. Another example of such flexibility is in trauma situations in which the best visualization of a fracture may be on some very nonstandard oblique reformatted image plane (see below).

Scanning Details. Another frustrating technical subtlety is that most of the cervical region is represented by a relatively small diameter, whereas the lower

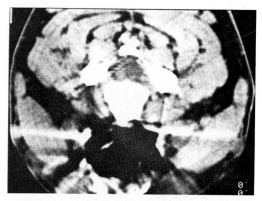

Figure 5.19. Streaking artifact from airway. Notice that the cervical vertebral body is sharply defined and without streaking artifact of motion. When patients swallow, speak, or cry during the scan phase, however, the movement of the larynx and trachea can cause confusing streaks. (From Rothman SLG, Glenn WV Jr: *Multiplanar CT of the Spine*. Rockville, MD, Aspen Systems, 1985, p 396.)

do not agree with its use as routine. First, much additional information that is purported to be provided by use of intrathecal contrast material is also obtainable from detailed sagittal and coronal sequences. Second, the use of contrast material often confuses the picture. Clearly, when the cord is the center of diagnostic attention, use of intrathecal contrast is absolutely appropriate. This is the exception, not the rule, however, with regard to routine cases. A more detailed discussion in terms of cervical scanning protocols and some of the "tricks of the trade" are provided elsewhere (17).

MR

Imaging Concept

Pulse Sequences and Tissue Appearances. Adequate interpretation of MR images of the spine presupposes a basic grasp of the physical principles of MR as well as of the fundamentals of the composition of body tissues. Acquiring this knowledge need not be frightening or hopelessly complicated.

The key to determining how a particular anatomical structure will appear in a MR image is an understanding of the pulse parameters or "pulse sequence" utilized to obtain the MR signal. A pulse sequence is a series of controlled radiofrequency signal transmissions that occur in repetitive cycles of finite time called the "repetition time" or TR. These radiowave signals are emitted by the scanner and absorbed by the patient.

The MR imager, however, not only is sending radio signals but also is capable of receiving them in a controlled fashion, in much the same way a car radio can be turned on or off and tuned to any station at will. At certain times during the cycle of radiowave emissions, the MR imager is "tuned into" receiving radio signals (whose ultimate origin is the patient) rather than emitting them. This concept is related to the "echo time" or TE. The TE is a measure of the exact point in the pulse sequence cycle when this "listening in" occurs. It is important to understand TR and TE, since both are major factors in determining what the images will look like. The typical pulse sequence I utilize in spine imaging consists of a TR equal to 2 seconds and two TEs equal to 30 and 60 msec, respectively. This will produce two images at each slice location that will appear quite different and contain unique diagnostic information, as is shown in Figure 5.20.

In spine imaging, the first spin echo

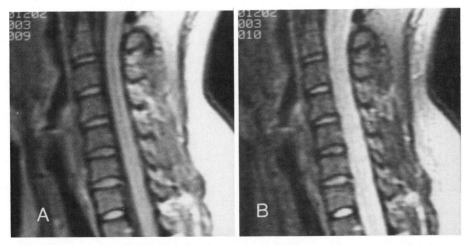

Figure 5.20. First and second spin echo MR images of the same anatomic slice. These two distinct images are from two different echo delay times (30 and 60 msec) during which the MR scanner was gathering data. The two sagittal images show midsagittal cervical views of the central canal. Notice that in **A** (first echo) the cervical cord is directly visualized, whereas in **B** (second echo) the CSF has become white and, therefore, has masked the cord.

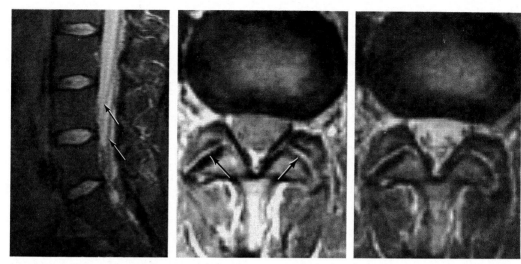

Figure 5.21.   MR "myelogram" effect. The sagittal view (*left*) represents as MR slice to the left of midline in which the CSF is white and nerve roots are dark vertical shadows (*arrows*), similar to the nerve root shadows one would expect on a lumbar myelogram. The two axial views (*center* and *right*) show the lumbar central canal and subarachnoid space at L3-L4. The second echo image (*right*) shows white CSF and intradural rootlets as negative "defects." The myelogram effect is simply the appearance of white CSF similar to that on an iohexol or iopamidol myelogram.

image (Fig. 5.20*A*) is usually best for evaluating the NRCs facet joints, vertebral bodies, and spinal cord. The bone marrow of the vertebral body appears relatively bright but not as intensely bright as does body fat. Fluid-containing structures and cortical bone are often very low in signal intensity (dark).

Images generated from TEs of at least 60 msec are called T2 or T2-weighted. Such a T2-weighted image is shown in Figure 5.20*B*. These images are much better at depicting fluid-containing structures and their boundaries (thecal sac) as well as the nerve roots and intervertebral discs. Choosing a long TR/TE will usually render cerebrospinal fluid (CSF) a very bright white while also delineating the nerve roots contained within, thus simulating a contrast myelogram (Fig. 5.21). Osseous structures are usually poorly defined on T2-weighted images.

The choice of pulse sequence parameters in MR imaging is not to be considered a trivial or rote procedure. Even though some "routine" sequences have been established for practical purposes, a thorough knowledge of the clinical question to be evaluated may suggest significant variations.

In summary, both T1- and T2-weighted images are important for a complete evaluation of the cervical spine.

Recommendations for Scanning Technique

Slice Thickness and Scanning Intervals. State-of-the-art cervical MR imaging allows for 3-mm-thick sections that are obtained with a surface coil. What is a surface coil? Two types of surface coils used in cervical spine MR imaging are shown in Figure 5.22. They act to increase spatial resolution by functioning as a focusing antenna. Sagittal sections are directly acquired, usually with small 1.5-mm interslice gaps. Contiguous slices would enable a slightly more complete examination, although this acquisition mode implies potential tradeoffs in image quality and in scanning times. My choice of parameters is, in part, a reflection of the present capabilities of the General Electric Signa system operating at a field strength of 1.5 T, as well as my own experience and that of other investigators pioneering the MR examination of the spine (18–25).

The following represents a complete protocol used in my practice. The sagittal acquisition is generally treated as the primary spine imaging sequence. It is usually done in multislice mode with a 24-cm field of view and a 256 x 128 acquisition matrix. This provides in-plane resolution of 0.9 x 1.8 mm/pixel. A secondary axial sequence of images is acquired by utilizing a 16-cm field of view and 256 x 128 matrix, with in-plane resolution of 0.6 x 1.25 mm/pixel. In the axial plane, I obtain 5-mm-thick sections (for more signal) with 1-mm interslice gaps. When properly performed, this protocol should leave little to the imagination.

Choosing an appropriate pulsing sequence is extremely important in MR imaging. Although there are no time-tested or proven protocols, a dual spin echo pulse sequence (TR of 2000 msec; TEs of 30–35 and 60–70 msec) produces high signal anatomic definition with the early spin echo and a definite CSF "myelogram effect" with the late spin echo. From a practical standpoint, i.e., time per study, this has proven a very good compromise between pulsing sequences with short TR (faster) and long TR (more signal, long scan times). This protocol is not "written in stone" and is altered occasionally due to severe time constraints or, when the patient can only tolerate a very short examination, due to pain or claustrophobia. The utilization of variable echoes (e.g., TEs of 25 and 90 msec) is appealing and is gaining acceptance. If the two echoes are chosen carefully, acquiring more is superfluous.

Surface Coils. The use of surface coils in MR imaging is absolutely integral to a complete study and produces images with spatial resolution comparable to that produced by CT. Attention to technique is even more important in MR than CT, however. The coil—whether round, rectangular, rigid, or flexible—must be meticulously positioned to ensure maximum response in the central portion of the spine segments being evaluated. In addition, the patient's spine must be as straight as possible on the coil to avoid confusion in image interpretation. Generally, very short TR (150-msec) coronal or sagittal images are acquired as "scout views" to check the position of the coil and to prescribe appropriate primary sagittal slice locations.

RECOMMENDED CT AND MR FILM ORGANIZATIONAL STRATEGIES

In a recent monograph on CT spine case film formats (7) there were identified six "ideal" film format features, although at

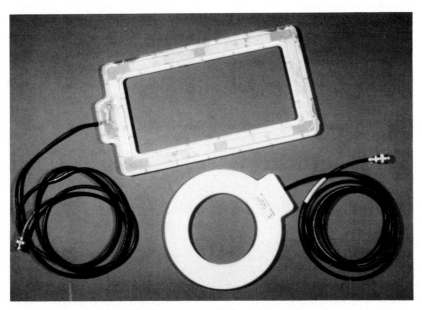

Figure 5.22.   Two types of surface coils. The *upper coil* is the rectangular or license plate type surface coil. The *bottom coil* is the circular type that provides for obtaining data from an even smaller anatomic area (i.e., temporomandibular joint, orbit, etc.).

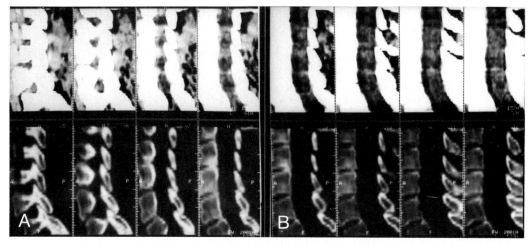

Figure 5.23.   Proposed CT film format. These images are organized to read left to right, with the *top row* representing soft tissue and the *bottom row* the same images windowed for bone detail. This particular case illustrates normal cervical CT anatomy in a movie strip-like format. Placing the bone window and soft tissue window photographs together on the same film exploits image cognition. Adjacent bone window and soft tissue sequences provide a comprehensive understanding of anatomy, which is difficult to match when these images are presented on different films and placed on separate illuminator panels.

the same time the avoidance of confusion was stressed. Even though this monograph was illustrated with lumbar case examples, the lessons apply equally well to the imaging of the cervical spine. The "ideal" film format features were:

1. Digital localizing image
2. Soft tissue and bone window photography
3. Composite groupings of images
4. Reformatted sagittal and/or coronal images
5. Consistent prone or axial image orientation
6. Full-field axial views

The films shown in Figures 5.23 and 5.24 represent the type of CT image organization I routinely use for cervical cases. Wherever possible, these same features are also utilized in MR cervical case organization. One similarity is that both examinations treat the sagittal image sequences as primary. Sagittal images are organized and numbered from left to right. Two sets of sagittal images are presented. For CT, these are left-to-right soft tissue and matching left-to-right bone window images. For MR, the two sagittal sequences are left-to-right first echo (T1-weighted) and matching sec-

ond echo (T2-weighted) images. These two sets of images are photographed as top and bottom rows of images, respectively. Axial images are similarly treated CT, i.e., prone-oriented, cranial to caudal sequences of soft tissue and matching bone window images (reading left to right from the films). MR axials often consist of just one sequence done with partial saturation pulsing. They are presented prone (like CT) and organized from cranial to caudal (again like CT). Coronal CT images are to left-to-right rows, proceeding posterior to anterior, with matching rows of soft tissue (top row) and bone detail (bottom row). Coronal images are rarely obtained in cervical MR studies.

An objective grading form is incorporated into the standard cervical CT and MR written consultation reports. Structures graded included left NRCs, disc and/or anulus margins, central canal, and right NRCs (in that order). An example of the cervical CT reporting form is shown in Figure 5.25. As explained at the bottom of that reporting form, the anatomic grades 1–3 represent variations of radiographic "normal," whereas grades 4 and 5 represent radiographically moderate and severe "abnormal" findings, respectively. A similar format is used for cervical MR examinations.

Case Examples Showing Current Uses of CT and MR

IMAGING OF CERVICAL TRAUMA

In cervical trauma, conventional radiography defines gross bony spinal integrity and alignment. Major fractures or dislocations are obvious on properly obtained plain films. Ligamentous injury without fracture can also be evaluated with careful use of fluoroscopic examination as well as flexion and extension films. Frequently with use of these procedures, however, the extent of cervical trauma is underestimated. Recent advances in thin section CT multiplanar reformation have increased the util-

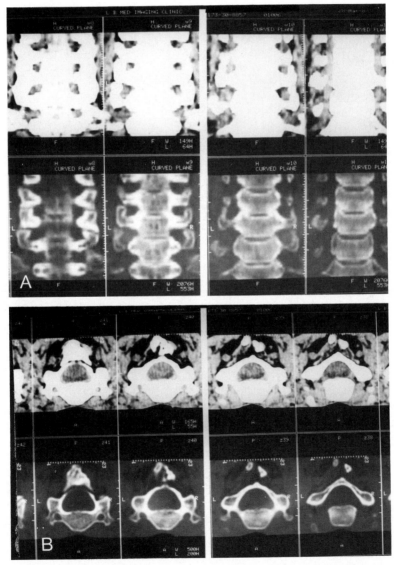

Figure 5.24. Proposed CT film format. (Coronals, **A**, Axials **B**) The axial film represents an easy reading left-to-right sequence organized as the sagittals were in Figure 5.23. Images proceed from cranial to caudal and represent normal cervical CT images from the same case as in Figure 5.23. The patient was originally scanned from caudal to cranial, therefore the images are numbered accordingly. Again, there is an analogy to strips of movie film.

ity of CT, so that it has now supplanted conventional tomography in the evaluation of spine trauma. Some historical lessons (i.e., imaging tricks) have been adapted from the experiences of neuroradiologists doing high-detailed x-ray diagnosis of the sella and temporal bone. Very simply, they learned that with polytomes there is cog-

CT/MPR CERVICAL SPINE EXAMINATION REPORT (c)
William V. Glenn Jr., M.D., Inc.

Patient #: 123456
Date: 3/6/87

Patient Name: John Doe

REFERRING PHYSICIAN:
XYZ, M.D.
Long Beach, CA 90732

Indications: 45 year old male with neck pain radiating into the right upper extremity/shoulder. No history of prior surgery. Referring physician requests assessment of possible bulging or herniated cervical disc, central canal stenosis (congenital or acquired), cervical nerve root canal entrapment of nerve roots, or degenerative changes such as endplate ridging, Luschka joint osteophytes, and/or articular facet hypertrophy.

Findings (When Used "NRA" Means No Radiographic Abnormality)

C2/3: NRA; C3/4: NRA, slight motion artifact on reformatted images; C4/5: Slight (Gr.2) disc/annulus bulge per axial image #33,34. Slight (Gr.2) reduction but not stenosis left nerve root canal and central canal. Mild (Gr.3) reduction but not stenosis right nerve root canal due to lateral extension of endplate ridging. See bone window sagittal #15; C5/6: Severe (Gr.5) disc herniation (right) per sagittal image #11, coronal #8, and axial #26,27. Moderate (Gr.4) stenosis central canal, worse to right of midline. Would predict large central & right myelographic abnormality. Slight reduction both nerve root canals; C6/7: Left NRC/foramen shows Moderate-Severe (Gr.4-5) stenosis due to significant endplate riding and Luschka joint sclerosis and spurring per bone window axial #15. See also left sagittal #4-6, special attention bone window sagittal #5. More centrally there is Mild (Gr.3) endplate ridging across anterior margin of canal, resulting in Mild (Gr.3) reduction but not stenosis central canal dimension, per axial image #15; C7/T1: NRA;

SUMMARY STATEMENT: EXAM ABNORMAL. At C5/6 there is Severe (Gr.5) disc herniation (right) which would would cause a significant myelographic abnormality. At C6/7 there is Moderate-Severe (Gr.4-5) stenosis left nerve root canal/foramen, due to a combination of endplate ridging and Luschka joint sclerosis/hypertrophy. No abnormal paraspinal masses. Vertebrae are normally aligned.

	Lt NRC	DISC	Canal	Rt NRC
C2/3	1	1	1	1
C3/4	1	1	1	1
C4/5	2	2	2	3OR
C5/6	2	5Rt	4Rt	2
C6/7	4-5OR	3OR	3	1
C7/T	1	1	1	1

Key Images: SAG(ST:4-6,11) (BW:5,15)
AX(ST:15,26,27,33,34) (BW:15) COR(ST:8) (BW:)

Interpretations Assume Grades 1-3 Considered Variations of Radiographic Normal; Grades 4 & 5 are Radiographically Abnormal Interpretations SUBJECTIVE & without detailed clinical knowledge of patient; Referring Physician Must Correlate Results Carefully!
Examination: This HIGH RESOLUTION CT/MPR study has contiguous 1.5 mm axial images C7-T1 to C4, with complete reformatted Sagittal/Coronal sequences (same area). Survey images: C2-3, C3-C4 and C7-T1. All image photos: Soft Tissue and Bone Window detail.
Graded Findings and Abbreviations: 1=Normal 2=Slight 3=Mild 4=Moderate 5=Severe F=Fused
SP=Spur OR=Osteophytic Ridging SL=Sublux NF=Not Fused *=Soft Tissue IJ=Irregular Joint SN=Schmorl's
Node FH=Flavum Hypertrophy LAM=Laminectomy HL=Hemilaminectomy VC=Vacuum Change DN=Deg. Narrowing

Figure 5.25. Cervical CT reporting form. This written consultation report is divided into sections for indications, summary, graded findings, and the examination details. The graded findings facilitate a very rapid glance at which levels and which structures are radiographically "abnormal" as indicated by moderate (Gr. 4) or severe (Gr. 5) notations.

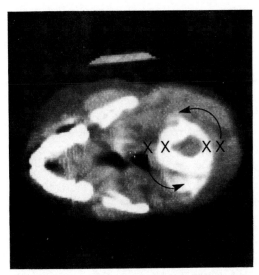

Figure 5.26.   Rotatory dislocation of C1-C2. This early first-generation CT picture has very limited resolution but still shows that the head is rotated 90° to the long axis of the body. Facets are totally dislocated. The spinal canal is significantly reduced. (From Geehr, et al: *Comput Tomogr* 2:79–97, 1978.)

nitive efficiency and convenience associated with organizing radiographic pictures into highly coned, numbered sequences of images at standardized intervals in multiple perspectives. The CT/multiplanar reconstruction filming techniques emphasized here are virtually identical but in a CT context.

In Figure 5.26 is shown a 1976 first-generation CT scan of C1-C2 rotatory dislocation in which routine radiographs and conventional tomograms revealed no fracture. In these same routine radiographs and tomograms is also shown an appropriate relationship of the anterior C1 arch to the C2 dens. This boy had been riding down a hill on a sled that crashed into a tree. The patient had sudden severe neck pain and turned his head to the right where it became stuck at approximately 90° to the long axis of his body. This case is important because even with very early limited CT resolution it demonstrates a 90° rotatory subluxation which is generally believed to require visual separation of the C1 arch from the C2 dens. After appropriate reduction and fixation there was an uneventful recovery.

The axial images in Figure 5.27 are from a patient who had no major neurological deficit but who complained of neck pain for 2 years after being hit by a train. Several sets of routine radiographs from several different occasions were reported as normal. The axial images shown here are subtly abnormal because no rotation is supposed to occur between occipital condyles and C1. There is 13° of rotation between C1 and the plane of the maxillary sinuses. The relationship of the C2 dens to the anterior arch of C1 is normal. Thus the rotation is apparent on the axial images, but the cause is not. Thin section sagittal reformations demonstrate two occult fractures: compression of the left occipital condyle and compression of the right lateral mass of C1 (Fig. 5.27). This did not require surgical intervention, but the correct diagnosis was very important because of the medical-legal implications of a definable anatomic injury.

Figure 5.28 demonstrates a complicated Jefferson fracture, with the axial views showing bursting of the C1 arch on the right with the posterior fracture component in a fairly typical location adjacent to the lateral mass. The anterior fracture line through the anterior arch also involves an avulsed tubercle. Sagittal reformatted views demonstrate displacement of the dens superiorly into the foramen magnum; coronal views demonstrated bilateral lateral C1 mass dislocations that are hallmarks of this disorder.

In Figure 5.29, the hangman's fracture lines traverse the neural arch at its insertion into the lateral masses. For evaluating fracture healing, the sagittal views shown here are extremely important. This is a relatively common motor vehicle type injury that fortunately is self-decompressing, with patients often avoiding serious neurological consequences.

Fractures of the C2 dens are difficult to evaluate in the axial plane because they mostly occur perpendicular to the long axis of the dens, also in an axial plane. The abnormality demonstrated in the sagittal views in Figure 5.30 were easily seen on plain films. The importance of CT in this case was that it excluded extradural hematoma or additional tiny bone fragments that might have been undetected by routine radiographs but for which CT is exquisitely sensitive.

Midcervical trauma can be grossly di-vided by extension rather than flexion vec-tor forces that produce such injuries. Force-ful extensions cause fracture of posterior

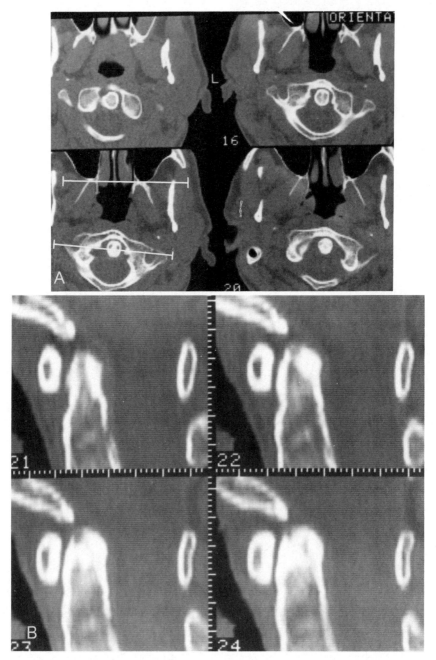

Figure 5.27. Traumatic craniooccipital subluxation. Axial images (**A**) show C1 rotated 13° clockwise from the maxillary sinuses (i.e., skull base). This should not occur. Axial images do not show any fracture. Midline sagittal views (**B**) are completely normal; there is no abnormal separation of the dens from the C1 arch. Sagittal views (**C** and **D**) show left and right atlantooccipital joints, respectively; there is compression fracture of the C1 left lateral mass (*arrow*) and compression fracture of the right occipital condyle (*arrow*). Neither of these abnormalities could be demonstrated on the routine axial CT perspective. (From Rothman SLG, Glenn WV Jr: *Multiplanar CT of the Spine*. Rockville, MD, Aspen Systems, 1985, pp 405 – 406.)

elements with little vertebral body fragmentation. Although very challenging radiographically, these fractures are ex-

tremely important clinically because of their potential of producing devastating spinal cord injury with little or no vertebral in-

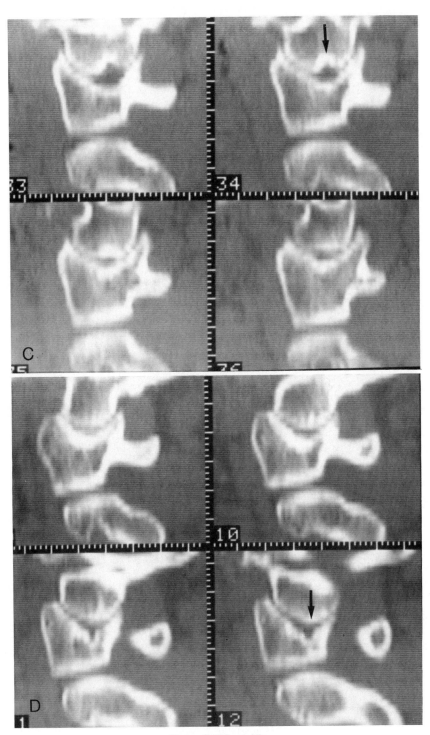

Figure 5.27C and D.

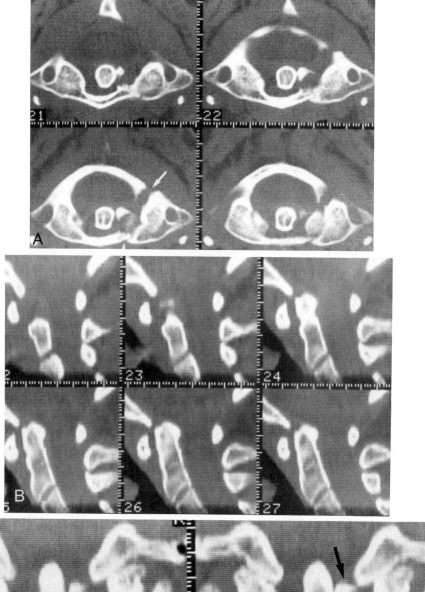

Figure 5.28.   Jefferson fracture of C1. Axial views (**A**) show typical posterior and anterior ring fractures (*arrow*). There is abnormal separation of the C2 dens and the C1 anterior arch. The tubercle is torn loose. Sagittal views (**B**) show the C2 dens to be displaced posteriorly and slightly superiorly. Coronal views (**C**) show the bilateral offset of the C1 facets, i.e., both laterally displaced. Notice also a dislocated fragment (tubercle) that has been torn away from the right lateral mass (*arrow*). (From Rothman SLG, Glenn WV Jr: *Multiplanar CT of the Spine.* Rockville, MD, Aspen Systems, 1985, p 407.)

jury. In Figure 5.31 are shown axial scans illustrating irregularity of the C3 articular process on the left. Oblique reformatted images show superior facet fracture. Although lateral mass fractures are difficult to diagnose on axial CT views, oblique sagittal and curved coronal reformations eliminate this difficulty.

Another extension injury is demonstrated in Figure 5.32, CT scans of a young patient who fell from a surf board and was hit on the head, subsequently complaining of neck pain with routine x-rays reported as normal. In the 2 weeks following injury, there was increased tingling in the fingers of the left hand. CT demonstrated bilateral

neural arch fractures at the junction with the lateral masses (Fig. 5.32A–C), the equivalent of a C6 hangman's fracture. Note that in this case in spite of the complex bony pathology involved in the fracture, the left-sided disc herniation shown in Figure 5.32D was most likely the cause of the patient's presenting symptoms.

The other broad category of midcervical injuries involves flexion forces that usually cause vertebral compression. These are generally diagnosed easily on routine radiographs, with the subtleties of such injuries best seen on CT. The CT images in Figure 5.33 reveal compression of C5 with loss of normal lordotic curvature but with-

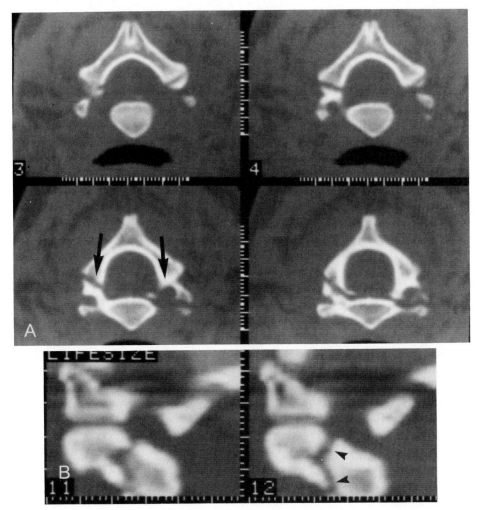

Figure 5.29. Hangman's fracture of C2. Axial views (**A**) demonstrate the bilateral neural arch fractures just posterior to the C2 vertebral body (*arrows*). Sagittal views (**B**) show the left arch fracture (*arrowheads*). (From Rothman SLG, Glenn WV Jr: *Multiplanar CT of the Spine.* Rockville, MD, Aspen Systems, 1985, p 408.)

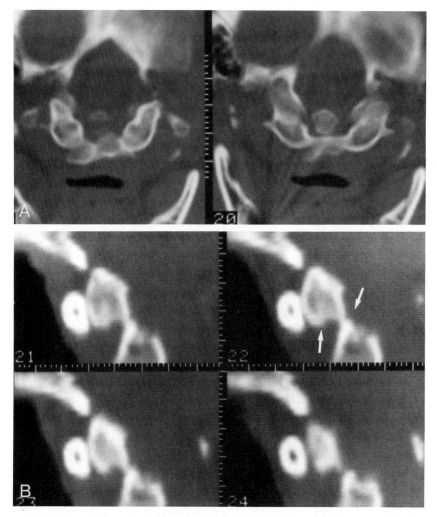

Figure 5.30. Fractured base of C2 dens. Axial views **(A)** show malalignment of C1 and C2, but without a history the diagnosis of fracture would be difficult. Sagittal views **(B)** clearly identify 50% spinal canal narrowing plus fracture dislocation at the base of the C2 dens (*arrows*). (From Rothman SLG, Glenn WV Jr: *Multiplanar CT of the Spine.* Rockville, MD, Aspen Systems, 1985, p 409.)

out dislocation. The vertebral body is fractured but not fragmented. The neural arch is intact. Best visualization is provided in the lateral or sagittal reformatted CT image. More severe trauma is demonstrated in Figure 5.34 in which sagittal reformation (Fig. 5.34*A*) shows a separated bony "teardrop" fracture of C6, with the C7 vertebra appearing normal. The axial scans (Fig. 5.34*B*) demonstrate an element of the vertebral body bursting with fragmentation. Because the neural arch is also fractured, this injury is considered unstable. Coronal reformations (Fig. 5.34*C*) show the linear

central component of fracture extending from C6–C7. Oblique views (Fig. 5.34*D*) show not one but probably two levels of neural arch fractures. The complexity of these types of cervical injuries is very well illustrated in this case. The important lesson, which is repeated in every similar trauma situation, is the *safety factor* that is achieved by taking high-resolution scans in one position and then "repositioning" the CT image data in various important viewing perspectives. To continually reposition the injured patient into difficult oblique orientations for low-quality portable cervical films in an emergency room (ER) setting has some very obvious and serious potential liabilities.

This lesson was learned from imaging of our very first serious cervical trauma patient who presented quadriplegic in the ER following a relatively "minor" whiplash incident on one of Los Angeles' busy freeways. The date was early 1977, and the EMI CT 5005 whole-body scanner used then is definitely not the 1988 high-resolution 1.5-mm scanner used today. The patient weighed over 250 lb. ER physicians ordered an emergency cervical CT scan largely because plain films in this very large and acutely injured patient were of extremely poor quality. His shoulders were so large that the portable x-ray ER equipment could barely make a decent film. Moving him from place to place was too dangerous for anything but a portable x-ray generator and simple anteroposterior (AP) and lateral cervical views. ER physicians requested the emergency CT scan, but because of his massive shoulders the patient could not be placed very far into the scanning gantry. It was only on the C4-C5 cuts (which were some of the last scans taken!) that the obvious serious encroachment shown in Figure 5.35 was noted. The patient had little or no margin for error in terms of any violent flexion or extension movements of the cervical spine. The central canal was already seriously compromised by preexisting ossification of the posterior longitudinal ligament (OPLL) which left less than 50% of the normal cross-sectional area for the cervical cord. This whiplash incident demonstrated the cord's extreme vulnerability. Subsequent surgery for anterior cord decompression did not alter the patient's quadriplegia. The important lessons learned in this very early case were several. First, the CT technique can provide critical imaging without having to put a seriously injured patient in a variety of different positions. Second, the combination of the axial or cross-sectional view and the exquisite bone detail imaging provided by CT can quickly highlight any serious bony encroachments of the spinal canal that may place whiplash candidates at considerable risk. Third, large patients may be very difficult for portable x-ray equipment to penetrate but, conversely, may produce excellent-quality CT images, provided the patient fits into the scanner. Some of the best CT images of the abdomen are obtained in large patients whose internal fatty tissues provide a soft dark background (fat on CT is dark), thereby making organs and major vessels stand out with much better contrast.

The extreme end of the trauma spectrum is illustrated by the case demonstrated in Figure 5.36 in which a CT scan was requested to evaluate increasing myelopathy (even after surgical decompression and fusion). The examination showed an intact fusion but very severe bony encroachment of the spinal canal. This was because the

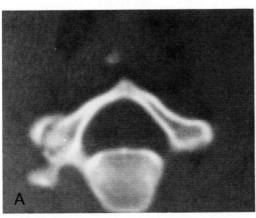
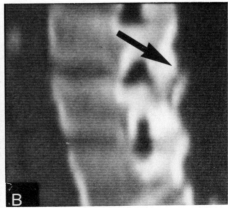

Figure 5.31.   Articular process fracture. The axial view (**A**) shows only irregularity of the C3 lateral mass. The oblique reformation (**B**) shows flattening and fragmentation of the superior articular process (*arrow*). (From Rothman SLG, Glenn WV Jr: *Multiplanar CT of the Spine*. Rockville, MD, Aspen Systems, 1985, p 411.)

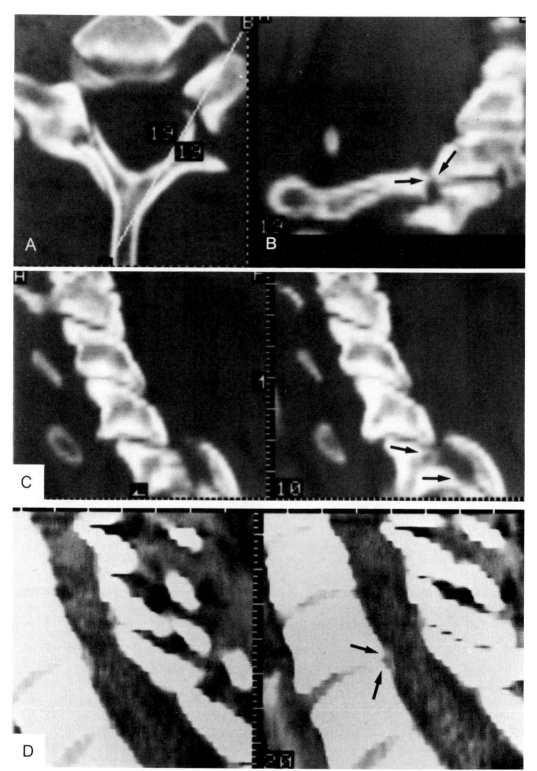

Figure 5.32. Hangman's fracture of C6. Axial views (**A**) plus the oblique (**B**) and sagittal (**C**) reformations show the bilateral neural arch fractures located at the insertion of the neural arches into the lateral masses. At the level above this fracture, however, there was a left-sided disc herniation (**D**) which clinically was considered to be consistent with the patient's signs and symptoms. (From Rothman SLG, Glenn WV Jr: *Multiplanar CT of the Spine.* Rockville, MD, Aspen Systems, 1985, pp 412–413.)

vertebral body was in two fragments, one displaced forward and the other displaced posteriorly into the spinal canal with a resulting severe reduction in central sagittal diameter.

DEGENERATIVE CHANGES OF CERVICAL NRCs

One of the clear advantages of thin section CT imaging in the cervical region is the capability it affords in evaluating osteoarthritic ridging and spurring in judging the effects that these bony overgrowths have on central canal and the NRCs or foramina. As disc spaces narrow and nuclear material becomes dessicated, annular fibers may be stripped from their bony attachment, producing spurs and ridges. Further degenerative reduction in disc space height results in changes of uncinate processes that ride high above the vertebral endplates. The

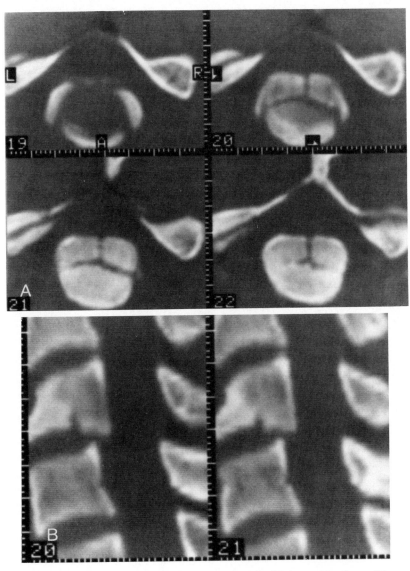

Figure 5.33.   C5 flexion fracture. Axial views (**A**) show an inverted Y-shaped fracture of the vertebral body with an intact normal-appearing neural arch. Sagittal views (**B**) optimally demonstrate the compression of C5. (From Rothman SLG, Glenn WV Jr: *Multiplanar CT of the Spine.* Rockville, MD, Aspen Systems, 1985, p 414.)

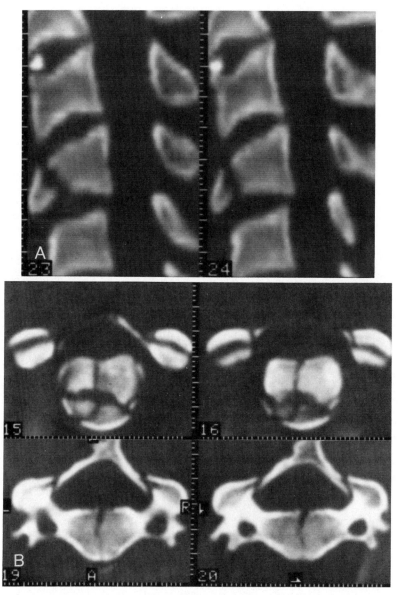

Figure 5.34. C5 and C6 compression fractures. Sagittal views **(A)** show that C5 and C7 are intact. There is a compression or teardrop fracture of C6. The superior endplate of C5 is depressed. Sagittal views also indicate loss of normal lordosis but no subluxation. Axial views **(B)** show that the C5 body has been split into four primary pieces (see *axial image #15*) and that the C6 body has bilateral neural arch fractures plus a fracture cleft in the midsagittal plane (see *axial image #20*). Coronal views **(C)** indicate a vertical fracture cleft continuous between C5 and C6. Oblique reformations **(D)** demonstrate fractures at the insertions of the posterior arches of both C5 and C6. (From Rothman SLG, Glenn WV Jr: *Multiplanar CT of the Spine.* Rockville, MD, Aspen Systems, 1985, p 416.)

normal uncinate processes are smooth, shoulder-like curved ridges along the superior posterolateral surfaces of vertebral bodies. They are capped with cartilage medially, and they normally demonstrate 1–2 mm of radiographic lucency between the upper cortical margin or uncinate process and the adjacent inferior vertebral endplate as shown in Figure 5.37.

With degenerative disc space narrow-

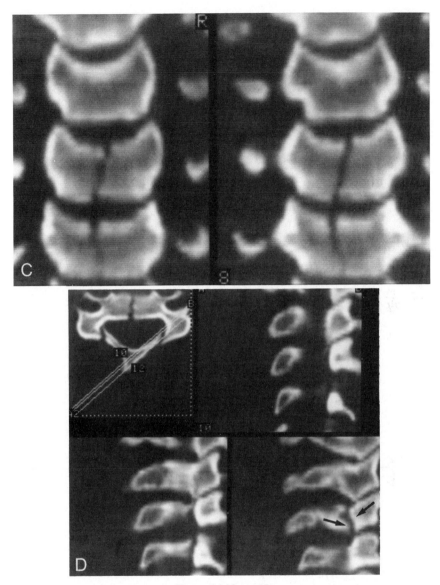

Figure 5.34C and D.

ing, the uncinate processes lie progressively closer to and eventually come into direct contact with adjacent endplates, resulting in hyperostotic ridging and spurring from this bony contact. Such ridges extend posteriorly and compress the lateral portion of the spinal canal or extend posterolaterally to compress exiting nerve roots. They may also extend laterally to compress the vertebral artery. The example of coronal bone window images demonstrated in Figure 5.39 shows an important spectrum of these changes from the four joints at two different levels in the same patient. In Figure 5.38 is demonstrated severe lateral canal and NRC compression by large spurs. One such spur is from an uncinate process, and a parallel mate is from the inferior endplate above. The observation that the medial two thirds of the NRC or foramen is narrowed and stenotic is important information to any surgeon contemplating an interdiscal approach because it may be difficult or impossible to visualize

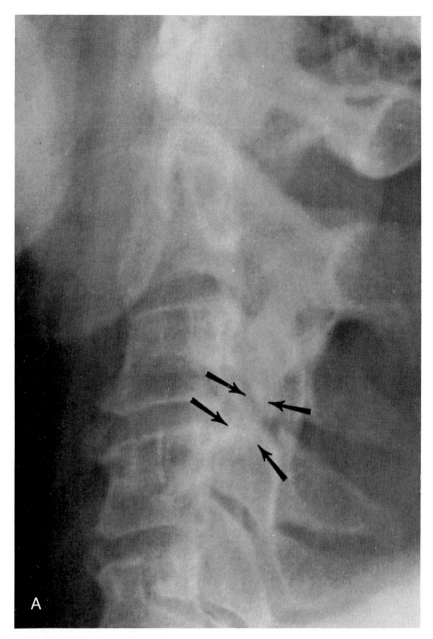

Figure 5.35.   Whiplash and cord compromise. Lateral cervical radiograph (**A**) shows severe anterior canal encroachment from two large ossifications (*arrows*) in a patient with OPLL. Whiplash in this case caused cord compression and quadriplegia. Axial images (**B**) show the lateral perspective. Surgical decompression (**C**) did not alter this patient's permanent cord damage; the patient died a few months following the injury.

the lateral extent of the uncinate ridge. I have seen several cases in which even major central decompression was inadequate for relieving cervical radiculopathy caused by far lateral uncinate ridging and/or spurring.

DEGENERATIVE FACET JOINT CHANGES

Figure 5.40*A* demonstrates severe destructive arthritis of both facets with irregularity of articular processes, bone scle-

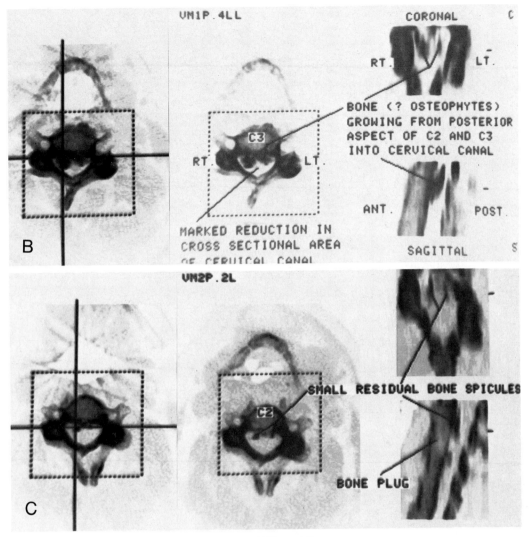

Figure 5.35B and C.

rosis, and cystic degeneration. The NRC or foramen is compressed by a combination of endplates extending to the apex of the joint as well as by uncinate spurs. The example shown in Figure 5.40*B* is from a patient with compression fracture at C7 where, because of subsequent neck pain, CT scan was obtained and demonstrated severe localized degenerative arthritis. It is not clear why some of these patients develop severe articular arthritis and some do not. What is clear, however, is that these are symptoms following the anatomic changes and, therefore, must be (to the extent possible) defined by CT.

Although CT is our current gold standard for evaluating cervical stenotic changes, as MR continues to be refined, there is much promise that this imaging technique will also provide evaluation of stenosis. Some of our worst and most difficult cases have given us an opportunity to understand what the future of MR may hold. The ability to noninvasively evaluate cervical cord changes directly following severe flexion or extension cervical forces will make the fu-

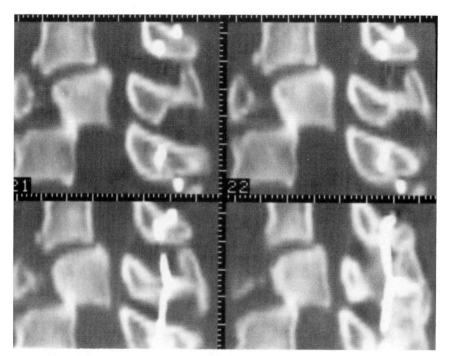

Figure 5.36. Stabilized burst fracture of C5. Sagittal images show severe postoperative central canal stenosis due to retropulsion of the posterior fracture fragment into the central canal. The posterior wire fusion is intact. (From Rothman SLG, Glenn WV Jr: *Multiplanar CT of the Spine*. Rockville, MD, Aspen Systems, 1985, p 417.)

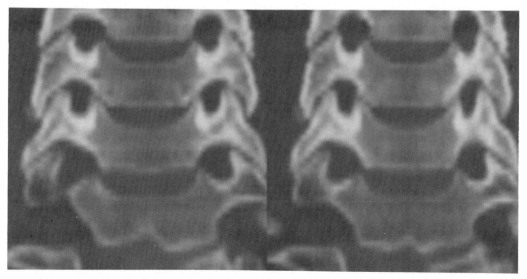

Figure 5.37. Normal uncinate processes. Bone window coronal CT reformations demonstrate normal uncinate processes bilaterally at C3-C4, C4-C5, and C5-C6.

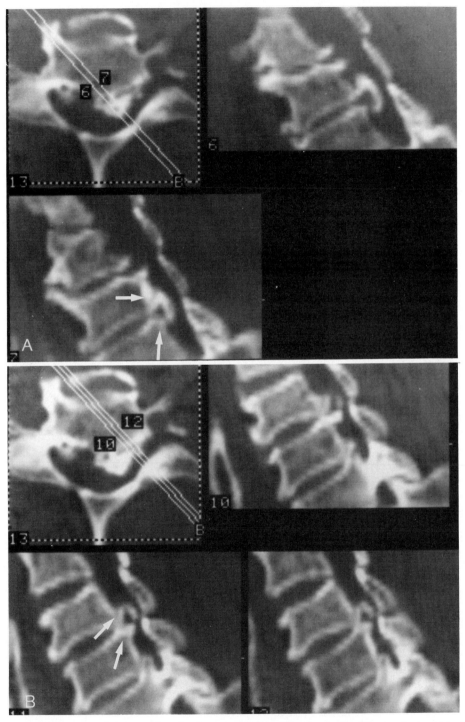

Figure 5.38.   Cervical endplate and uncinate spurs. Two adjacent sets of oblique reformations show a patient with a large pair of degenerative ridges or spurs (*arrows*). These cause stenosis of the central canal, lateral recess, and medial aspect of the NRC. (From Rothman SLG, Glenn WV Jr (eds): *Multiplanar CT of the Spine*. Rockville, MD, Aspen Systems, 1985, p 434.)

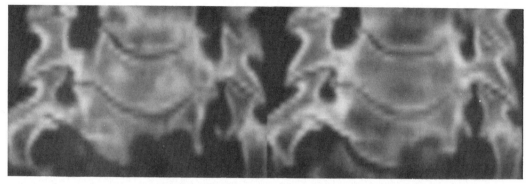

Figure 5.39. Endplate and uncinate spurs. These bone window coronal reformations show one stenotic NRC or foramen on the left and portions of two stenotic NRCs or foramina on the right. The cause is bony overgrowth and ridging involving the joints of Luschka and the endplates, with lateral extension causing the presumed neural encroachments.

ture contributions of cervical MR imaging extremely attractive.

CERVICAL STENOSIS

Causes of central canal and lateral recess encroachment in the cervical spine are not unlike their lumbar counterparts: disc herniation, osteoarthritic endplate ridging, and apophyseal joint hypertrophy and/or spurring. As in lumbar MR or CT scanning, the best view for central canal and lateral recess stenosis is basically the axial view. Why? Because the axial perspective is a cross-section of the tubular structure (central canal) being compressed. Depicting cervical NRC or foraminal encroachment is somewhat different, however. This canal or foramen is essentially another tubular structure that is smaller and much differently oriented than the central canal. CT is definitely superior to MR for reasons of bone detail and thin, contiguous reformatted slices. Oblique reformatted views are essential in order to get a true tunnel view of the NRC. The difficulty (or inconvenience) of generating and comparing separate left and right oblique cervical reformations has recently been overcome by novel use of the curved plane image manipulation concept discussed under "Future Developments." In the following several paragraphs, representative examples of cervical stenosis are given, with a distinct emphasis on CT imaging for any stenotic problem off the midline. MR, how-

ever, is the cervical imaging modality of choice for evaluation of suspected cord abnormalities or central disc problems.

A normal frame of reference provided earlier in this chapter shows the axial, sagittal, and coronal views of a wide-open cervical central canal, lateral recesses, and NRCs or foramina. Several examples of high-resolution CT bone detail images that show where there is central canal stenosis, lateral recess, and NRC stenosis from endplate and uncinate ridges or spurs are already reviewed.

Another type of stenotic situation in which high-detail bone CT reformations are very helpful is cervical subluxations. Subluxation is defined for imaging purposes as a partial dislocation of one vertebral segment on another. In Figure 5.41 is shown significant anterior displacement of C3 on C4 in a patient with cervical rheumatoid arthritis. It is very obvious from this case that the critical canal measurement must be taken in the sagittal plane. Axial image measurements would be incorrect. Furthermore, the measurement of interest is from the ventral surface of one lamina to the upper posterior endplate margin of the next lower vertebral body (as shown in Figure 5.41).

Three cases of cervical rheumatoid disease (and stenosis) causing very severe changes are demonstrated in Figure 5.42. Each of the latter cases is worse than the previously shown case but demonstrates the routine miscalculation of a stenotic central canal when the axial images alone are

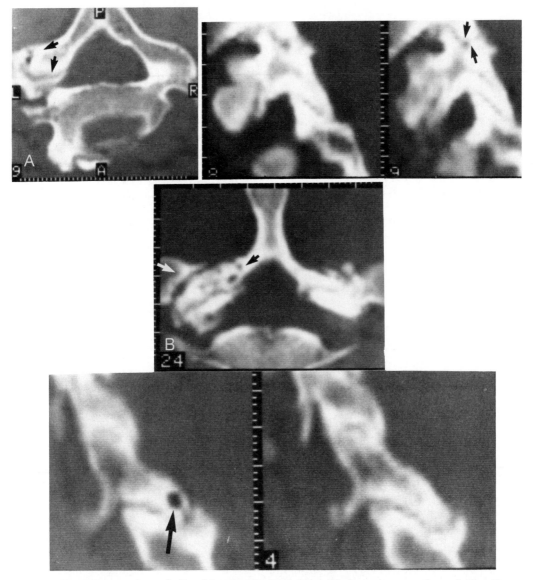

Figure 5.40. Degenerative arthritis of the facets. Axial views **(A)** show degenerative arthritis with more involvement of the left facet complex than the right. Images from a second patient **(B)** reveal localized posttraumatic arthritis of the left facet, shown here in the sagittal perspective. There is a joint space narrowing, irregularity, and degenerative cyst formation.

used as the primary reference. In Figure 5.43 is shown one example of NRC stenosis in severe rheumatoid disease. Judging patency of individual cervical NRCs can be a very tedious undertaking, even with availability of multiplanar CT imaging.

In Figure 5.44 are schematically represented some of the remarkably complex altered relationships that must be analyzed carefully with fully reformatted CT image sequences if the various and frequent stenotic changes in cervical rheumatoid disease are to be accurately demonstrated. It would not be overly dogmatic to state categorically that complex cervical cases such as these simply cannot be accurately analyzed with axial CT images alone. This entire subject is covered fully elsewhere (28).

Examples of high-resolution cervical scanning and three different causes of central canal and/or lateral recess stenosis are shown in Figures 5.45–5.47. In Figure 5.45 are examples of solid interbody fusion at C5-C6 but with a bone plug that protrudes into the central canal to the left of midline. Symptoms were relieved when this bone "spur" was removed. In Figure 5.46, severe central canal and right lateral recess stenosis due to ossification of the posterior longitudinal ligament is shown. As seen in the sagittal view, the OPLL involves several cervical segments. In the third example (Fig. 5.47) are demonstrated the stenotic changes that can accompany the diffuse idiopathic skeletal hyperostosis syndrome.

Future Developments

CT: THE POTENTIAL OF THREE-DIMENSIONAL IMAGING

The potential of three-dimensional imaging with CT is a topic unto itself, which can only be briefly summarized in this chapter. There has been much progress recently. Our coverage illustrates the range of current three-dimensional imaging possibilities.

The list of viewing capabilities beyond axial CT images is both long and increasingly useful in terms of routine clinical contributions. Because of (a) the thinner directly scanned images with CT than with MR (1–1.5 mm versus 3–5 mm) and (b) the much higher bone edge definition with CT than with MR, the following list applies primarily to cases imaged by CT. This may change in the future and may also include cases imaged by MR.

1. Reformatted orthogonal sagittals
2. Reformatted orthogonal coronals
3. Reformatted oblique sagittals
4. Reformatted curved coronals
5. Reformatted curved sagittals
6. Videotape sequences of capabilities listed under 1–5
7. Surface-shaded three-dimensional views (internal and external)
8. Stereo pair presentations of capability listed under 7
9. Dynamic videotape presentations of capabilities listed under 7 and 8
10. Hand-held models of bone edges

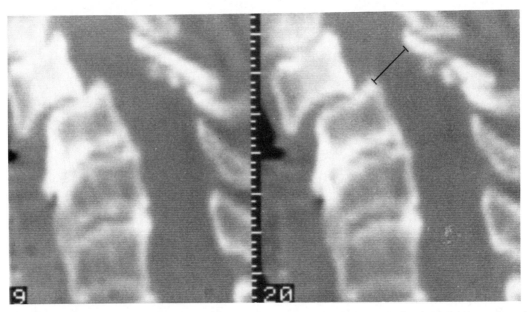

Figure 5.41.   Rheumatoid subluxation. Sagittal reformations demonstrate narrowing and degeneration of the C4 disc space with more than 5 mm of subluxation. The narrowest diameter of the canal is between the body of C4 and the lamina of C3 (*bars*). (From Rothman SLG, Glenn WV Jr: *Multiplanar CT of the Spine*. Rockville, MD, Aspen Systems, 1985, p 442.)

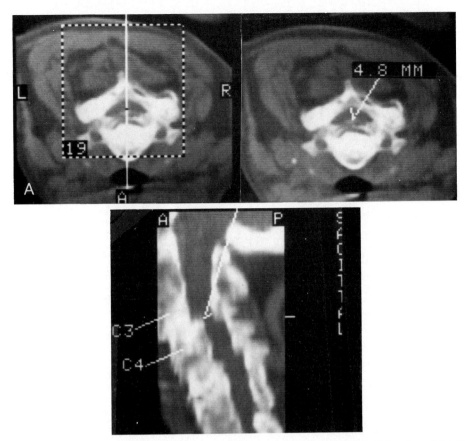

Figure 5.42. Three cases of cervical rheumatoid arthritis and stenosis. **A.** C3-C4 subluxation. *Axial slice #19* with a midsagittal reference line indicates the position of the reformatted sagittal image. Note that the axial measurement of the midsagittal AP canal diameter is 4.8 mm, whereas the more accurate oblique measurement from the sagittal view is 3.5 mm. **B.** Rotatory subaxial subluxation at C3. *Axial image #24* shows the adequate axial canal measurement of 13.5 mm. The reformatted sagittal image shows the correct and severely stenotic midsagittal AP dimension of 3.5 mm. Such misrepresentation of actual central stenosis on axial images is the rule, not the exception, in severe cases of cervical rheumatoid disease. **C.** Axial and sagittal views of subaxial staircase subluxation. Note the extreme stenosis at its narrowest spot is 1.5 mm of clearance in a patient who (remarkably) could still walk. These three cases do not represent maximum high-resolution scanning protocol but rather earlier 1980–1982 5-mm-thick axial images obtained every 2.5 mm. (From Rothman SLG, Glenn WV Jr: *Multiplanar CT of the Spine*. Rockville, MD, Aspen Systems, 1985, pp 464–466.)

Reformatted Orthogonal Sagittals and Coronals. Examples of reformatted orthogonal sagittals and coronals have been seen throughout the last section of this chapter. They are routinely used in our practice, on every single case.

Reformatted Oblique Sagittals. The most important use for reformatted oblique sagittals is in the "gun barrel" view for demonstrating cervical NRCs or foramina. From Rauschning's cryosectional anatomic work (13, 15, 26, 27) it has become abun-

dantly clear that the endplate ridging that encroaches on lumbar NRCs has even more critical stenotic potential in cervical NRCs. The reason is twofold. First, the exiting nerve root passes much closer to the endplate ridges in the cervical spine. Second, cervical NRCs are considerably smaller than their lumbar counterparts and have joint of Luschka degenerative changes that also contribute to the lateral recess and foraminal bony encroachments.

Reformatted Curved Coronals.

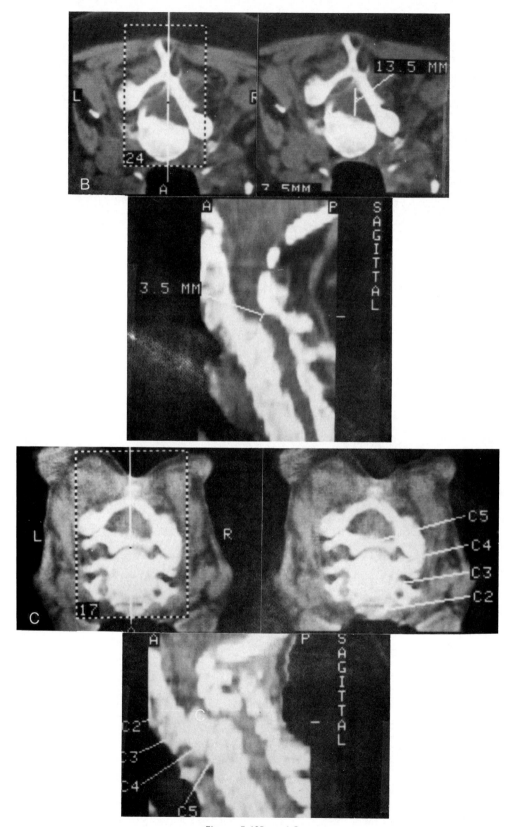

Figure 5.42B and C.

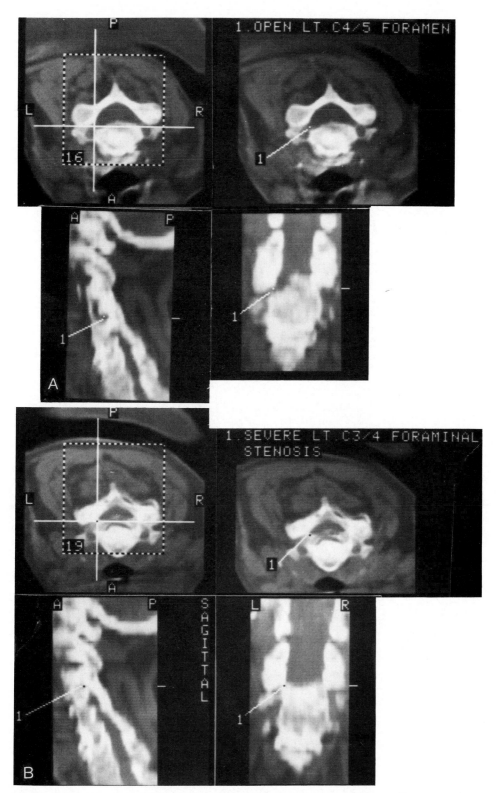

Figure 5.43. Cervical foraminal stenosis in rheumatoid arthritis. These multiplanar CT views of a severely stenotic C3-C4 foramen demonstrate that it often requires all three perspectives to have an adequate representation of just what is going on with regard to NRC or foraminal stenosis. (From Rothman SLG, Glenn WV Jr: *Multiplanar CT of the Spine*. Rockville, MD, Aspen Systems, 1985, p 467.)

Reformatted curved coronals have been routinely used in lumbar spine cases since their introduction several years ago (28). One advantage to using this view is to "straighten out" the lordotic curvature and allow longer visualization of lumbar nerve roots (as shown in Fig. 5.48). Another advantage is the ability to see and compare multiple lumbar NRCs simultaneously; this was often impossible with regular orthogonal coronal images. These advantages also apply to the cervical spine but in a slightly different (additional) manner. Recently, the curved plane capability has been extended in order to simplify the comparison of multiple cervical NRCs. By using an axial reference image as in Figure 5.49 and then defining an anteriorly curved family of images, it is possible to obtain the same gun barrel oblique sagittal perspective but with the added advantage of having left and right NRCs in the same image. This

very new technical development has just recently been reported and is not yet in routine clinical use (29).

Videotape Sequences Videotape sequences are a recent development (30). The goal with use of these is to simplify the transfer of visual information from its source (scanner/computer/radiologist) to its intended audience (referring physicians/surgeons). Normally this is done via film. But these films, no matter how well organized, must present image sequences in either horizontal rows or vertical columns of images. And in so doing, the viewer has absolutely no appreciation for the otherwise perfect registration (superimposability) of one image over another. The result with film is to introduce confusion and require the expenditure of additional time by forcing the viewer to reassemble the image sequence in his or her mind. By capturing the perfectly registered sequence of images

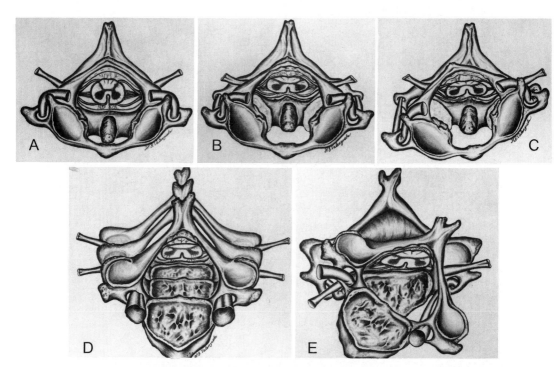

Figure 5.44. Mechanical abnormalities requiring careful analysis in cervical rheumatoid disease. **A.** Normal relationship of atlas on axis. **B.** Axial view of symmetric anterior subluxation of C1 and C2. **C.** Axial view of asymmetric rotary subluxation of C1 and C2. **D.** Axial view of staircase subluxation of C3, C4 and C5. **E.** Axial view of extreme rotary subluxation of C3 and C4. (From Kaufman R. In Rothman SLG, Glenn WV Jr: *Multiplanar CT of the Spine.* Rockville, MD, Aspen Systems, 1985, chap 15, pp 454–457.)

on videotape, one after another, it becomes easier to perceive the sequence as a whole, and it will take substantially less time than reviewing the same images from film. If there is audio narration of the video image sequences, the key findings in the official written consultation report will be absorbed more easily and quickly if the words used in the audio narration match the written report.

Surface-Shaded Three-Dimensional Views and Stereo Pair Presentations. Surface-shaded three-dimensional views and stereo pair presentations represent variations on the manner of presenting the same bone edge data. Some exam-

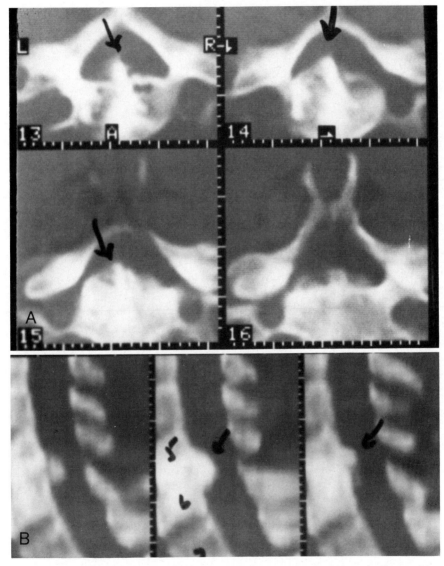

Figure 5.45.   Solid cervical interbody fusion with residual central canal stenosis. The problem here is malpositioning of the interbody bone plug such that it protrudes into the left anterior aspect of central canal, resulting in moderate central stenosis. Stenotic symptoms were relieved when this protruding bone was removed. (From Rothman SLG, Glenn W V Jr: *Multiplanar CT of the Spine*. Rockville, MD, Aspen Systems, 1985, pp 448–449.)

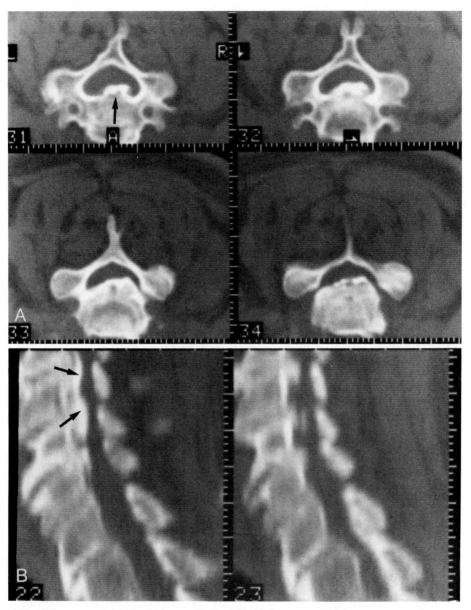

Figure 5.46.   OPLL causing central canal stenosis. The posterior longitudinal ligament over several segments is ossified, resulting in severe multilevel stenosis of the central canal. (From Rothman SLG, Glenn WV Jr: *Multiplanar CT of the Spine*. Rockville, MD, Aspen Systems, 1985, p 443.)

ples of this capability had been previously reported (1), while others have only recently been reported (29). The options are: (*a*) single versus stereo pair displays and (*b*) external versus internal spinal canal or NRC views. A stereo pair display is simply two single views with an angular separation in perspective of 8–12°. The examples shown in Figure 5.50 show external and internal stereo pair displays of a highly stenotic C5-C6 cervical NRC. The stereo pairs presented here are for cross-eyed viewing; a simple and inexpensive viewer is under development for the large percentage of those who have never learned cross-eyed stereoscopy. Such a viewer (made essentially of cardboard) will significantly increase the number of people who are able to appreciate the incremental clinical value in terms of depth effect that the stereo perspective provides.

Dynamic Videotape Presentations of Single or Stereo Surface-Shaded Images. Dynamic videotape presentations of single or stereo surface-shaded images are virtually identical to videotape sequences of sagittal or coronal reformatted sequences. The equipment is identical. The only difference is the type of image sequence being captured and subsequently narrated.

Hand-Held Models of Bone Edges. Data can be transformed into sagittal reformations, surface-shaded three-dimensional views, and stereo pairs of surface-

shaded three-dimensional views and then into a hand-held model. Such diagnostic models, in my opinion, represent probably the most useful and cost-effective form of three-dimensional imaging that could be provided to the referring physician for his or her inspection and/or discussion with a patient.

With very careful sagittal sequences, is the surface-shaded three-dimensional perspective really needed? Currently the answer is unknown. My suspicion is that full appreciation of routine multiplanar sagittal sequences decreases the need for three-dimensional imaging. This is a hunch based on considerable technical and clinical experience in three-dimensional imaging. A hunch, however, is not a scientifically proven fact.

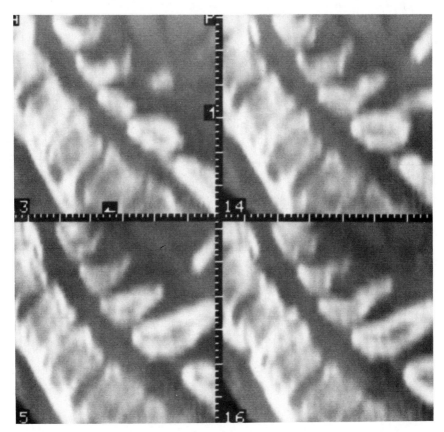

Figure 5.47. Diffuse idiopathic skeletal hyperostosis causing central canal stenosis. This case represents the exuberant excess bone formation characteristic of Forestier's disease with ossification of the anterior longitudinal ligament as well as multilevel central canal stenosis, due here to the significant endplate osteoarthritic ridges. The cervical NRCs or foramina at multiple levels (not shown) were also stenotic. (From Rothman SLG, Glenn WV Jr (eds): *Multiplanar CT of the Spine.* Rockville, MD, Aspen Systems, 1985, p 442.)

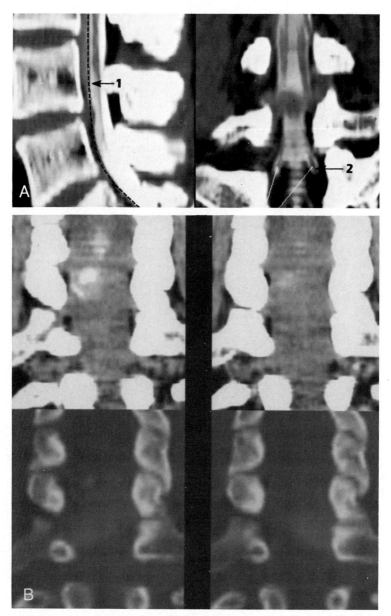

Figure 5.48. Reformatted curved coronals (standard). The usual form of curved coronal imaging (shown in this figure) is where the user specifies a curved line by placing "dots" along the posterior margins of the vertebral bodies as visualized from a reference sagittal image. The computer then replicates a family of parallel curves (user supplies number and spacing), and the curved coronal image sequence is generated. The single reference line on the reference sagittal and resulting curved coronal image is from a lumbar examination with intrathecal metrizamide. The images at the bottom of this figure represent a pair of soft tissue curved coronal cervicals with matching bone window images.

Another hunch, equally unproven, is that the potential of three-dimensional imaging is overshadowed by the potential of hand-held diagnostic models of the same three-dimensional information. An informal market survey (WV Glenn Jr, unpublished data) was conducted at the meeting of the International Society for Study of the

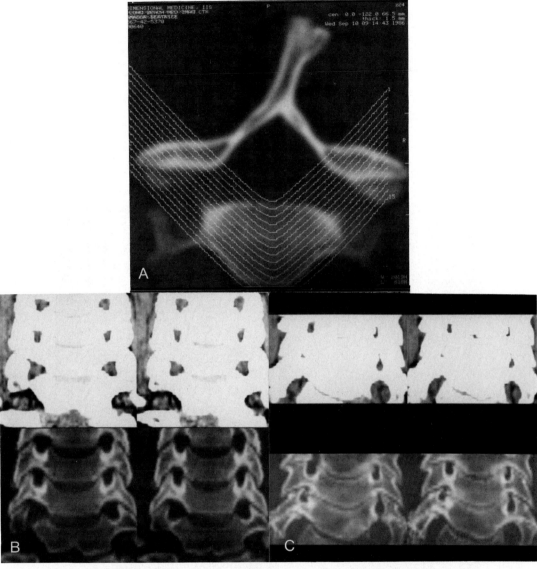

Figure 5.49. Reformatted curved coronals (extended capability). This is a new version with the same capability, here adapted to optimum oblique sagittal viewing of cervical NRCs and, in this case, of both NRCs at once! The user essentially defines one anterior curved line on an axial reference image rather than on the usual sagittal reference image. Next, a family of curved reference lines and their respective images are generated. The result is a combination of both the left and right oblique sagittal images described previously for optimum viewing of cervical NRCs. The difference (and convenience) is that both the left and right NRCs can be visualized and compared in the same sequence of images. (From Glenn WV Jr, Amador R: *Case Histories in MPR and 3-D Imaging: Complex Cervical Nerve Root Canal (NRC) Stenosis.* Minneapolis, Dimensional Medicine, 1986.)

Lumbar Spine (Sidney, Australia, 1985) during which 25 well-known spine surgeons were asked whether they preferred sagittal reformatted images, sagittal three-dimensional images, or a crude (!) hand-held model. Each choice consisted of the *same data* presented in three related but different ways. The very obvious preference, if a "complicated case" was assumed, was that the three-dimensional model justified

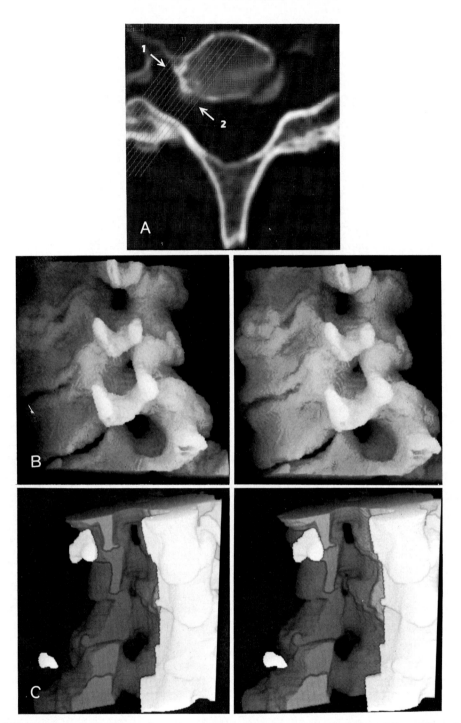

Figure 5.50. Surface-shaded three-dimensional views and stereo pair presentations. **A.** Two different single surface-shaded external NRC views 8° apart. *Arrows* in the reference axial image indicate the external and internal viewing perspectives for these stereo three-dimensional pairs. **B.** External surface-shaded views. Note the highly stenotic NRC or foramen in the middle. **C.** Internal views of the same stenotic cervical NRC. The surface-shading computer-processing algorithm has rendered the closer structures lighter (whiter) and the more distant or deeper structures darker. The axial data for these images were from a high-resolution G.E. 9800 CT scanner using 1.5-mm-thick slices obtained every 1.5 mm. (From Glenn WV Jr, Amador R: *Case Histories in MPR and 3-D Imaging: Complex Cervical Nerve Root Canal (NRC) Stenosis.* Minneapolis, Dimensional Medicine, 1986.)

additional expense (2:1 over three-dimensional imaging) with required availability in 3–5 days at an incremental cost of approximately 80% the original CT examination cost. For those favoring three-dimensional imaging, the justified incremental cost was approximately 50% the original CT cost, also in the 3–5-day time frame. In our practice, this would mean that the surgeons comprising this survey would recommend that the complicated case should have an $850–950 multiplanar CT examination and then an additional $650–700 diagnostic model (first choice) or $425–475 three-dimensional imaging (second choice). I believe the former should be produced at probably $75–150 cost with a "retail" value of $350–450, well below the surgeon-approved estimates. The three-dimensional should have a retail value of $150–250, also considerably lower than the survey suggested.

MR: MORE RESOLUTION, MORE SPEED, DETAILED SOFT TISSUE EVALUATIONS, AND SPECTROSCOPY

MR imaging is currently entering a "second level" of technical advancements which include the advent of "contrast agents," spectroscopy, and ultrafast imaging. The ultrafast acquisitions and new pulse sequences are likely to have particular relevance for spine evaluation and will facilitate new modes of image analyses and presentation. The first MR spinal three-dimensional holograms may be available not far in the future.

Conclusion

This chapter is an attempt to provide a "snapshot" of the present state of the art in terms of MR and CT imaging capabilities. The contents are admittedly very lengthy and represent considerable personal opinion on many related issues. Just because MR and CT scanners represent enormous capital investments and two remarkable evolutions of imaging technology, it does not follow that the actual operation of these widespread instruments is anywhere near optimum for spine-related problems. Far from it. The good news is

that virtually every high-resolution MR or CT scanner is capable of producing the types of studies that are contained in this chapter. The bad news is that most facilities routinely perform minimal type examinations. That is the frustrating part. Clearly written educational material for referring physicians has only recently become available. Sufficient experience with state-of-the-art CT and MR vis-à-vis the limitations of myelography is only just beginning to surface. Likewise, there is also some convincing cost-effect proof that proper CT the first time around is better than myelography and improper CT together.

Because of unnecessary diversity in scanning protocols and film organization, there is confusion about the capabilities of CT and MR imaging. Whether the organization of visual information in MR and CT spine imaging will get better or worse will depend in large part on the influence exerted by referring physicians (predominantly orthopaedic surgeons). Reducing the diversity may require a careful, coordinated standardization effort involving contributing medical subspecialists as well as third party payers. The idea of standardization is neither new nor particularly popular. Manufacturers have a vested interest in dissimilarity. The various users have comfortable patterns and habits of usage. To change or to conform is to overcome inertia.

The MR and CT imaging capabilities discussed herein will, it is hoped, find more and more routine application. Clearly, there has been rapid technological progress during the past decade. The future relative utilization of these two imaging modalities can only be determined by the referring subspecialists who order the examinations and whose patient management decisions are guided, in part, by the results of the imaging tests. The future of MR and CT spine imaging is in the hands of these referring physicians.

Acknowledgements

I would like to thank and personally acknowledge Richard Amador, CRT, Joel Levine, MD, Keith Burnett, MD, and Robert McCormick, CRT, for contributing their expertise and objectivity to this chapter.

References

1. Glenn WV, Rhodes ML, Altschuler EM, Wiltse LL, Kostanek C, Kuo YM: Miltiplanar display (MPD) computerized body tomography (CBT) applications in the lumbar spine. *Spine* 4(4):282–352, 1979.
2. Carrera GF, Haughton VM, Syvertsen A, Williams AL: Computed tomography of the lumbar facet joints. *Radiology* 134:145, 1980.
3. Kirkaldy-Willis WH, Heithoff K, Bowen CT, Shannon R: Pathological anatomy of lumbar spondylosis and stenosis, correlated with the CT scan. In Post MJD (ed): *Radiographic Evaluation of the Spine: Current Advances with Emphasis on Computed Tomography.* New York, Masson, 1980.
4. Brant-Zawadzki M, Miller EM, Federle MP: CT in the evaluation of spine trauma. *AJR* 136:369–375, 1981.
5. Glenn WV: *The Lumbar Spine — Recent Developments*, Spine Monograph #1, lab materials for "CT scanning of the lumbar spine: how to read the films," American Academy of Orthopaedic Surgeons Summer Institute, New York City, September 13, 1985.
6. Glenn WV, Burnett K, Rauschning W: *Magnetic Resonance Imaging of the Lumbar Spine: Nerve Root Canals, Disc Abnormalities, Anatomic Correlations, and Case Examples*, Spine Monograph #4. General Electric Medical Systems Division, April 1986.
7. Glenn WV: *Organizing Lumbar Spine CT Images: A Proposed Format Which Combines Several Currently Available Display and Photo Options*, Spine Monograph #2. Los Angeles, Foundation for Advanced Medical Display Technology, March 1986.
8. Glenn WV: *The Lumbar Spine — Recent Developments*, Spine Monograph #3, reading lab workbook for CT scanning of the lumbar spine: how to read the films. Los Angeles, Foundation for Advanced Medical Display Technology, March 1986.
9. Glenn WV: *Overview — CT/MPR of the Lumbar Spine*, Videolecture #1. Los Angeles, Foundation for Advanced Medical Display Technology, January 1986.
10. Glenn WV: *CT Grading of Lumbar Structures:* Part I, *Discs—Sagittal*; Part II, *Lateral Recessed—Axial*; Part III, *Central Canal—Axial*, Videolecture #2. Los Angeles, Foundation for Advanced Medical Display Technology, January 1986.
11. Glenn WV: *CT Grading of Lumbar Structures: Normal and Abnormal Neural Foramen—Sagittal View*, Videolecture #3. Los Angeles, Foundation for Advanced Medical Display Technology, January 1986.
12. Glenn WV: *CT Grading of Lumbar Structures: The Normal and Abnormal Zygapophyseal Joints—Axial View*, Videolecture #4. Los Angeles, Foundation for Advanced Medical Display Technology, January 1986.
13. Glenn WV, Rauschning W: *Spine and Peripheral Joint Anatomy*, Videolecture #5: demo of laser Video Disc #1. Los Angeles, Foundation for Advanced Medical Display Technology, January 1986.
14. Glenn WV: *Issues in Lumbar CT Scanning* (from Glenn WV, Rothman SLG: *G.E. Medical Systems Report*), Videolecture #6. Los Angeles, Foundation for Advanced Medical Display Technology, January 1986.
15. Glenn WV, Rauschning W: *Normal Lumbar Anatomy* (from: *Spine and Peripheral Joint Anatomy*, Laser Video Disc #1), Videolecture #7. Los Angeles, Foundation for Advanced Medical Display Technology, March 1986.
16. Glenn WV: *Review of "An Impossible Lumbar CT Case,"* Videolecture #8. Los Angeles, Foundation for Advanced Medical Display Technology, July 1987.
17. Rothman SLG, Glenn WV: *Multiplanar CT of the Spine.* Baltimore, University Park Press, 1984.
18. Chafetz NI, Genant HK, Moon KL, Helms CA, Morris JM: Recognition of lumbar disk herniation by NMR. *AJR* 141:1153–1156, 1983.
19. Han JS, Kaufman B, El Yousef SJ: NMR imaging of the spine. *AJR* 141:1137–1145, 1983.
20. Modic MT, Weinstein MA, Pavilicek W, Starnes DL, Duchesneau PM, Boumphrey F, Hardy RJ Jr: NMR of the spine. *Radiology* 148:757–762, 1983.
21. Edelman RR, Shoukinas GM, Stark DD, Davis KR, New PFJ, Saini S, Rosenthal DI, Wismer GL, Brady TJ: High resolution surface-coil imaging of lumbar disk disease. *AJR* 144:1123–1129, 1985.
22. Modic MT, Pavilicek W, Weinstein MA, Boumphrey F, Ngo F, Hardy RJ Jr, Duchesneau PM: MR imaging of intervertebral disk disease: clinical and pulse sequence considerations. *Radiology* 152:103–111, 1984.
23. Pech P, Haughton VM: Lumbar intervertebral disk: correlative MR and anatomic study. *Radiology* 156:699–701, 1985.
24. Burnett KR, Levine JB, Seiger L: MRI evaluation of the cervical spine at high field strength. *Appl Radiol* 14:6:47–55, 1985.
25. Burnett KR, Levine JB: MRI of lumbar disc disease: clinical observations with high resolution surface coils at 1.5 T. *Appl Radiol* in press.
26. Rauschning W: Detailed sectional anatomy of the spine. In Rothman SLG, Glenn WV Jr (eds): *Multiplanar CT of the Spine.* Baltimore, University Park Press, 1985, chap 3.
27. Rauschning W: Computer tomography and cryomicrotomy of lumbar spine specimens. A new technique for multiplanar anatomic correlation. *Spine* 8:170–180, 1983.
28. Rothman SLG, Glenn WV Jr: *Multiplanar CT of the Spine.* Rockville, MD, Aspen Systems, 1985.
29. Glenn WV, Amador RA: *Case Histories in MPR and 3-D Imaging: Complex Cervical Nerve Root Canal (NRC) Stenosis.* Dimensional Medicine, 1986.
30. Glenn WV: *Videotape Pilot Study—Narrated Video Consultation Reports.* Los Angeles, Foundation for Advanced Medical Display Technology, 1986.

6

Fractures and Dislocations of the Cervical Spine

STEPHEN M. FOREMAN, DC, DABCO

Motor vehicle accidents are responsible for the vast majority of cervical spine fractures and dislocations, which is not surprising given their force and frequency. Some studies have reported that as many as 80% of all cervical fractures are the direct result of these accidents (1). The sudden movement of the cervical spine is often accentuated by the combined effects of cervical mobility and cranial weight. The weight of the cranial area is intensified by the centrifugal force generated during the accident. The resultant hyperflexion or hyperextension may cause either ligamentous or osseous damage, depending on the force of the injury. The specific biomechanics of the injury are complex and are detailed in Chapter 1.

Other factors may intensify the force of the injury and produce a greater degree of trauma than expected. Preexisting changes such as ankylosing spondylitis, rheumatoid arthritis, or diffuse idiopathic skeletal hyperostosis may alter the normal flexibility of the area and predispose the patient to fractures (2, 3). The cervical area, in these conditions, is usually osteoporotic from disuse. This, too, contributes to the severity of the injury.

Arthritic and degenerative processes, such as those mentioned previously, contribute to and complicate cervical fractures. These processes restrict motion and produce a secondary osteoporosis which may cause the vertebral column to break "like a pencil." The resultant fracture may extend

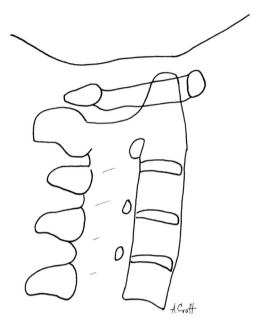

Figure 6.1. Line drawing of a lateral view of the cervical spine with ankylosing spondylitis. The thin layer of ossification around the intervertebral disc makes this area more susceptible to fractures.

tion exposure through the shoulder area. Improper technique, such as overpenetration or underpenetration, may also cause the examiner to miss an injured area.

The second reason for overlooked trauma is failure to radiograph the patient after a "minor" accident. Patients who present with cervical pain, especially those who have also suffered head trauma, should be radiographed. It is not uncommon for the ambulatory patient to present with articular or compression fractures. It is often difficult, if not impossible, to totally exclude the presence of fractures on the physical examination.

Lastly, the examiner may lack the interpretive skills necessary to evaluate such injuries (4). Total familiarity with the osseous and soft tissue manifestations that may be encountered on cervical radiographs is essential. For a complete review of the posttraumatic signs, see Chapter 4.

Fractures and dislocations of the cervical

through both anterior and posterior elements. The injuries associated with ankylosing spondylitis will occur through the disc, since the thin vertical osteophytic fusion is weaker than the vertebral body, thus localizing the fracture in that area (Fig. 6.1).

The fracturing associated with ankylosing spondylitis may be contrasted with that seen in diffuse idiopathic skeletal hyperostosis. The bridging osteophytic process in the latter condition forms a thick, calcific armor in front of each intervertebral disc level. The osteophytes are thin at the middle of each vertebral level, which makes this area more susceptible to fracturing. The fractures in both conditions may cause neurological complications, pseudoarthrosis, or even death.

An examiner's failure to recognize a cervical fracture or dislocation may result for one of several reasons. First, the examiner may use improper radiographic technique. The position and the width of the patient's shoulders often produce obliteration of the C7 area, resulting in a missed fracture or dislocation. This can be corrected by using a swimmer's view and/or an overpenetra-

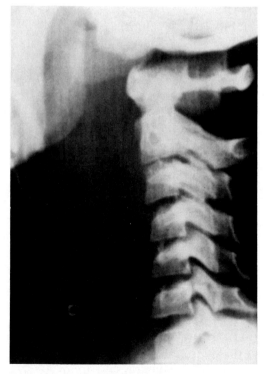

Figure 6.2. Lateral view of the cervical spine demonstrates a large retropharyngeal hematoma and an abnormal distance between the atlas and the occiput.

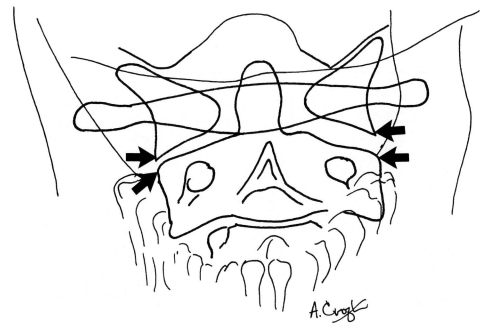

Figure 6.3.   Line drawing of AP open mouth view. The lateral margins of the atlas and the axis (*arrows*) should be equal.

spine may be classified by a variety of methods (5). I prefer to divide the injuries by anatomical area into those of the upper and those of the lower cervical spine. The radiographic examination outlined in Chapter 4 should be sufficient to demonstrate the majority of injuries to be discussed.

Occiput Injuries

An occipital dislocation is a rare clinical condition, in that it usually causes death by respiratory paralysis. Those patients who do survive the initial trauma often suffer from quadriparesis or similar damage. Radiographically this condition will usually appear as a dislocation of the occiput and a large retropharyngeal hematoma (Fig. 6.2).

Fractures of the occiput are rare. Spencer et al. (6) reported only seven cases in their review of the literature. The stresses applied to the area will typically cause the atlas to fracture first, thereby sparing the occipital condyles.

Atlas Injuries

FRACTURES

Fractures of the atlas usually occur in either the neural ring or the lateral masses. First reported in 1920, the Jefferson (7) or "burst" fracture is a traumatic rupture of the neural ring of the atlas. The broken areas are typically located in both the anterior and the posterior arches and are usually confirmed by inspection of the anteroposterior (AP) open mouth view (Fig. 6.3). The widening of the retropharyngeal space will also be apparent on the lateral view.

This injury occurs when the patient strikes his or her head on the car roof or into the windshield. The mechanism of injury is an axial load placed on the vertex of the patient's skull. The vertical load literally compresses the lateral masses of the atlas between the articulating surfaces of the occiput and the axis. The slope of these articular surfaces will separate or "burst" the neural ring and force the lateral masses laterally (Figs. 6.4 and 6.5). The shifting of the lateral masses causes an overlapping of

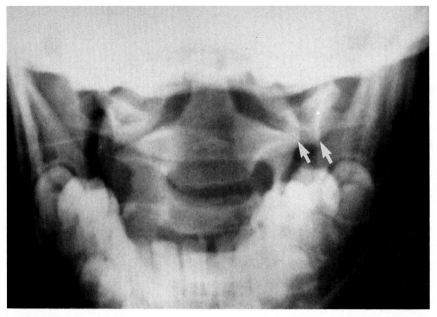

Figure 6.4.   AP open mouth view of a 7-year-old boy. Note that the lateral mass of the atlas is even on the left and offset on the right (*arrows*).

the articular margins, as is described in Chapter 4.

A false positive for fracture may be indicated on the AP open mouth view, which should lead the examiner to search for a

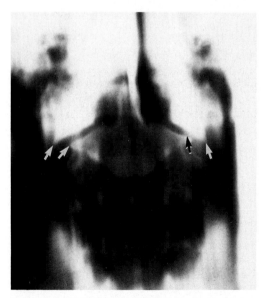

Figure 6.5.   Tomogram of the upper cervical spine. The disparity between the atlas and the axis is well demonstrated bilaterally.

Jefferson fracture. The false positive or "pseudospread" is attributed to a disparity in the growth rate between the atlas and the axis and is most commonly seen in children around 4 years of age (8).

Surprisingly, a Jefferson fracture does not typically cause a great deal of neurological encroachment or deficit (7). The lack of neurological deficit stems from decompression of the neural ring, which is induced by trauma. This mechanism is quite similar to the clinical improvement seen after a laminectomy. The symptoms, if any, will usually arise as a result of the hematoma associated with the osseous fracture or the callus formation produced during the healing process. The most common symptoms during healing include posterior scalp numbness or retroauricular pain due to irritation of the C2 nerve root as it passes the healing area (7).

A Jefferson fracture is considered highly unstable and is treated with Halo traction immobilization for a minimum of 6–8 weeks. The period of treatment is followed by support with a rigid or semirigid cervical collar for an additional 8 weeks. After the 4 months of external support, range of motion exercises to restore biomechanical function may be begun. A final evaluation with computed tomography must be considered in order to assess the degree of healing before cervical manipulation can be considered.

Untreated posterior arch fractures usually heal without complications. Pseudoarthrosis may develop at the fracture site, however, and cause chronic instability of the area. One case has been reported in which the posterior arch was fractured, formed a pseudoarthrosis, and 2 years later became entrapped on the posterior border of the foramen magnum (9) (Fig. 6.6A and B).

DISLOCATIONS

The shape and the location of the atlantoaxial joint make it susceptible to a variety of fractures and dislocations. There are four major varieties of dislocations that occur in this area.

Dislocations Associated With Odontoid Fracture

The odontoid process serves as a vertical stabilization post around which the atlas revolves and as an anchor that restricts the anterior and the posterior movement of the atlas. Instability of this process places this area in great neurological jeopardy.

Some atlas dislocations are the result of type II or type III fractures of the dens. This fracture-dislocation complex does not usually cause severe neurological damage. Anterior dislocation of the atlas on the axis (Fig. 6.7A and B) may cause compression of the spinal cord between the posterior arch of C1 and the posterior surface of the body of the axis.

Posterior atlas dislocations may also arise in type II and type III fractures. The spinal cord is compressed between the posterior aspect of the odontoid process and the spinolaminal junction of the axis.

Treatment of these injuries consists of surgical reduction and immobilization with a Halo appliance. This treatment is usually continued until stabilization is achieved.

Anterior Dislocation Due to Rupture of the Transverse Ligament

The transverse ligament is responsible for limiting the forward movement of the atlas. A traumatic rupture of this structure will allow anterior movement of the atlas

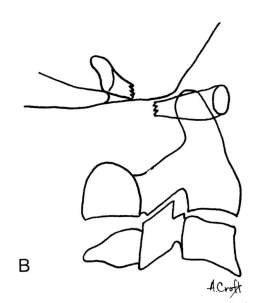

A

B

Figure 6.6. Line drawings of the upper cervical spine area. **A.** Demonstrates a nondisplaced fracture of the posterior arch of the atlas, and the view below indicates the final position of the posterior arch within the foramen magnum. **B.** Later examination revealed that the posterior arch had not healed and had become entrapped within the foramen magnum.

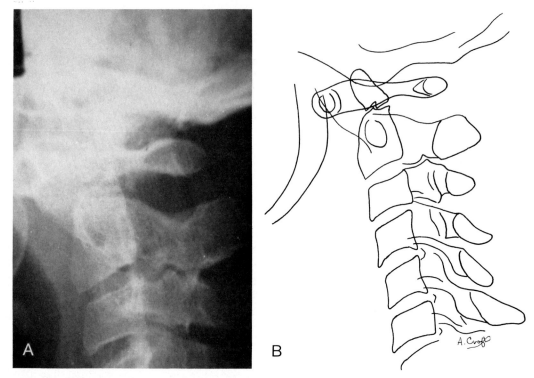

Figure 6.7. A. Lateral view of the C1-C2 complex. Anterior dislocation of the atlas on the axis has caused a narrowing of the spinal canal which is demonstrated by a widening of the atlantodental interval. **B.** Line drawing of **A.**

on the axis. This positional change typically causes a greater degree of neurological damage than occurs with other atlantal dislocations or fractures. During the dislocation, anterior movement of the atlas forces the spinal cord into the stationary odontoid process, resulting in high-level spinal cord damage. The resulting upper motor neuron lesion produces symptoms such as pathological reflexes and extremity muscle spasticity (10).

Unfortunately, many of these patients fail to recover and expire because of the severity of the spinal cord injury. Those patients who do survive must undergo posterior stabilization at the C1-C2 level because of the poor healing found in the transverse ligament. The area may be stabilized by a variety of methods. Wiring the spinous processes at C1 and C2 together immobilizes the area quite well. Visualization of the dislocation is revealed by an increased atlantodental interval. A discus-

sion of this radiographic sign is found in Chapter 4.

On rare occasions, a patient may present with a gradual onset myelopathy due to an anterior dislocation of unknown origin. This idiopathic dislocation is clinically significant and, unless it is recognized and surgically stabilized, is associated with a poor long-term prognosis. The postoperative prognosis is excellent on account of the lack of acute trauma and subsequent brainstem damage (11).

Because of a congenital absence of the transverse ligament, some conditions predispose a patient to an anterior atlas dislocation. The most common example of this is seen in Down's syndrome. Approximately 10% of patients with this syndrome lack a transverse ligament (12). Acquired conditions such as rheumatoid arthritis (13), arthritis resulting from *Yersinia* infection, (14), and Reiter's syndrome (15) may also predispose the patient to instability. The synovial pannus formation seen in these conditions may result in localized hyperemia that weakens or ruptures the transverse ligament. Osseous damage in the form of erosions affecting the odontoid process may also be seen (Fig. 6.8A and B). Linear or computed tomography may be employed to detect small or questionable areas of damage. The weakened transverse ligament will usually allow excessive movement of the atlas on flexion and extension lateral views. For a complete discussion of atlantodental interval measurements, see Chapter 4.

Posterior Dislocation

Posterior dislocation is a seldom-seen injury resulting from cervical hyperextension combined with a blow under the chin. This mechanical combination causes the anterior arch of the atlas to move up and over the odontoid process, finally coming to rest behind the odontoid process (Fig. 6.9).

This injury results in tearing or stretching of both the anterior and posterior longitudinal ligaments. Bleeding into the retropharyngeal space will be seen in addition to the osseous dislocation. The vertical

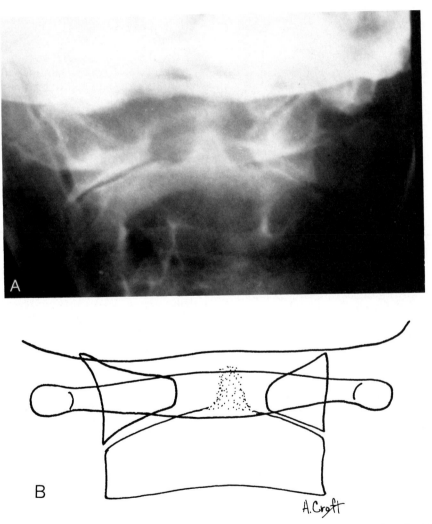

Figure 6.8.   A. AP open mouth view reveals severe erosions on the odontoid process. This patient is suffering from rheumatoid arthritis. **B.** Line drawing of **A.**

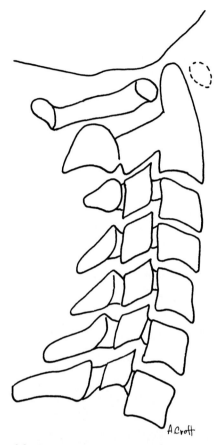

Figure 6.9 Line drawing of the upper cervical spine. The original anterior arch position is represented by the *dotted line*. The final atlas position is posterior to the odontoid process.

traction occurring during the accident may damage the ligamentous structures and cause instability and no dislocation. Jamshidi et al. (16a) reported on one patient in whom the dislocation occurred the day after the accident while the patient was recovering in the hospital.

Treatment of posterior dislocation consists of continual traction with cranial tongs, which raises the atlas which is then repositioned to its original position (16a). Surgical stabilization may then be needed as a follow-up procedure.

Rotational Dislocation

It has been demonstrated that the primary function of the atlas is to provide rotation of the cranium on the cervical spine. Injuries that result in overrotation may cause a tearing of the articular capsule that surrounds the atlantoaxial joint. The transverse ligament may or may not be ruptured (Fig. 6.10), depending on the force and direction of injury.

The dislocation arises when the atlas is rotated beyond its normal limit. The articulating surface on the inferior portion of the lateral mass is rotated anteriorly and drops inferiorly along the superior edge of C2. On clinical presentation, the patient's head is usually rotated, and he or she is unable to return to the neutral or opposite position. Treatment consists of traction for reduction and of immobilization for repair.

Axis Injuries

Because of its atypical shape and high location within the cervical unit, the axis is suceptible to a variety of fractures. These fractures are typically located within either the pedicles or the odontoid process. The vertebral body and spinous process, because of their location, seldom sustain fracture. Fractures of the spinous process or vertebral body usually occur at the C5–C7 level.

HANGMAN'S FRACTURE

The hangman's fracture, also known as a "traumatic spondylolisthesis," is a bilateral pedicle fracture of C2. This colorful injury was initially recognized as the cause of death in a judicial hanging. The person's sudden demise in these cases was caused by a combination of respiratory paralysis and strangulation.

The hangman's fracture associated with vehicular trauma, unlike its judicial counterpart, does not usually result in sudden death unless there is severe spinal cord or brainstem damage. The size of the patient's spinal canal at the level of the axis, combined with the instant decompression afforded with a hangman's fracture, usually allows the patient to escape with few neurological complications. It would seem that the rope makes all of the difference!

The radiographic presentation of a hangman's fracture may be quite variable. Some of the fractures may be well aligned and nondisplaced. A small radiolucent line on the superior surface of the pedicle may be the only osseous sign of injury (Fig. 6.11). Other patients may present with a large displacement of the two segments. Cases have been reported in which the vertebral body of C2 moved forward and came to rest directly anterior to the body of C3 (7). This complete dislocation resembled a grade 5 spondylolisthesis or "spondyloptosis" of the L5 vertebral body.

Statistically, hangman's fracture is not common. Roda et al. (7) in their survey found that this fracture represents only 7% of all cervical fractures. The injury is the result of an axial load on the vertex of the patient's head while the cervical spine is in extension. This is usually seen after the patient strikes his or her head against the windshield after a sudden deceleration (Fig. 6.12). The use of the cross-chest seat belt helps prevent these fractures.

Confusion may arise in the radiographic evaluation of children after trauma. The synchondrosis between the dens and the posterior arch is a normal structure that may be mistaken for a fracture. This growth area may persist until the child is 7-years-old. This entity may be differentiated from a fracture in several ways. First, the synchondrosis is never visible on the neutral lateral view, only on oblique views. Second, congenital defects in this area are rarely seen on the lateral view (8, 9) and should not be mistaken for a fracture. And third, a retropharyngeal hematoma will not be seen.

The treatment of these fractures often requires immobilization with a Halo appliance. The treatment protocol follows that for the Jefferson fracture closely.

ODONTOID FRACTURES

Fractures of the axis vary in their clinical significance and treatment, depending on the location and degree of displacement of the fragments. Anderson and D'Alonzo (16b) have classified fractures of the odon-

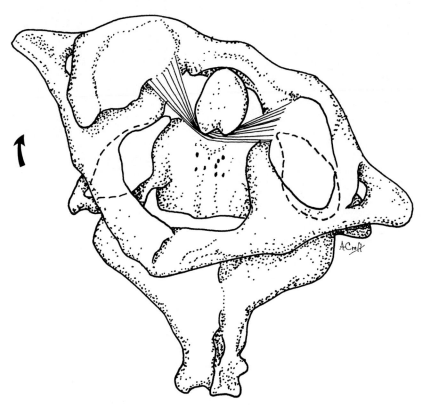

Figure 6.10. Axial line drawing of the atlas on the axis. The atlas has rotated enough to dislocate but has not rotated enough to rupture the transverse ligament. *Arrow* indicates direction of atlas rotation.

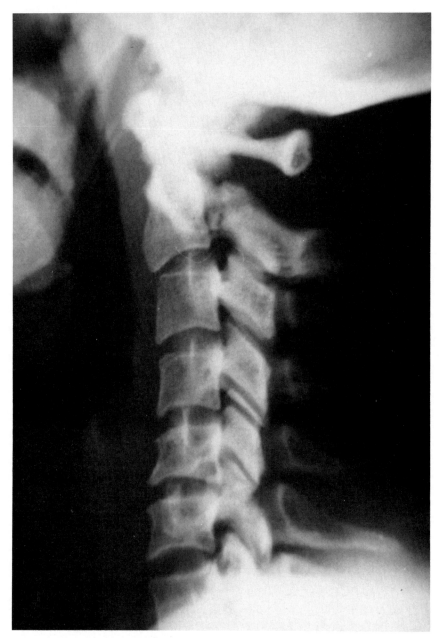

Figure 6.11.   Lateral view of the cervical spine. A thin radiolucent line on the pedicles of C2 represents a hangman's fracture. Note the absence of a retropharyngeal hematoma.

toid into three types (I–III) according to their location.

Type I

A type I fracture is a rare avulsion of the superior aspect of the odontoid process, with the break running obliquely through the upper third of the process (Fig. 6.13). This unusual location is attributed to excessive tension on the alar ligaments during trauma. Care should be exercised when the AP open mouth view is being evaluated, as the patient's front incisors may be superimposed over the superior aspect of the

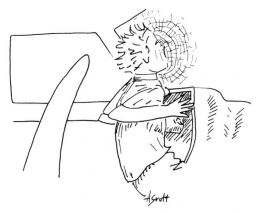

Figure 6.12. A hangman's fracture in the making.

odontoid and effectively obscure the type I fracture.

The existence of the type I avulsion has been questioned in the past (17, 18). Some believe that the fracture will only be seen if occipitoatlantal dissociation occurs. The fracture, despite its controversial etiology, is stable in nature and tends to heal without complication. Treatment is usually uncom-

plicated and will often consist of a hard cervical orthosis for 4–6 weeks.

This rare entity may be confused with a developmental defect known as the ossiculum terminale. Guidelines for a differential diagnosis between the two conditions are covered in Chapter 4.

Type II

Type II fractures are far more common and clinically significant than type I lesions. These fractures are located at the base of the odontoid and should be classified as to their degree of displacement as well as to their location. The displacement of the odontoid must be measured in terms of angulation and translation (19). Angulation is characterized by a deviation of the longitudinal axis of the dens in relation to the posterior cortex of the body (Fig. 6.14). Translation is measured by the horizontal displacement of the base of the odontoid in relation to the posterior aspect of the axis (19) (Fig. 6.15). Translation and angulation may be anterior, posterior, or both.

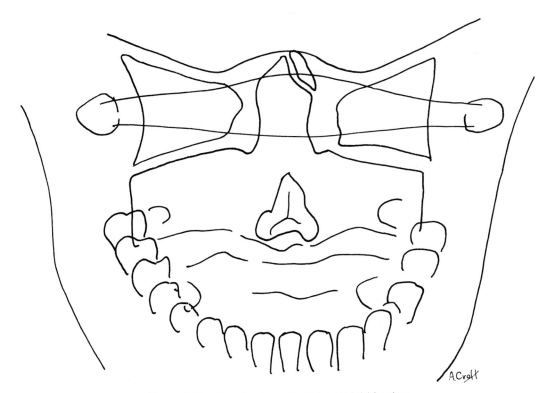

Figure 6.13. Line drawing of type I odontoid fracture.

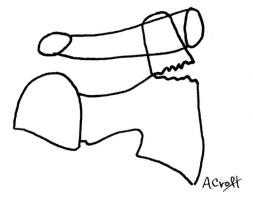

Figure 6.14.   Line drawing of posterior angulation of the odontoid process after a type II fracture.

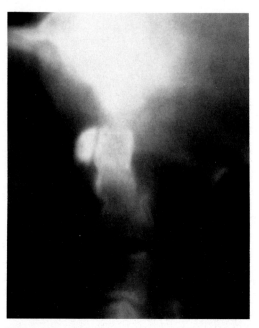

Figure 6.15.   Tomogram of translation. Note that the base of the odontoid is shifted anteriorly, but the odontoid is not angulated.

Translation is an important consideration in both the treatment and prognosis of type II fractures. The horizontal movement seen on the initial study correlates with the high rate of non-union that occurs with these fractures. Schatzer et al. (20) reported a non-union rate of 64% in their review of 37 patients. When translation was 5 mm or more, the non-union rate was 100%. This non-union may be clinically expressed as an area of necrotic bone. The pathophysiological mechanism is quite similar to that seen in fracture of the scaphoid bone of the wrist.

Treatment of type II fractures can be conservative, but surgical intervention is usually chosen because the rates of union may be quite low in the nonsurgical group. One

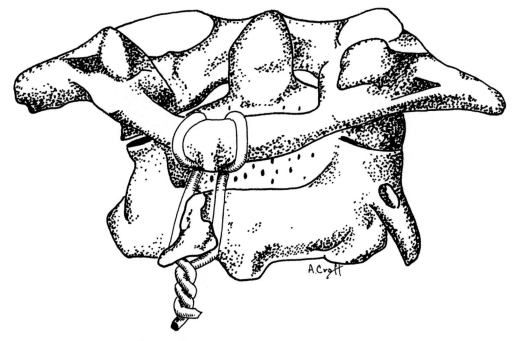

Figure 6.16.   Line drawing of Gallie procedure.

study reviewed the success rate of the non-surgical group and found that it varied 5–64% (20). These low and unreliable results make many physicians choose the more predictable surgical alternative.

Anterior displacement of the odontoid is often treated with surgical constructs, which counteracts the tendency for displacement. This is, in effect, surgically induced traction. Most of these procedures utilize posterior stabilization with wire. The Gallie procedure (21) is a typical example in which a wire is looped around the arch of C1 and then passed underneath the spinous process of C2 (Fig. 6.16). This procedure is able to provide stabilization, and the patient usually has to only wear a collar in the postoperative period.

Anterior displacement of the odontoid is less likely to result in neurological deficits than is posterior displacement. Posttraumatic stabilization of posterior displacements is usually achieved with a combination of block bone graft and immobilization and traction with a Halo device (19).

Type II fractures may be confused with an os odontoideum. Differentiation between the two entities is discussed in Chapter 4.

Type III

A type III fracture involves the body of the axis and is clinically different from the type II lesion. A type III or low odontoid fracture is distinguishable from the type II fracture, in that it disrupts the neural ring of the axis (22). This condition is serious, unstable, and weakens the neural canal. The incidence of the type II and type III fractures is approximately the same.

Radiographically, the type III fracture may demonstrate a variety of changes. The odontoid may be either nondisplaced or displaced with both severe angulation and translation. The detection of this injury on an AP open mouth view is difficult at best. The nondisplaced variety may only be suspected by prevertebral swelling anterior to the affected area.

Axial views, via computed tomography, may not disclose some of the type III fractures. The use of sagittal reconstructions should greatly increase the diagnostic yield.

Lower Cervical Spine Injuries

Vehicular accidents are a common source of trauma to the lower cervical spine and may cause a wide variety of fractures and dislocations. Allen et al. (5) have described mechanisms for lower cervical spine fractures which are termed injury vectors. Forces that produce the initial tissue or osseous strain are called major vectors. Forces that produce strain on the cervical spine from a second direction are called minor vectors.

Major vectors, consisting of either extension or flexion, are typically produced by the sudden acceleration or deceleration of the vehicle. The major vector of injury produces two directions of force within the cervical spine at the same time. For example, hyperflexion produces traction along the ligamentum nuchae and, simultaneously, compression along the anterior edge of the vertebral bodies. In hyperextension the converse is true. The section of the spine, approximately along the posterior longitudinal ligament, that does not experience either compression or extension is termed the neutral axis. The minor vector accentuates the major vector and helps determine whether the injury will arise from the compression or traction force being applied to the spine.

COMPRESSION FRACTURES

Compression fractures at the anterior edge of the vertebral bodies may be caused by a hyperflexion motion alone or in combination with a vertical compression. The stability of these fractures is dependent upon the degree of vertebral compression and the presence of posterior ligamentous damage. The major vector is flexion, and the minor vector is compression, which combined cause varying degrees of anterior vertebral damage. These fractures have been classified, based on degree of damage and potential instability evidenced radiographically, into five groups (5).

Compressive Flexion Stage 1

Compressive flexion stage 1 injuries are often seen in the ambulatory patient and are

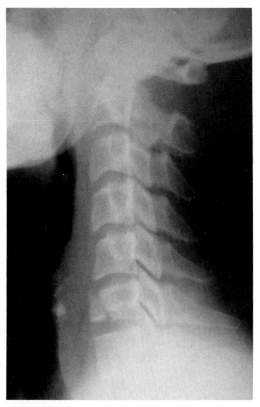

Figure 6.17. Small fracture at C6. The anterior corner of C6 is beginning to beak.

rior corner of the vertebral body. The compressive change or "beaking deformity" seen on the lower corner of Figure 6.17 is characteristic of the lesion. The two areas of compression will usually cause a difference in height of at least 3 mm between the anterior and the posterior border of the vertebral body.

It is at this point that the intervertebral disc comes into play in the production of further damage. The nucleus pulposus serves as a fulcrum over which the vertebral body is forced. This fulcrum acts as a wedge and will cause a vertical fracturing through the vertebral body. It is not unusual to see an increased concavity of the inferior endplate, even at this early stage.

Compressive Flexion Stage 3

Compressive flexion stage 3 lesions demonstrate a continuation of the damage initiated by the nucleus pulposus and seen in stage 2. The hallmark finding is an oblique fracture extending from the inferior endplate, through the centrum, to the superior

commonly encountered in the clinical setting. Neutral lateral radiographs will demonstrate a slight compression or blunting of the anterior-superior vertebral border. Little, if any, increase is to be expected in the size of either the retrotracheal or the retropharyngeal space. The biomechanics of the cervical unit make many of these fractures appear in the lower cervical spine rather than in the C1–C3 area. There is usually no disruption of the posterior ligamentous complex.

Clinically, the patient with this injury will usually not present with any abnormal neurological findings. The symptomatic picture will often consist only of decreased range of motion and constant pain.

Compressive Flexion Stage 2

Compressive flexion stage 2 lesions demonstrate, in addition to the stage 1 changes, compression of the anterior-infe-

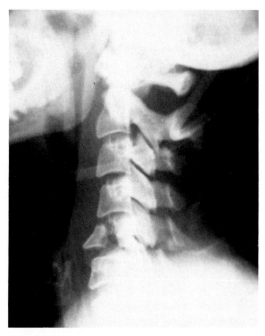

Figure 6.18. Lateral view of the cervical spine shows fracturing of the superior and inferior endplate of C5. An oblique, superior to inferior vertebral body fracture is present.

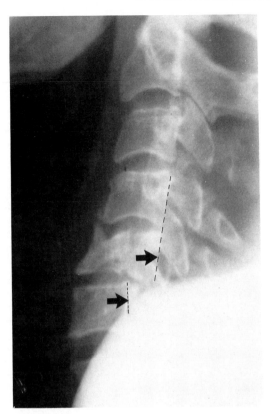

Figure 6.19. Lateral view of the cervical spine shows a stage 4 injury. The neural canal is compromised. The posterior vertebral line (George's line) is altered.

endplate (Fig. 6.18). The stability of the segment is highly compromised. Computed tomography is mandatory at this point.

Damage to the posterior ligamentous complex is likely but cannot be ruled out on the neutral lateral film. Flexion and extension views will be required to demonstrate the osseous separation of the spinous processes.

Compressive Flexion Stage 4

Compressive flexion stage 4 and stage 3 injuries have a similar radiograhic appearance. The chief difference between the two stages is the posterior displacement of the vertebral body fragments into the neural canal, which is only seen in stage 4. The degree of posterior displacement is usually small, not more than 3 mm. This is usually clinically apparent, but computed tomography will determine the number, size, and location of the various fragments (Fig. 6.19). Posterior ligamentous damage is to be expected at this stage.

Compressive Flexion Stage 5

There is no difference in the osseous appearance between compressive flexion stage 3 and stage 5 fractures. The change in neurological damage is caused by an increase in the degree of posterior displacement.

POSTERIOR ELEMENT DAMAGE

Tearing and stretching of the ligamentum nuchae and interspinous ligaments occur during hyperflexion. What causes this damage to occur posteriorly instead of anteriorly, as was just seen in compressive flexion injuries? The differentiating feature seems to be a minor vector. In most posterior element injuries, the minor vector consists of a blow to the back of the head, in contrast to a compressive minor vector in which the force is directed to the front of the head.

Allen et al. (5) have classified these distractive flexion injuries, based on radiographic changes, into four distinct groups. The minor vector, consisting of a blow to the occiput, is considered to apply a distractive or tractional force on the posterior cervical spine.

Distractive Flexion Stage 1

Clinical correlation of the information gained during the history with regard to the mechanism of injury must be applied to the radiographic picture in distractive flexion stage 1 injuries. The neutral lateral radiograph may show a widening or subluxation of the facets, and the vertebral movement is usually sufficient to allow for compression of the anterior-superior border of the vertebral segment immediately below the facet subluxation. The radiographic appearance of the fracture is identical to that seen in stage 1 compressive flexion injuries.

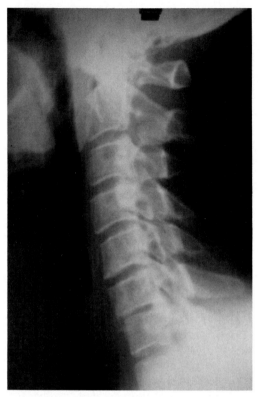

Figure 6.20. Lateral view shows a slight displacement of C6 on C7. This was later confirmed as a unilateral facet dislocation.

Distractive Flexion Stage 2

Distractive flexion stage 2 lesions demonstrate as a typical unilateral facet dislocation. This type of injury often contains a rotation component, causing the majority of damage to occur unilaterally. The unilateral dislocation requires a disruption of the interspinous and capsule ligament on the affected side (23). Complete disruption of the posterior ligamentous complex is rare at this stage.

Widening of the posterior disc height is to be expected in stage 2 injuries. There is often an anterior displacement of the affected segment in relation to the vertebrae directly below. This anterior movement is approximately 20–25% of the AP size of the vertebral body (Fig. 6.20).

Distractive Flexion Stage 3

Distractive flexion stage 3 injuries demonstrate as a bilateral dislocation of the posterior facet. The vertebral body is typically displaced approximately 50%. Most of these stage 3 injuries occur at the C5 and C6 levels. Injuries at the lower C7 and T1 levels are quite rare (24).

In stage 3 injuries, the posterior elements are stretched, and it is at this point that a complete tearing of these structures may occur. The biomechanics of this injury are discussed later.

Distractive Flexion Stage 4

Distractive flexion stage 4 injuries are distinguished by a wide and total dislocation of the vertebral segments (Fig. 6.21). The failure of the posterior ligamentous structures occurs at approximately the same moment that the posterior facets dislocate. There is no osseous resistance after dislocation, and the disc is usually sheared, tearing the anterior longitudinal ligament in the process (25) (Fig. 6.22).

Experimental studies have attempted to

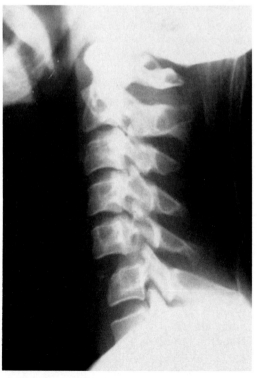

Figure 6.21. Lateral view shows wide separation of the intervertebral disc. This represents a total dislocation of the vertebral segments.

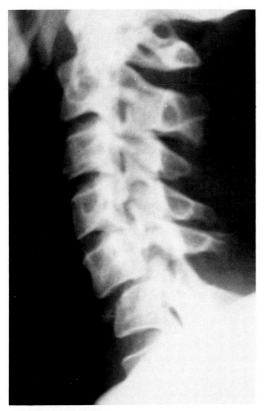

Figure 6.22. Neutral lateral view of the same patient as in Figure 6.21 shows total disruption of the posterior ligament complex.

reproduce flexion dislocations in the laboratory. Bauze and Ardran (25) were able to cause distractive flexion stage 4 dislocations after applying a vertical load of 135 kg (297 lb). This load seems quite low if the force produced in vehicular accidents and the weight of the human body are taken into consideration.

Treatment usually requires an extensive amount of stabilization. In the past, attempts were made to rely on interbody fusion as the sole means of correction, but it was found that posterior wire stabilization was also needed, as there was a high incidence of failed fusion (23).

Extension Injuries_____

Hypertension, a primary destructive force in a typical accident, results in cervical acceleration/deceleration syndrome. The

biomechanical implications of such an injury are found in Chapter 1. The major vector of extension injuries produces traction along the anterior longitudinal ligament and compression between the spinous processes. The minor vectors of compression and distraction may once again be applied to the biomechanical components of the injury.

COMPRESSIVE EXTENSION INJURIES

In extension injuries, the posterior facets act as a fulcrum. The minor vector serves to accentuate the pressure on either the anterior or the posterior side of the fulcrum. Compression minor vectors cause damage to the posterior elements. The distractive minor vectors apply the forces along the anterior longitudinal ligament. Allen et al. (5) have classified the compressive extension injuries into five groups.

Compressive Extension Stage 1

Compressive extension stage 1 injuries demonstrate as a unilateral fracture through

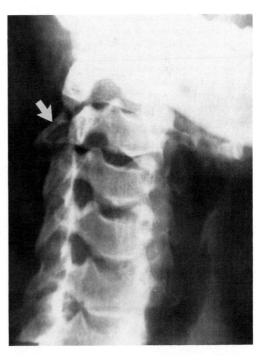

Figure 6.23. Oblique view of the cervical spine demonstrates a unilateral fracture of the articular facet (*arrow*).

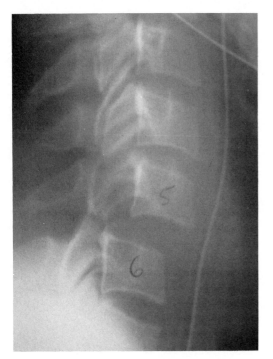

Figure 6.24.   Severe dislocation of C5 on C6 is visualized. The radiopaque line anterior to the vertebral bodies represents a nasogastric tube.

either the lamina or the articular facet (Fig. 6.23). Displacement is not seen, and the visualization of this injury may be quite difficult. Woodring and Goldstein (26) reviewed a series of patients and found that 87.5% of the articular facet fractures would have been missed when only AP and lateral cervical films were utilized. Tomography in the lateral position was found to demonstrate a large majority of these ''hidden'' fractures.

Compressive Extension Stage 2

Compressive extension stage 2 lesions demonstrate stage 1 characteristics at multiple, contiguous levels. There is usually a rotational component to the position of the head at the time of injury.

Compressive Extension Stages 3 and 4

Compressive extension stage 3 and stage 4 injuries demonstrate logical progressions of the anterior movement that began with the stage 2 fracture. The anterior vertebral movement may vary and is totally dependent on the degree of ligamentous injury.

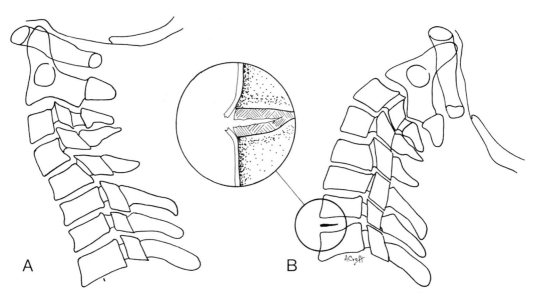

Figure 6.25.   **A.** Line drawing of a neutral lateral view shows the normal appearance of the disc spaces. **B.** Line drawing of extension view reveals the formation of a lucent cleft in the C7-T1 disc space. The *inset* illustrates the anatomical changes responsible for the cleft.

Compressive Extension Stage 5

Compressive extension stage 5 lesions are identical to stage 4 lesions, except for displacement. The stage 5 lesion demonstrates as a complete dislocation of the vertebral segments secondary to the complete disruption of both the anterior and the posterior longitudinal ligament (Fig. 6.24).

DISTRACTIVE EXTENSION INJURIES

The major vector of extension may be coupled with a minor distractive vector usually caused by a blow to the face or chin. It is not uncommon for the patient to present with lacerations on his or her face. The facial injury should alert the examiner to the possibility of cervical trauma.

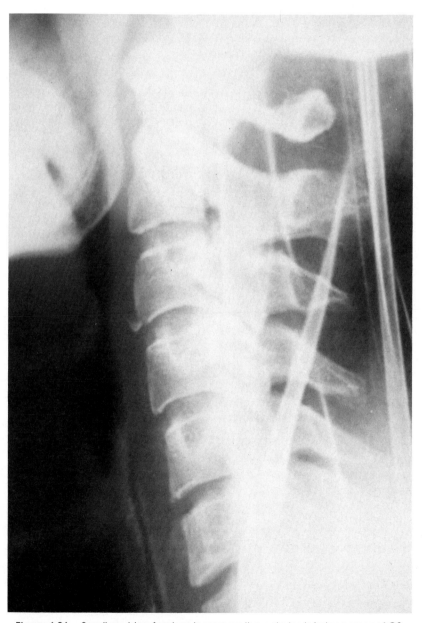

Figure 6.26.   Small avulsion fracture is seen on the anterior-inferior corner of C3.

The majority of extension injuries involve the soft tissue rather than the osseous structures. The hyperextension forces do not confine themselves to the paravertebral ligament. Injuries to the trachea and esophagus have also been reported. Two stages of distractive extension have been classified.

Distractive Extension Stage 1

Distractive extension stage 1 injuries demonstrate as failure of the anterior longitudinal ligament. There is often damage of the disc at the point of ligamentous rupture. The changes may be subtle. Some cases may only demonstrate a lucent cleft at the anterior border of the affected level (Fig. 6.25A and B). More severe stage 1 injuries may widen the entire anterior border of the affected area.

This vacuum phenomenon or lucent cleft sign should not be mistaken for the nitrogen that accumulates within the clefts of degenerative discs. The clefts are usually located within the center of the discs, whereas the vacuum phenomenon arising from trauma is relegated to the anterior portion of the disc.

Fractures may also occur in stage 1 injuries. The majority of these are small avulsion fractures projecting off of the inferior vertebral corner (Fig. 6.26). Bleeding into the retropharyngeal space is to be expected. The posttraumatic alignment is good, with no posterior displacement of the vertebra demonstrated above the injured disc.

The presence of an avulsion fracture, as seen in Figure 6.26, must alert the physician to the possibility of hyperextension dislocation. Edeiken-Monroe et al. (27) conducted a study of hyperextension dislocations and found that each case demonstrated diffuse prevertebral swelling and normally aligned vertebrae. Sixty-five percent of these patients also presented with an avulsion fracture on the anterior-inferior corner that is wider than tall.

Distractive Extension Stage 2

Distractive extension stage 2 injuries demonstrate the same changes as stage 1

Table 6.1.
Cervical Spinal Canal Sizes as Determined by Eismont et al. (31)

Level	Average (mm)	Range (mm)
C1	23.9	17–29
C2	20.8	15–26
C3	18.5	14–23
C4	17.8	14–21
C5	17.8	14–22
C6	17.7	14–21
C7	17.9	14–22

injuries. The only difference is the posterior displacement of the vertebral body. On the neutral lateral view, the posterior movement rarely is more than 3 mm.

Neurological Effects

Fractures and dislocations of the cervical spine can have a wide variety of effects on the patient's neurological status. The findings may range from minimal nerve root symptoms to quadriplegia. It is often quite difficult to predict the patient's neurological status by using only the combined vector stages as guides. The major factor in these injuries is the size of the spinal canal, as it varies from person to person and directly correlates with the degree of injury.

Various studies that have sought to establish the normal limits of spinal canal size have been performed (28–31). Eismont et al. (31) conducted a retrospective study of 98 patients who suffered a closed cervical spine fracture or dislocation. Their findings concerning spinal canal sizes, which are listed in Table 6.1, are consistent with those from previous studies. Despite the varied factors that may affect the neurological status of the patient, Eismont et al. (31) found a strong and direct correlation between the size of the patient's spinal canal and the degree of damage suffered. For a complete discussion of the clinical presentation of neurological injuries, see Chapter 9.

Summary

1. Fractures of the cervical spine may be divided into those occurring in the upper and those occurring in the lower cervical areas. Upper cervical fractures are typically unstable because of the disruption of either the neural ring or the odontoid process. Lower cervical fractures may be either stable or unstable, depending on the degree of injury of the vertebral body.

2. The area of damage to the lower cervical spine, either anterior or posterior longitudinal ligament, is totally dependent upon the major and minor vectors of forces applied during the accident.

3. The atlas, due to its unusual shape and function, is particularly susceptible to a variety of dislocations. An atlas fracture is usually of the burst configuration.

References

1. Walter J, Doris P, Shaffer M: Clinical presentation of patients with acute cervical spine injury. *Emerg Med* 13(7):512–515, 1984.
2. Murray GC, Persellin RH: Cervical fractures complicating ankylosing spondylitis: a report of eight cases and a review of the literature. *Am Med* 70:1033–1041, 1981.
3. Foo D, Bignami A, Rossier AB: Two spinal cord lesions in a patient with ankylosing spondylitis and cervical spine injury. *Neurology* 33:245–249, 1983.
4. Scher AT: Unrecognized fractures and dislocations of the cervical spine. *Paraplegia* 19:25–30, 1981.
5. Allen BL, Ferguson RL, Lehmann TR, O'Brien RP: A mechanistic classification of closed indirect fractures and dislocations of the lower cervical spine. *Spine* 7(1):1–27, 1982.
6. Spencer AJ, Yeakley JW, Kaufman HH: Fracture of the occipital condyle. *Neurosurgery* 15(1):101–103, 1984.
7. Roda JM, Gastro A, Blazquez M: Hangman's fracture with complete dislocation of C2-C3. *J Neurosurg* 60:633–635, 1984.
8. Suss RA, Zimmerman RD, Leeds NE: Pseudospread of atlas. False sign of the Jefferson fracture in children. *AJR* 140:1079, 1983.
9. Kahanovitz N, Mehringer MC, Johanson PH: Intercranial entrapment of the atlas complicating an untreated fracture of the posterior arch of the atlas. *J Bone Joint Surg* 63A(5):831–832, 1981.
10. Powers B, Miller M, Kramer R, Martinez S, Gehweiler J: Traumatic anterior atlanto-occipital dislocation. *Neurosurgery* 4(1):12–17, 1979.
11. Cloward RB: Progressive idiopathic anterior dislocation of the upper cervical spine with severe myelopathy. *Surg Neurol* 21:579–587, 1984.
12. Peuschel SM, Scola FH, Perry C, Pezzulo JC: Atlantoaxial instability in children with Down's syndrome. *Pediatr Radiol* 10:129–132, 1982.
13. Redlund-Johnell I: Posterior atlantoaxial dislocation in rheumatoid arthritis. *Scand J Rheumatol* 13:337–341, 1984.
14. Vilppula AH, Jussila TU, Kukko AM: Atlantoaxial dislocation in an 18 year old female with *Yersinia* arthritis. *Clin Rheumatol* 3(2):239–241, 1984.
15. Moilanen A, Yli-Kerrtula U, Vilppula A: Cervical spine involvements in Reiter's syndrome. *ROFO* 141(1):84–87, 1984.

16a. Jamshidi S, Dennis M, Azzam C, Karim N: Traumatic posterior dislocation without neurological deficit: case report. *Neurosurgery* 12(3):211–212,, 1983.
16b. Anderson LD, D'Alonzo RT: Fractures of the odontoid process of the axis. *J Bone Joint Surg* 56A:1663, 1974.
17. Rothman RH, Simeone FA (eds): *The Spine*. Philadelphia, WB Saunders, 1975.
18. Selecki BR, Williams HBL: *Injuries to the Cervical Spine and Cord in Man*, Australian Medical Association, Mervyn Archdall medical monograph no 7. New South Wales, Australian Medical Publishing, 1970.
19. Levine AM, Edwards CC: Treatment of injuries in the C1/C2 complex. *Orthop Clin North Am* 17(1):31–44, 1986.
20. Schatzker J, Rorabeck CH, Waddell JP: Fractures of the dens (odontoid process): an analysis of 37 cases. *J Bone Joint Surg* 53B:392, 1971.
21. Gallie WE: Fractures and dislocations of the cervical spine. *Am J Surg* 46:495–499, 1939.
22. Harris JH Jr, Burke JT, Ray RD, Nichols-Hostetter S, Lester R: Low (type III) odontoid fractures: a new radiologic sign. *Radiology* 153:353–356, 1984.
23. O'Brien P, Schweigel J, Thompson W: Dislocations of the lower cervical spine. *Trauma* 22(8):710–714, 1982.
24. Pick R, Segal D: C7-T1 bilateral facet dislocation. A rare lesion presenting with the syndrome of the acute anterior spinal cord injury. *Clin Ortho Rel Res* 150:131–135, 1980.
25. Bauze RJ, Ardran GM: Experimental production of forward dislocation in the human cervical spine. *J Bone Joint Surg* 60B(2):239–245, 1978.
26. Woodring JH, Goldstein SJ: Fractures of the articular processes of the cervical spine. *AJNR* 139:341–344, 1982.
27. Edeiken-Monroe B, Wagner LK, Harris JH Jr: Hyperextension dislocation of the cervical spine. *AJR* 146(4):803–808, 1986.
28. Hasimoto I, Tak YK: The true sagittal diameter of the cervical spinal canal and its diagnostic significance in cervical myelopathy. *Neurosurgery* 47:912–916, 1977.
29. Payne EE, Spillane JD: The cervical spine—an anatomical study of 70 specimens (using a special technique) with particular reference to the problem of cervical spondylosis. *Brain* 80:571–596, 1957.
30. Wolf BS, Khilnani M, Malis L: The sagittal diameter of the cervical spine with spondylosis. *J Mt Sinai Hosp* 23:283–292, 1956.
31. Eismont F, Clifford S, Goldberg M, Green B: Cervical sagittal spinal canal size in spine injury. *Spine* 9(7):663–666, 1984.

7

Developmental Anatomy

ARTHUR C. CROFT, DC, MS, DABCO

"You should show first the spine of the neck with its tendons like the mast of a ship with its shrouds without the head; then make the head with its tendons which give it its motion upon its axis."

Leonardo da Vinci (1452–1519)

Anatomy of Embryonic and Early Childhood Musculoskeletal System

After fertilization, the successful zygote becomes loosely embedded into the nurturing wall of the endometrium in preparation for a rather extensive ontogeny—one that, as my professor of zoology once said, "neatly recapitulates phylogeny." After several cell divisions, the zygote becomes known as a morula. Continuing this rapid development, the morula then passes into the stage during which it is known as the blastocyst, at about 5 days of life. The early blastocyst is purely unilaminar and still lies attached in the uterine cavity. By the seventh day, implantation into the uterine wall has occurred.

Two weeks after fertilization, a now bilaminar embryonic disc forms. This disc consists of two distinct layers: ectodermal on the dorsal side and entodermal on the ventral side. At the caudal end of the embryo, a primitive groove forms, and cells from the rostral end of this groove in an area known as the primitive node begin to invaginate into the groove and separate the entoderm and ectoderm to form a new layer, the mesoderm. This new layer then condenses to form the notochord. As this occurs, the ectodermal layer is rapidly folding into a neural tube and primitive brain (Fig. 7.1).

Adjacent to the notochord, mesodermal tissue begins to form segmented somites or metameres, which are now visible through the thin ectodermal covering (Fig. 7.2). These somites continue to form in a craniocaudal direction until eventually 42–45 pairs are present. They represent early body segmentation and ultimately will differentiate into bone, muscle, and skin. The cells

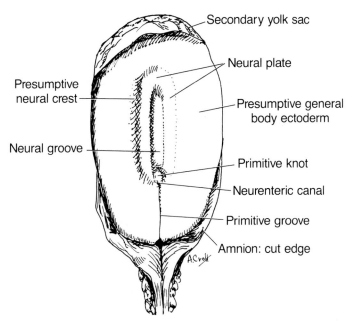

Figure 7.1. Human embryo at about 3 weeks. The amnioembryonic vesicle has been opened to illustrate early stages of differentiation. (Adapted from Warwick R, Williams PL: *Gray's Anatomy*, Br ed 35. Philadelphia, WB Saunders, 1973, p 82.)

of the ventromedial portion of the somite become mesenchymous and migrate medially. They are destined to become the axial skeleton and are referred to appropriately as the sclerotome (from the Greek *sclero* meaning hard). The dorsolateral cells of the somite make up the dermatome and eventually become the dermis. The medial aspect is made up of spindle-shaped cells known as the myotome. These will become the striated muscle of the body (Fig. 7.3).

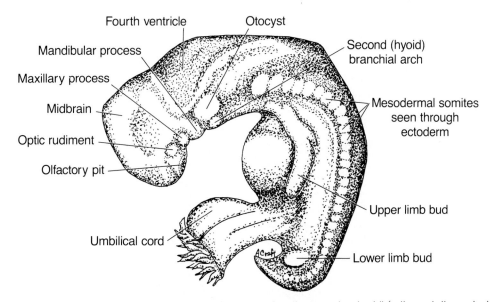

Figure 7.2. Human embryo at the end of the fifth week. Somites are clearly visible through the ectoderm (Adapted from Warwick R, Williams PL: *Gray's Anatomy*, Br ed 35. Philadelphia, WB Saunders, 1973, p 122.)

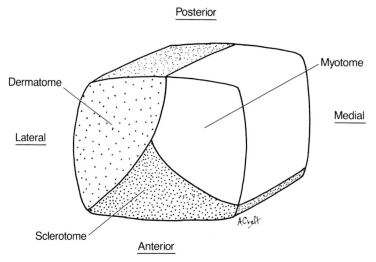

Figure 7.3. Schematic representation of the somite. Eventually 42–45 pairs of somites will differentiate into sclerotome, myotome, and dermatome, making up the bone, muscle, and skin, respectively, of the developing embryo.

VERTEBRAE

The skeletal development passes through two stages. The first is the blastemal stage characterized by a mesenchymal condensation. The second is a cartilaginous stage in which chondrification occurs, replacing the mesenchymal cells. This cartilaginous vertebral column is later ossified. In some bones (e.g., facial and cranial bones), this intermediate step does not occur.

The earliest "skeleton" is formed by the notochord which is covered with a notochordal sheath and is nonsegmented, run-

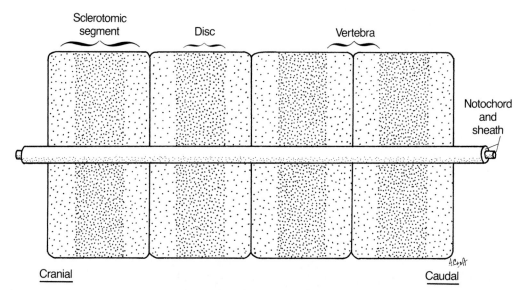

Figure 7.4. Schematic representation of the developing spinal column. Proliferating sclerotomal cells migrate medially and engulf the notochord. The sclerotome divides to form the vertebrae and the intervertebral discs, with the vertebrae being formed by two adjacent segments. (Adapted from Warwick R, Williams PL: *Gray's Anatomy*, Br ed 35. Philadelphia, WB Saunders, 1973, p 111.)

ning rostrally beyond the limits of the future bony spine as far as the hypophysis and eventually becoming part of the occiput and the sphenoid. This notochordal skeleton is later engulfed by the proliferation of sclerotomal cells that migrate medially and ventrally, eventually surrounding the notochord. Still segmented, these sclerotomic segments eventually separate into two parts. The cephalad portion of one sclerotomic segment and the caudad portion of another will fuse to form the centrum or body of a vertebra, whereas the central portion of each sclerotome will become the intervertebral disc. Within each disc the residual notochord expands to form the nucleus pulposus that, under normal conditions, is all that remains of the original notochord (Fig. 7.4).

By end of the eighth week, the process of chondrification is complete and the final stage, ossification, begins. For practical purposes, the cervical vertebrae may be categorized as either typical or atypical. C3–C6 are considered the "typical" vertebrae, whereas the atlas, axis, and C7 are considered "atypical" vertebrae.

The typical vertebra is ossified from three primary ossification centers located in the centrum and at each root of the transverse processes. The process of ossification then proceeds outward from the centrum, forward into the pedicles, backward into the laminae and spinous process, upward and downward into the articular facets, and lat-

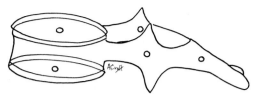

Figure 7.6.   Five secondary ossification centers (*circles*) appear in the cartilagenous portions of the typical vertebrae at puberty. These occur at both epiphyseal plates, the tip of each transverse process, and the tip of each spinous process.

erally into the transverse processes (Fig. 7.5). These centers first appear in the cervical vertebrae.

The primary ossification center in the centrum is, at times, actually two centers. When one fails to develop, a wedge-shaped vertebra and consequent spinal curvature result.

At puberty, five secondary ossification centers appear in the cartilaginous portions of the vertebrae: one in the tip of each transverse process, one in each epiphyseal plate of the body superiorly and inferiorly, and one at the tip of the spinous process (Fig. 7.6). If two secondary ossification centers are present in the spinous process, the process will develop bifid (Fig. 7.7).

The *atlas* is generally formed from three centers. The first two appear in early fetal life and are situated in the area of the lateral masses. These develop anteriorly and posteriorly, ultimately fusing in the posterior arch at about age 3 or 4 years. At the end of the first year of life, a third center ap-

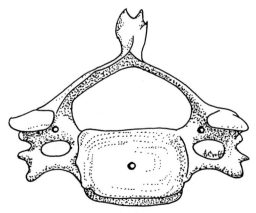

Figure 7.5.   The typical vertebra is ossified from three primary centers which are located in the centrum and at the roots of the transverse processes (*circles*).

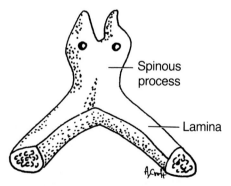

Spinous process

Lamina

Figure 7.7.   Lamina and spinous process of typical cervical vertebra. A bifid spinous process is the result of two separate ossification centers at the spinous process (*circles*).

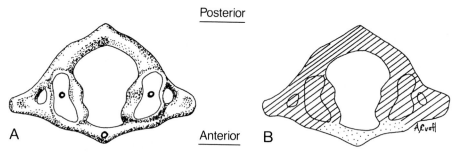

Posterior

Anterior

Figure 7.8. Three ossification centers of the atlas vertebra (C1) (*circles* in **A**). Those of the lateral masses eventually unite at the posterior arch, contributing the *shaded area* in **B**. The *stippled area* in **B** represents the contribution of the anterior arch ossification center.

pears in the anterior arch and grows outward to meet the original two (Fig. 7.8).

The *axis* (C2) is formed from five primary and two secondary centers. Early in uterine life, two centers are formed in the neural arch, as is seen in the typical vertebra. By about 5 months, another center becomes active in the centrum—again characteristic of a typical vertebra. Shortly thereafter, two additional centers form in the dens (which actually represents the centrum of the atlas) (Fig. 7.9). These centers develop in a cephalad direction and meet the first of two secondary centers which forms around the second year of life. This ossification center is frequently visible as a horizontal line on x-ray films and may be seen in children as late as age 11 years. In trauma cases, this must be distinguished from fracture and, when present, is usually referred to as the "ossiculum terminale" (Fig. 7.10). If this ossification center persists into adult life, it is known as the "os odontoideum" and, although at one time thought to be quite

rare, has been reported with greater frequency in recent years (1), especially in comorbid conditions such as Down's syndrome, Klippel-Feil syndrome, Morquio's syndrome, and spondyloepiphyseal dysplasia. Os odontoideum must be distinguished from fracture. This condition usually results in atlantoaxial instability (Fig. 7.11).

A broad cartilaginous band separates the body or centrum of the axis from the dens. This corresponds to the "intervertebral disc" and is referred to as the "subchondral synchondrosis." It usually disappears (ossifies) by age 3 years, but a thin radiolucent line simulating a fracture may persist into early adolescence, and the center may remain cartilaginous until advanced age. This occurs in about one third of normal adults (2) (Fig. 7.12). The other secondary ossification center of the axis forms as an epiphyseal plate at the caudad portion of the body of the vertebra (Fig. 7.9).

In the *seventh cervical vertebra*, separate

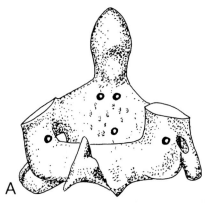
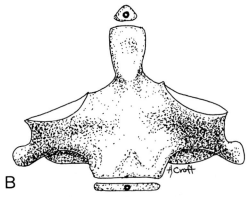

Figure 7.9. The axis vertebra (C2) is formed from five primary ossification centers (*circles* in **A**) and two secondary ossification centers (*circles* in **B**).

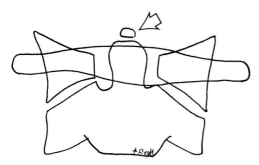

Figure 7.10. Line drawing illustrating the radiographic appearance of the ossiculum terminale (*arrow*). A normal finding in children under age 11 years, it must be differentiated from fracture in trauma cases.

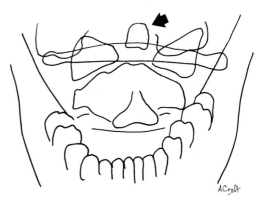

Figure 7.11. Line drawing illustrating the radiographic appearance of the os odontoideum (*arrow*). This developmental anomaly may be associated with atlantoaxial instability and must be distinguished from fracture in trauma cases.

ossification centers form the costal processes. If these ossification centers fail to unite, they may grow anteriorly and laterally, forming cervical ribs (Fig. 7.13). In Figure 7.14, the relative contributions of the various portions or primary ossification centers of the typical cervical vertebra are indicated.

In general, the secondary ring ossification centers or epiphyseal discs fuse with the primary centers by age 25 years. The central portion of the cartilaginous endplate does not ossify but remains cartilaginous.

As development continues into adult life, further notable changes take place. By early childhood, the original notochordal cells that went to make up the nucleus pulposus

are beginning to be replaced by fibrocartilage. By age 12 years, this process is said to be complete, and as time passes, the gelatinous matrix of the nucleus is gradually replaced with a dense, relatively desiccated and less resilient fibrocartilage. This is now less resistant to injury.

The cervical spine joints of Luschka (also known as the uncovertebral joints) lie at the margins of the vertebral bodies. These true joints begin to form in late adolescence or early adulthood. They may be developmental and are thought to be associated with the normal aging process. Extensive fissuring in the disc spaces is often associated with these joints of Luschka, and as

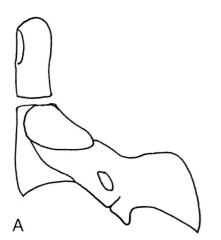

A

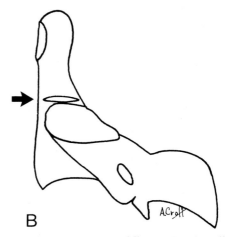

B

Figure 7.12. The subchondral synchondrosis separates the centrum of the axis (C2) from the dens (**A**). It usually ossifies in the child by age 3 years but may persist into adulthood as a cartilaginous remnant (*arrow* in **B**).

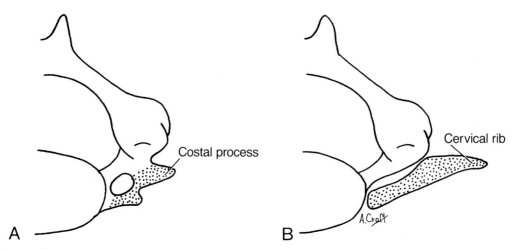

Figure 7.13. In the seventh cervical vertebra, a separate ossification center forms the costal process (*stippled area* in **A**). When these centers fail to unite with other centers, a cervical rib may be formed (*stippled area* in **B**).

aging proceeds, so do the degenerative changes. This process is accelerated by injury or disease (3) (Fig. 7.15).

MUSCLES

`All striated muscle is derived from the myotome, except for some muscles of the head and neck and the limb buds. In the head, the tensor tympani, tensor veli palatini, and masticatory muscles (including the mylohyoid and anterior belly of the digastric) are derived from the mandibular arch. These muscles are supplied by the mandibular branch of the trigeminal nerve. The stapedius, stylohyoid, digastric (posterior belly), facial and epicranial, platysma, and auricular muscles are derived from the hyoid arch and are supplied by the facial nerve. The musculature of the pharynx, larynx, and soft palate form from the remaining arches and are supplied by the glossopharyngeal and vagus nerves.

Limb buds begin to appear early in the embryo in the latter part of the fourth week. The upper extremities predate the lower in their development by a short period of time—perhaps 3 days. The musculature of the extremities is developed in situ from a small proliferating mass of mesenchyme. There is no myotomic mesodermal migration into the limb bud once it is formed.

As the limbs take form, flexion creases develop at the elbow and wrist and at the knee and ankle. After the eighth week, the limbs, having attained the fetal position, begin to rotate so that in the upper extremity the preaxial border becomes lateral and the ventral surface becomes anterior. In the lower extremity the reverse is true: The preaxial border rotates medially, turning the dorsal surface to face anteriorly. The cutaneous nerve supply to the extremities

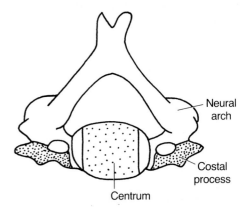

Figure 7.14. Line drawing illustrating the relative contributions of various portions of primary ossification centers in the typical cervical vertebra. The *lightly stippled area* is from the centrum, the *heavily stippled area* is from the costal processes, and the *unshaded area* is from the neural arches. (Adapted from Warwick R, Williams PL: *Gray's Anatomy*, Br ed 35. Philadelphia, WB Saunders, 1973, p 111.)

can largely be explained by this limb rotation phenomenon, in that the innervation to the lateral aspect of the upper extremity (which is the preaxial border) is derived from the upper segments of the brachial plexus, whereas the more medial border innervation comes from the lower brachial plexus.

In the rest of the axial skeleton, the myotome divides into both posterior and anterior parts which are then innervated by posterior and anterior rami, respectively, of their corresponding spinal nerve. The former remains posterolateral to the spinal column, and the latter migrates anteriorly (Fig. 7.16). Migration distance may be quite significant, such that muscles derived from anterior myotomal mesoderm, e.g., the serratus posterior, may have posterior attachments but receive their innervation from the anterior primary rami (Fig. 7.17). Originally, the paraspinal muscles of the neck and back are strictly segmental and run only from one vertebra to the next. As development proceeds, however, these individual muscle segments begin to fuse together and organize into much larger, longer, and more complex muscle groups which eventually become multilayered.

Tendons develop independently in mesenchyme and are connected with muscles only secondarily.

SKIN

The dermis is derived from the somatic layer of mesoderm as well as from the dorsolateral aspects of the mesodermal somites (Fig. 7.16). The epidermis along with

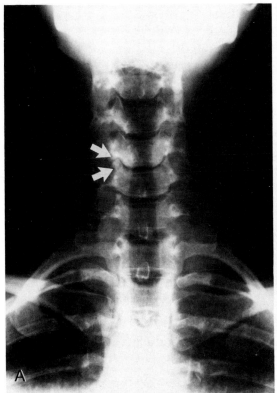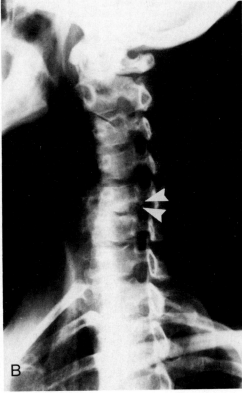

Figure 7.15. The joints of Luschka or the uncovertebral joints appear to be developmental. Degenerative changes parallel the aging process and are accelerated by injury or disease. This patient sustained an acceleration/deceleration injury 5 years prior to these films and manifests typical posttraumatic degenerative changes. At the joints of Luschka, exuberant, proliferative bony growth can be seen along with marked subchondral sclerosis (*arrows* in **A**) and consequent neuroforaminal encroachment (*arrowheads* in **B**).

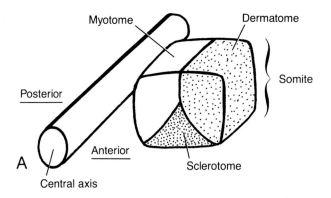

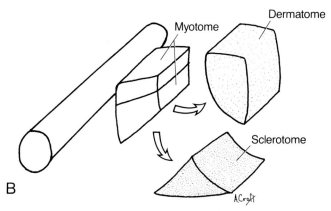

Figure 7.16. **A.** Primitive somite illustrated in relation to the central axis. **B** and **C.** As its constituent parts begin to differentiate and migrate, the myotome divides into posterior and anterior segments. **D.** These become innervated by posterior and anterior primary rami, respectively.

its specialized components, such as hair, nails, sweat glands, and sebaceous glands, originates from the ectoderm.

JOINTS

In the early stages of development, the axial and peripheral skeleton exist only as condensed, nonsegmented, amorphous masses of mesoderm. From within these aggregations of cells, individual centers are formed. These are the early chondrification and ossification centers that rapidly begin to shape and form the skeletal structures of cartilage and bone, respectively.

As this development proceeds, small rests of mesenchymal cells fail to undergo bony or cartilaginous metamorphosis and persist as plates of "interzonal mesenchyme" interposing between adjacent skel-

etal structures. These plates will form the future joint—be it fibrous, synchondrosis, symphysis, or synovial (Fig. 7.18).

All joint components will spring from this interzonal mesenchyme, including fibrous connective tissue, hyaline cartilage, or synovium (depending on the type of joint involved). Other intraarticular structures, such as tendons, ligaments, discs, and menisci, are probably also derived from this tissue.

SPINAL CORD AND NERVE ROOTS

As the embryo develops, certain other structures, which are illustrated in Figure 7.19, begin to form. These include the neural plate and adjacent cells that will become the neural crest. The notochordal plate lies beneath the neural groove which is seen in

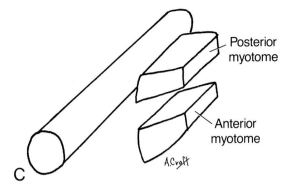

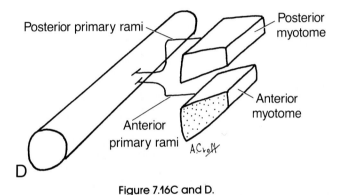

Figure 7.16C and D.

the midline of the neural plate. As development proceeds, the neural groove deepens and its dorsal edges begin to fold up and around, eventually meeting at the top and forming the neural tube with its central canal. This formation begins toward the end of the third week and is complete by the end of the fourth week.

The neural crest cells eventually migrate laterally to become the dorsal root ganglia. Virtually all of the sensory cells of the peripheral nervous system (both somatic and visceral) are derived from the neural crest. The cell bodies are located outside of the central nervous system.

The neural tube exists in a trilaminar form composed of ependymal, mantle, and marginal layers (Fig. 7.20). The ventral spinal nerve roots are formed by the anterior migration of axons from the anterior gray column within the mantle layer. These axons will form both the alpha efferent system, innervating the striated extrafusal muscle fibers, and the gamma efferent system, which has the intrafusal muscle fibers of the muscle spindles as its end organ.

The autonomic nervous system in the thoracic, lumbar and midsacral regions is formed by a segment of mantle layer in the dorsal part of the basal lamina. Laterally, a long group of cells initially becomes visible as a primary sympathetic trunk and later organizes into sympathetic chain ganglia. Axons from the lateral column follow the ventral root and then, via the white rami communicantes, enter the sympathetic ganglia. The basic organization is illustrated in Figure 7.21.

The combined spinal nerve is composed of both a ventral (motor) and dorsal (sensory) root. The ventral root grows out from the mantle layer, through the marginal layer

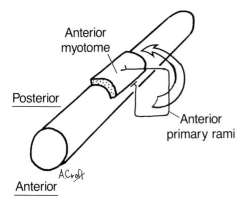

Figure 7.17. Some muscles derived from the anterior myotome segments migrate posteriorly, taking their anterior primary rami with them.

and external limiting membrane to enter the myotome at that level.

Anatomy of Adult Musculoskeletal System

BONE

The *skull* is usually composed of 22 bones. All but the mandible are firmly fused together. Of these 22 bones, 15 are said to belong to the cranium, and 7, to the face. The apex of the skull or cranium is known as the vertex, the back of the head is known as the occiput, the forehead is known as the frons, and the sides of the head are known as the tempora. The terms used to describe some other anatomical landmarks are indicated in Figure 7.22.

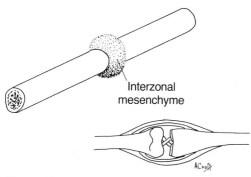

Figure 7.18. Various types of joints develop from interposing rests of mesenchymal cells known as interzonal mesenchyme. A synovial joint is illustrated.

The muscular attachments to the base of the skull necessary for this discussion are identified in Figure 7.23. Note that several muscles have purposely been omitted in this figure, including the tensor veli palatini, levator veli palatini, pterygoids, and masseter.

The cervical vertebrae can be categorized as either typical or atypical. The "typical" vertebrae comprise C3–C6, and the "atypical" vertebrae comprise C1, C2, and C7.

The C3–C6 vertebrae are made up of a heavier cylindrical axial support segment known as the *body*. The superior and inferior surfaces of this body are covered by cartilaginous endplates. Attached posteriorly to the body are two stout projections of bone known as *pedicles* which fuse with the two posterior *laminae* to form an enclosed protective arch known as the *vertebral arch*. The space inside the arch is referred to as the vertebral foramen, and when successive vertebrae are considered as a unit, this space is referred to as the vertebral canal. The canal encloses and protects the spinal cord and spinal nerves.

Several projections emanate from the vertebral arch. These serve as attachments for various muscle groups which act as levers for cervical spine motion. Projecting posteriorly from the fused laminae is the *spinous process*. Typically, spinous processes are short and bifid in nature. The *transverse processes* project laterally from the union of pedicle and laminae. These processes contain the *transverse foramen* through which the vertebral artery passes. In the cervical spine, these processes are actually compound, being formed by the union of the *posterior root* or *tubercle*, which is the true transverse process, and the *anterior root* or *tubercle*, which is the homolog of the rib. These roots are joined by the *costotransverse bar*. Projecting upward from the upper border of the laminae on each side are the *superior articular processes* (superior zygapophyses), and projecting below this border are the *inferior articular processes* (inferior zygapophyses). The union of these joints on adjacent vertebrae (i.e., the superior articular process of one vertebra articulating with the inferior articular process of the vertebra above) form synovial joints generally referred to as *facet joints* or *zygapophyseal joints*. The pedicles do not approximate the superoinferior dimension of the vertebral body as do the laminae. This is due to a shallow superior and deep inferior *ver-* *tebral incisure* which, when two vertebrae are attached, forms a potential space known as the *intervertebral foramen* (Fig. 7.24).

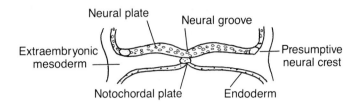

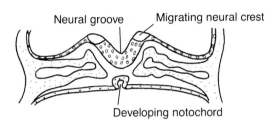

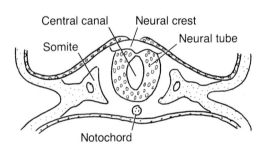

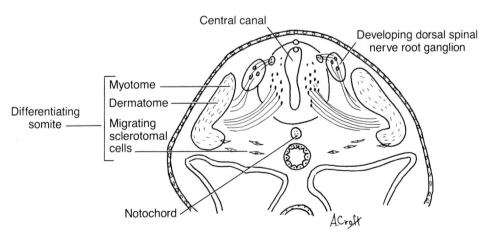

Figure 7.19. This series of schematic drawings illustrates important stages in the formation of the neural axis and mesenchymal structures. (Adapted from Warwick R, Williams PL: *Gray's Anatomy*, Br ed 35. Philadelphia, WB Saunders, 1973, p 84.)

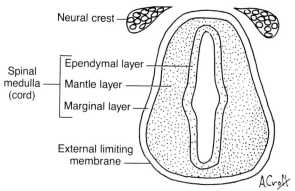

Figure 7.20. The completed neural tube is trilaminar, consisting of ependymal, mantle, and marginal layers. (Adapted from Crelin ES: *Ciba Clinical Symposia: Development of the Nervous System* (reprint). Summit, NJ, Ciba-Geigy, 1974, vol 26, no 2, p 24.)

Normally, two adjacent vertebrae are attached by four types of joints: the uncovertebral joints, the facet joints, the fibrous joints between laminae and spinous processes, and the fibrocartilaginous joint composed of the *intervertebral disc* which, while allowing a stable but extensive motion between the attached vertebrae, firmly unites them.

The first cervical vertebra is known as the *atlas*. It lacks a body but has an *anterior* and a *posterior arch*. At the ventralmost part of the anterior arch is the *anterior tubercle* to which are attached both ligaments and muscles.

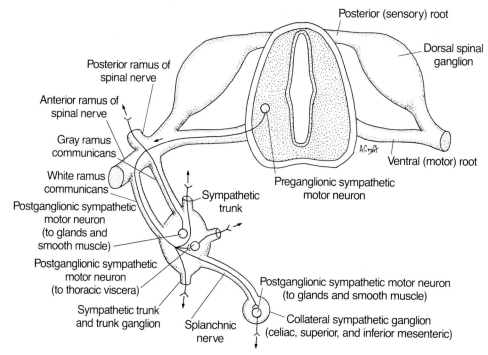

Figure 7.21. Organization of the sympathetic nervous system of the spinal cord, spinal nerves, and chain ganglia at 5–7 weeks of development. (Adapted from Crelin ES: *Ciba Clinical Symposia: Development of the Nervous System* (reprint). Summit, NJ, Ciba-Geigy, 1974, vol 26, no 2, p 25.)

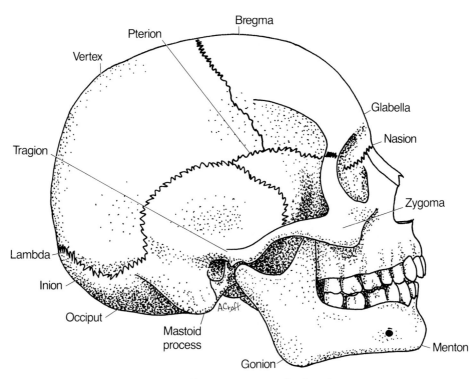

Figure 7.22.   Landmarks on the head.

Similarly, a *posterior tubercle* exists at the dorsalmost part of the posterior arch. This also serves as attachment for ligaments and muscles. Behind the anterior arch lies the *fovea dentis* or facet for articulating with the dens. The transverse processes are wider at this level than throughout the remainder of the cervical spine, with the exception of C7. In adult Caucasian men, this width varies from about 74 to 99 mm, and in adult Caucasian women, it ranges from 65 to 76 mm. This measurement is often useful in determining the sex of human remains not readily identifiable. The transverse process of the atlas contains a transverse foramen through which the vertebral artery runs to pass superiorly and posteriorly to the lateral masses and then over the posterior arch, creating a shallow sulcus known as the *groove* or *sulcus for the vertebral artery*. The first cervical spinal nerve lies between the artery and the bone in this groove (Fig. 7.25). The *arcuate foramen* (sometimes referred to as the posticus ponticulus or posterior ponticulus) is formed by calcification of the atlantooccipatal liga-

ments and appears as a crescent-shaped bone projecting from the superior aspect of the posterior arch of the atlas to the occiput. Through this foramen pass the vertebral arteries. These foramen may be incomplete and are a normal variant.

The *axis* or second cervical vertebra has an *odontoid process* or *dens* projecting cephalad from its body. This again is the rudiment of the body of the atlas. The superior articulating surfaces are mounted directly atop the body and pedicles, so it has no real superior articular processes. The configuration of these facets allows for a tremendous amount of rotation of the head on the neck, hence the name "axis." Also because of this arrangement, the second cervical spinal nerve emerges from behind the facet joint at this level, rather than in front of the facet joint, as is seen at all lower levels. The laminae here are thicker than those at any other level in the cervical spine and fuse posteriorly to form a large and prominent spinous process which serves as an important attachment of muscles, as is discussed later (Fig. 7.26).

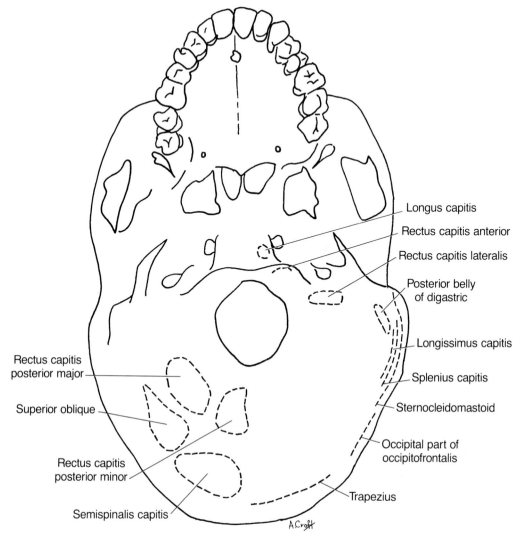

Figure 7.23.   Muscular attachments to the base of the skull. Several muscles have been omitted.

MUSCLE

For practical purposes, the neck can be divided into anterior and posterior halves. It can also be divided into anterior and posterior triangles along with several subsidiary triangles (Fig. 7.27).

In the superficial anterior portion of the neck, the *platysma muscle* is the cervical equivalent of the facial muscles. Its action is not important for this discussion, however. Deep to this lie the *suprahyoid muscles*, which include the stylohyoid, mylohyoid, and digastric muscles, and the *infrahyoid* or *strap*

muscles, which include the sternohyoid, omohyoid, sternothyroid, and thyrohyoid (Fig. 7.27A). These muscles act to move the larynx, tongue, hyoid bone, and mandible.

The *sternocleidomastoid muscle* arises from the sternum and from the clavicle and travels obliquely upward and posteriorly to insert into the mastoid process of the skull (Fig. 7.27B). Innervated by the eleventh cranial nerve (the accessory nerve), it serves as a powerful flexor of the neck, when both sides contract together, and as a lateral flexor of the neck and rotator of the skull, when acting alone.

Deep to the sternocleidomastoid mus-

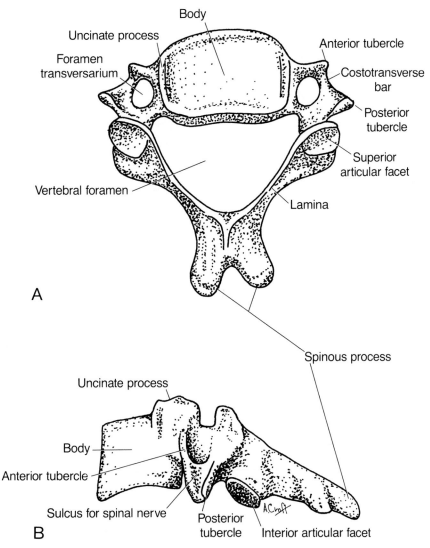

Figure 7.24. Landmarks of the typical cervical vertebra. **A.** Superior aspect. **B.** Inferior aspect. (Adapted from Warwick R, Williams PL: *Gray's Anatomy*, Br ed 35. Philadelphia, WB Saunders, 1973, p 234.)

cles lies the *scalene group* consisting of an anterior, middle, and posterior component. This group of muscles originates on the transverse processes and inserts into the first and second ribs. The *middle scalene* is usually the largest, and between it and the *anterior scalene* run the brachial plexus and subclavian artery. The *posterior scalene* is usually quite small. Occasionally, a very small *scalenus minimus* exists between the anterior and the middle scalene and may be responsible for certain compression neurop-

athies at the level of the brachial plexus (Fig. 7.28).

The *longus colli* and *longus capitis* run deep in the anterior cervical spine, bound closely to the anterior ventral bodies and transverse processes. They are flexors of the head and neck (Fig. 7.28). The *rectus capitis anterior* and *lateralis* arise from the lateral mass and the transverse process of the atlas, respectively, and insert into the basilar part of the occipital bone. The rectus capitis anterior serves as a flexor of the head, while

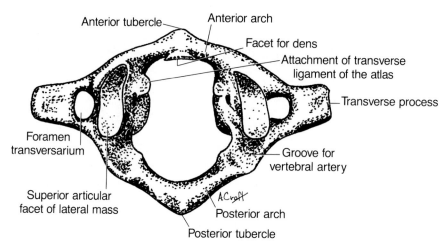

Figure 7.25. Anatomical landmarks of the atlas vertebra (C1). (Adapted from Warwick R, Williams PL: *Gray Anatomy*, Br ed 35. Philadelphia, WB Saunders, 1973, p 235.)

the rectus capitis lateralis serves as a lateral flexor of the head (to the same side) (Fig. 7.28).

In the posterior half of the neck, the *trapezius* is the most superficial muscle (remember there are two trapezius muscles). The trapezius originates from the superior nuchal line and the external occipital protuberance. It is attached to the ligamentum nuchae and, sweeping caudad, is further attached to the spinous processes of C7 and all of the thoracic vertebrae. From these points, the muscle runs laterally to its insertion on the clavicle, acromion, and spine of the scapula (Fig. 7.29). The *splenius capitis* and *splenius cervicis* arise from the

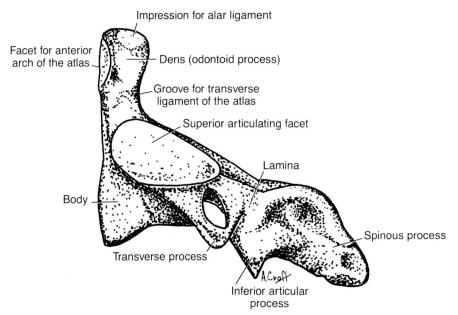

Figure 7.26. Anatomical landmarks of the axis vertebra (C2). (Adapted from Warwick R, Williams PL: *Gray's Anatomy*, Br ed 35. Philadelphia, WB Saunders, 1973, p 236.)

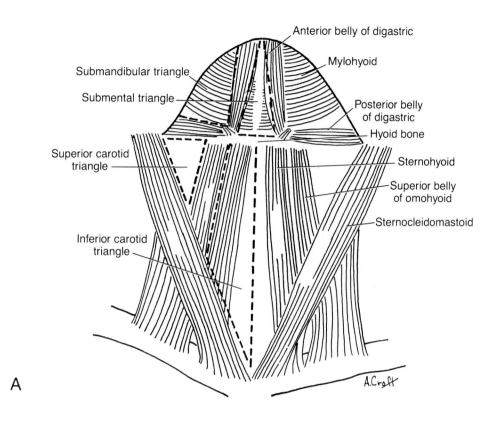

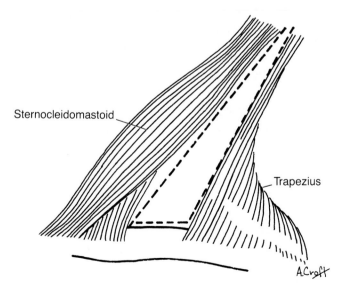

Figure 7.27.   **A.** Anterior triangle of the neck and its subsidiary triangles. **B.** Posterior triangle. (Adapted from Hollinshead WH: *Textbook of Anatomy*, ed 3. Philadelphia, Harper & Row, 1974, p 756.)

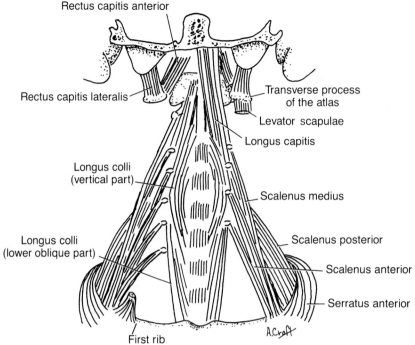

Figure 7.28.   Anterior and lateral muscles of the vertebral column. (Adapted from Warwick R, Williams PL: *Gray's Anatomy*, Br ed 35. Philadelphia, WB Saunders, 1973, p 509.)

ligamentum nuchae and spinous processes of the cervical and thoracic vertebrae and insert into the occipital and temporal bones and transverse processes of the upper cervical vertebrae, respectively (Fig. 7.30). Deep to the trapezius and sternocleidomastoid lies the *levator scapulae* with its origin on the transverse processes of the upper cervical vertebrae and its insertion into the superior angle of the scapula (Fig. 7.29).

The largest muscular system of the back is the *erector spinae* (formerly referred to as the *sacrospinalis*). It is represented by three major divisions: the *iliocostalis*, the *longissimus*, and the *spinalis*. These groups are further divided into subgroups. The uppermost part of the iliocostalis group, the *iliocostalis cervicis*, may insert as high as the seventh cervical vertebra, thus it is mentioned here. The rest of this group, however, is found below the level of the cervical spine (Fig. 7.30). The *longissimus cervicis* and *longissimus capitis* are both found in the cervical spine. The division of the longissimus cervicis runs from the transverse processes of the thoracic vertebrae to the

transverse processes of the cervical vertebrae, whereas the division of the longissimus capitis runs from transverse processes and articular processes to the mastoid processes of the temporal bone (Fig. 7.30). The smallest and most poorly defined division of the erector spinae is the spinalis group, of which only one, the *spinalis thoracis*, is relatively constant (Fig. 7.30).

The *transversospinalis muscles* are found deep to and medial to the erector spinae group and consist of the *semispinalis*, the *multifidi*, and the *rotatores* (or rotators, in English). The semispinalis group is subdivided into *thoracis*, *cervicis*, and *capitis*. These muscles are the largest of the transversospinalis muscles and span 4–6 vertebrae at a time. Muscles of the thoracis and cervicis, extend from transverse processes upward and medially to insert into the spinous processes, whereas those of the capitis division extend from transverse processes and articular processes to insert into the occiput.

Deep to the semispinalis run the *multifidi*. They run from the articular process of one vertebrae to the spinous process of the

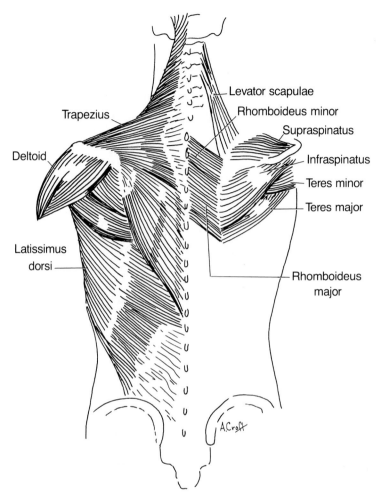

Trapezius

Deltoid

Latissimus dorsi

Levator scapulae

Rhomboideus minor

Supraspinatus

Infraspinatus

Teres minor

Teres major

Rhomboideus major

A.Croft

Figure 7.29. Posterior view of the superficial muscles of the back. Note that all receive innervation from cervical levels. (Adapted from Hollinshead WH: *Textbook of Anatomy*, ed 3. New York, Harper & Row, 1974, p 196.)

contiguous vertebra above or to the spinous process of two, three, or four vertebrae above (Fig. 7.31). Beneath the multifidi are found the *rotators* which are further subdivided into *long* and *short rotators*. The short rotators arise from the transverse process of a vertebra and insert into the spinous process of the vertebra above, whereas the long rotators insert into the vertebra two spaces above (Fig. 7.31). Unlike the multifidi, which tend to run together, each rotator has a distinct origin and insertion.

The small segmental muscles include the *intertransversarii* and the *interspinalis* (Fig. 7.32). The former are divided into anterior and posterior muscles.

The *suboccipital muscles* connect the atlas,

axis, and occiput posteriorly. This group consists of an *obliquus capitis inferior*, an *obliquus capitis superior*, a *rectus capitis posterior major*, and a *rectus capitis posterior minor*. The *suboccipital triangle* is formed by the obliquus capitis inferior, the rectus capitis posterior major, and the obliquus capitis superior (Fig. 7.33).

Movements of the head and neck can be categorized as flexion, extension, lateral flexion, and rotation. The following muscles are considered important in these motions:

Flexion

Longus capitis
Longus colli

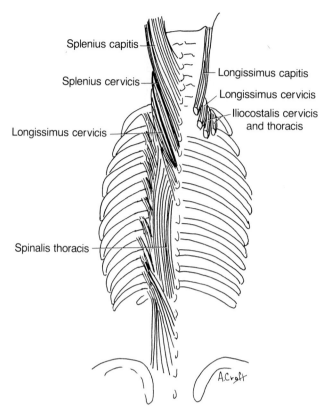

Figure 7.30. Posterior view of the deep muscles of the back. (Adapted from Hollinshead WH: *Textbook of Anatomy*, ed 3. New York, Harper & Row, 1974, p 327.)

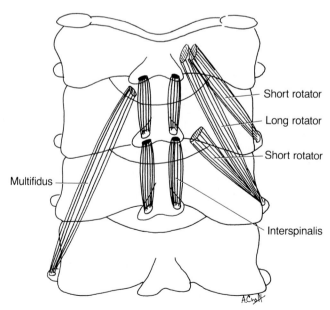

Figure 7.31. The rotator, interspinalis, and multifidus muscles of the cervical spine. The more superficial parts of the multifidus (illustrated) span two or three vertebrae. (Adapted from Hollinshead WH: *Textbook of Anatomy*, ed 3. New York, Harper & Row, 1974, p 332.)

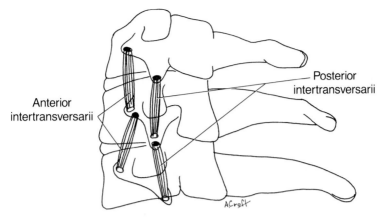

Figure 7.32. Lateral intersegmental muscles of the cervical spine. (Adapted from Hollinshead WH: *Textbook of Anatomy*, ed 3. New York, Harper & Row, 1974, p 332.)

Rectus capitis anterior
Sternocleidomastoid

Extension

Interspinalis
Longissimus capitis
Longissimus cervicis
Obliquus capitis superior
Rectus capitis posterior major
Rectus capitis posterior minor

Semispinalis capitis
Semispinalis cervicis
Splenius capitis
Splenius cervicis
Sternocleidomastoid
Trapezius

Rotation/Lateral Flexion

Iliocostalis cervicis
Intertransversarii

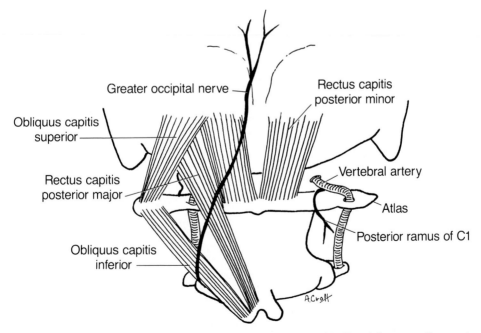

Figure 7.33. Suboccipital muscles. The suboccipital triangle is formed by the obliquus capitis superior, the rectus capitis posterior major, and the obliquus capitis inferior. (Adapted from Hollinshead WH: *Textbook of Anatomy*, ed 3. New York, Harper & Row, 1974, p 333.)

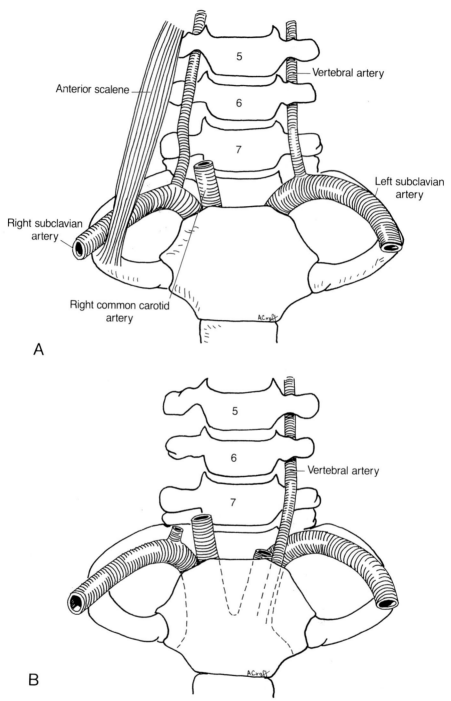

Figure 7.34. A and **B**. Some variations in the anatomy of the vertebral artery. (Adapted from Hollinshead WH: *Textbook of Anatomy,* ed 3. New York, Harper & Row, 1974, p 781.)

Levator scapulae	Obliquus capitis inferior	Splenius capitis
Longissimus capitis	Obliquus capitis superior	Splenius cervicis
Longus colli	Rectus capitis lateralis	Sternocleidomastoid
Multifidi	Scalene group	

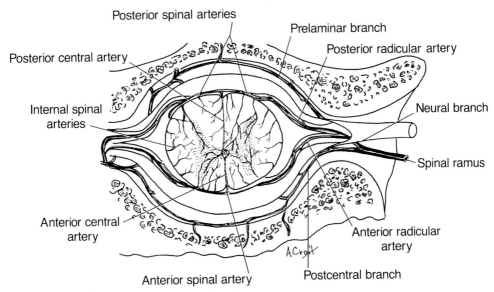

Figure 7.35.   Arterial supply of the spinal cord. (Adapted from Kaplan A: The central nervous system. In Netter FH (ed): *The Ciba Collection of Medical Illustrations*, vol I, *Nervous System*, ed 12. Summit, NJ, Ciba Pharmaceutical, 1977, p 53.)

VASCULAR ANATOMY

In the following discussion on the vascular anatomy of the cervical spine, only those aspects pertinent to cervical spine trauma are covered. For a more thorough discussion, see one of the standard textbooks on anatomy.

The *vertebral artery* arises from a posterosuperior position on the subclavian artery. The left side may arise from the arch of the aorta (9%). From here it runs cephalad and posteriorly to enter into the protective bony encasement of the vertebral column via the transverse foramen, usually at the level of the sixth cervical vertebra but occasionally at a higher level (it seldom enters at a lower level) (Fig. 7.34).

Once inside the transverse foramen, the vertebral artery courses upward through the cervical spine, finally emerging at the atlas just medial to the rectus capitis lateralis. From here it curves posteriorly and passes behind the lateral mass along with the ventral ramus of the first cervical nerve in the groove of the posterior arch. It then enters the vertebral canal beneath the posterior atlantooccipital membrane and, piercing the dura and arachnoid, runs medially to unite with the opposite artery to form the *basilar artery*. This union is usually at the lower border of the pons.

The upper spinal cord derives its blood supply from the vertebral artery as well as from individual spinal rami that enter each intervertebral foramen. As the vertebral artery enters the skull, it gives off branches which unite to form the *anterior spinal artery* which descends along the anterior aspect of the spinal cord. Wide variation in cord blood supply is the rule. The paired *posterior spinal arteries* are similarly formed from branches of the vertebral artery that originate at the level of the medulla oblongata. These arteries run down the posterior aspect of the spinal cord.

The *ascending cervical artery* is a branch of the *inferior thyroid artery*. Small branches of these arteries and of the vertebral arteries enter successive levels of the spinal canal through the intervertebral foramen. Here they branch into anterior and posterior rami: One runs cephalad and caudad, eventually anastomosing with adjacent levels to form two lateral chains on the posterior surfaces of the vertebral bodies; the other branches into anterior and posterior arteries that join the vertical-running anterior and posterior spinal arteries (Fig. 7.35). The spinal arteries and segmental branches that supply the spinal cord also serve as sources for the epidural connective tissue and nerve roots.

Just before forming the basilar artery, the

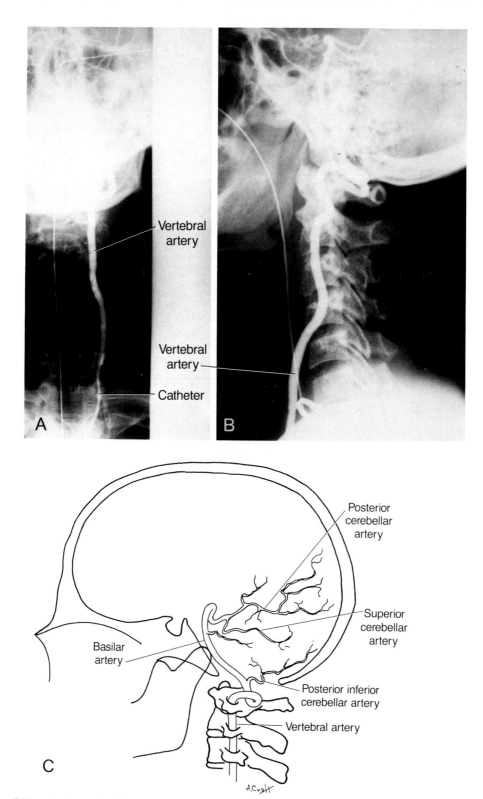

Figure 7.36. Angiography of the vertebral artery showing its normal course in the anteroposterior view (**A**) and the lateral view (**B**). Note that in this patient the artery enters the spine at the C4 level. **C**. Schematic representation of the normal course of the vertebral artery. (Adapted from List CF, Burge CH, Hodges FI: Intracranial angiography. *Radiology* 45:1, 1945.)

paired *posterior inferior cerebellar arteries* exit from the vertebrals to branch out and supply the lateral part of the medulla and to anastomose freely with other posterior fossa branches. Infarction due to occlusion of one of these arteries or to the parent vertebral artery may produce the so-called *lateral medullary syndrome* or *Wallenberg's syn-*

drome. The anterior spinal artery supplies the hypoglossal nucleus and nerve, the medial lemniscus, and the pyramidal tract. Infarction from occlusion of this artery will produce a *medial medullary syndrome*.

Figure 7.36 is an angiogram demonstrating the course of the vertebral artery in the neck. This example is somewhat atypical, in

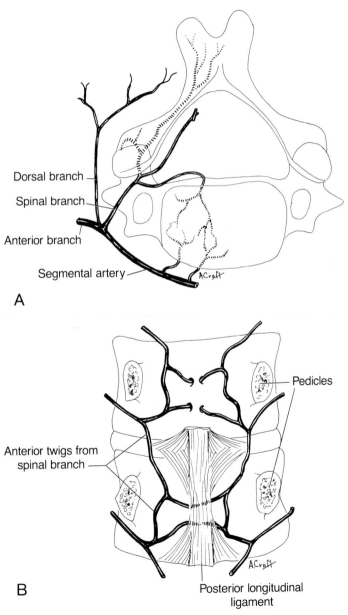

Figure 7.37.   The segmental artery and its branches which supply the vertebra are shown from the superior aspect (**A**) and the posterior aspect (**B**). Part of the posterior longitudinal ligament has been cut away. (Adapted from Hollinshead WH: *Textbook of Anatomy*, ed 3. New York, Harper & Row, 1974, p 313.)

that the artery usually enters the transverse foramen at the level of C6. The blood supply to the individual vertebra is derived from the aforementioned segmental arteries associated with them (Fig. 7.37).

Venous drainage takes place via *internal* and *external venous plexuses* which consist of rich networks of veins that ultimately anastomose and drain this area as the *intervertebral veins*. These plexuses are subdivided into *anterior* and *posterior external plexuses* and *anterior* and *posterior internal plexuses* (Fig. 7.38).

LIGAMENTS AND INTERVERTEBRAL DISCS

Intervertebral discs provide height and spacing to the vertebral column, thereby allowing the spinal nerves to exit safe and free from pressure or injury from their movable bony encasement.

The disc is composed of a tough outer zone of collagenous fibers and a broader inner zone of dense white fibrocartilaginous bundles that are arranged in concentric lamellae. Each lamella is slanted in an opposite direction. This crisscross pattern

provides both strength and compressibility—so much so that when a very heavy compressive load is applied to the healthy spine, the vertebrae will usually fracture before the disc will rupture.

In the cervical spine as in the lumbar spine, the discs are wider anteriorly than posteriorly, thereby contributing to the secondary lordotic curvatures. In general, they contribute about 25% to the vertical height of the spine, although the distribution between cervical, thoracic, and lumbar discs is not equal. Discs are numbered according to the vertebra above them. They are adherent to the hyaline cartilage endplates that cover the superior and inferior surfaces of the vertebral body and, with the exception of some peripheral supply from adjacent spinal arteries, are entirely avascular, deriving their nutrition by diffusion from spongy bone through the cartilaginous endplates.

Discs adhere strongly to the peripheral margins of the bony vertebra and to the anterior and posterior longitudinal ligaments. The tough outer part is referred to as the *anulus fibrosus*, and the inner mucoid or jelly-like substance is called the *nucleus pul-*

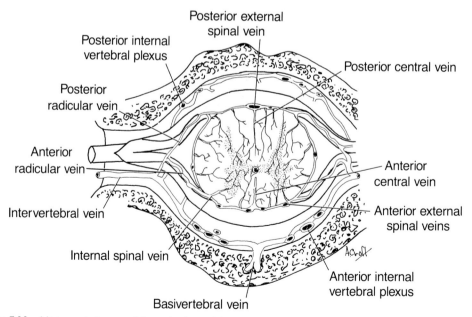

Figure 7.38. Venous drainage of the spinal cord. (Adapted from Kaplan A: The central nervous system. In Netter FH (ed): *The Ciba Collection of Medical Illustrations*, vol I, *Nervous System*, ed 12. Summit, NJ, Ciba Pharmaceutical, 1977, p 54.)

posus. This nuclear substance originates as primitive notochord. In early life, it contains 70–88% water, but as the person ages, the water content of the nucleus decreases and the mucoid material is gradually replaced with fibrocartilage derived probably from the cells of the anulus with some possible contribution from the cartilaginous endplates. Because of the high water content and diffusibility potential of the intervertebral disc, a man will lose approximately 0.75 inch of height by the end of the day just from the effects of gravity. This is replaced during sleep when gravity in the axial plane is negligible. The degeneration of discs also partly accounts for a gradual loss of stature with increasing age. The nucleus is located somewhat posterior to the center of the disc and serves an important biomechanical function in the kinematics of the cervical spine motion segment.

The *tectorial membrane* is the cephalic continuation of the *posterior longitudinal liga-ment.* It and the other ligaments under discussion are illustrated in Figures 7.39–7.44. It spans between the body of the axis and the base of the skull. The posterior longitudinal ligament runs along the posterior surface of the vertebral bodies, narrowing over the middle of the bone and expanding over the ends of the bodies and discs where it is anchored firmly, and, like its anterior counterpart the anterior longitudinal ligament, acts as a powerful stabilizer of the intervertebral joint. One of its major functions is to limit forward flexion of the neck. The *anterior atlantooccipital membrane* runs from the anterior margin of the foramen magnum to the anterior arch of the atlas (Fig. 7.40). Here it is continuous with the strong *anterior longitudinal ligament* which is firmly attached to the anterior tubercle and runs down the anterior surface of the entire spine, firmly attaching itself to the vertebrae and intervertebral discs. It, like its posterior counterpart, consists of fibers of

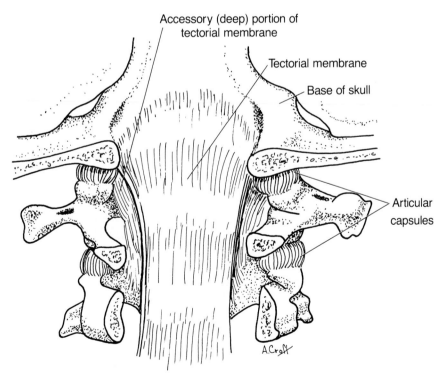

Figure 7.39.   Posterior view of the posterior aspect of the skull, atlas, and axis after removal of the posterior aspect of the skull and the laminae and spinous processes of the atlas and axis. (Adapted from Kaplan A: The central nervous system. In Netter FH (ed): *The Ciba Collection of Medical Illustrations,* vol I, *Nervous System,* ed 12. Summit, NJ, Ciba Pharmaceutical, 1977, p 25.)

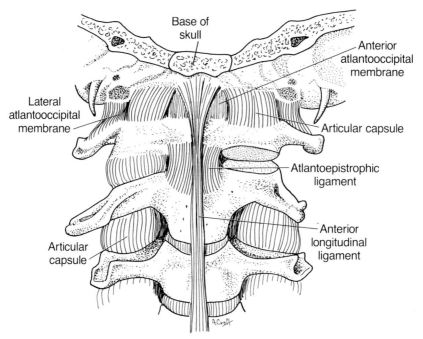

Figure 7.40.   Anterior view of the base of the skull and upper cervical spine. (Adapted from Kaplan A: The central nervous system. In Netter FH (ed): *The Ciba Collection of Medical Illustrations*, vol I, *Nervous System*, ed 12. Summit, NJ, Ciba Pharmaceutical, 1977, p 24.)

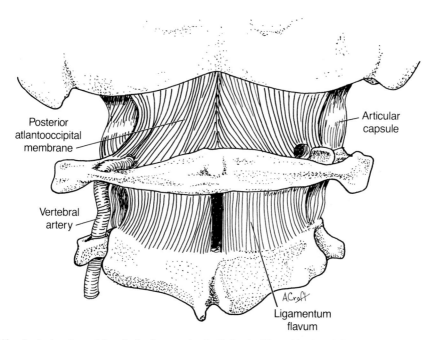

Figure 7.41.   Posterior view of the skull, atlas, and axis. (Adapted from Kaplan A: The central nervous system. In Netter FH (ed): *The Ciba Collection of Medical Illustrations*, vol I, *Nervous System*, ed 12. Summit, NJ, Ciba Pharmaceutical, 1977, p 24.)

variable length, with some spanning only one joint, while others (the most superficial) span four or five joints. It is thickest anteriorly. One of its prime functions is to limit extension of the neck.

Somewhat thinner than its anterior counterpart, the *posterior atlantooccipital membrane* runs between the posterior arch of the atlas and the base of the occiput (Fig. 7.41). The synovial joints, which include two atlantooccipital and three atlantoaxial joints (including the articulation between the dens and anterior arch of the atlas), contain a synovial lining and a fibrous joint capsule. Owing to the great demand for broad ranges of motion in the cervical spine, these joint capsules are somewhat lax and limit motion only slightly. Limitation of motion is the responsibility of other liga-

ments and the strong musculature of the neck.

Because of the posterior position of these joints in relation to the emergent spinal nerves, nerve root irritation and pain will often result when these joints hypertrophy by osteoarthritic proliferation or from local inflammation.

The paired *ligamenta flava* are strong ligaments that check forward flexion of the neck and act as powerful stabilizers. They are yellow because of their high elastic tissue content (elastin is deep yellow). They act to brake forward flexion gently, so that limits of joint motion are not reached abruptly. The paired ligaments run between adjacent laminae, almost filling the space completely (Fig. 7.41).

The *ligamentum nuchae* is homologous to

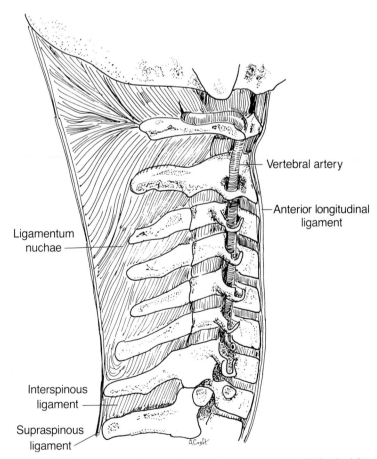

Figure 7.42.   Lateral view of the base of the skull and the cervical spine. (Adapted from Kaplan A: The central nervous system. In Netter FH (ed): *The Ciba Collection of Medical Illustrations*, vol I, *Nervous System*, ed 12. Summit, NJ, Ciba Pharmaceutical, 1977, p 24.)

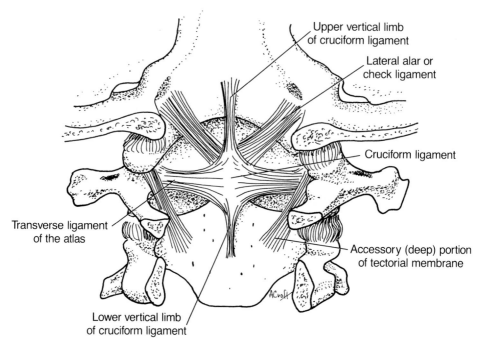

Figure 7.43.   Posterior view of the posterior aspect of the base of the skull, atlas, and axis deep to the tectorial membrane. (Adapted from Kaplan A: The central nervous system. In Netter FH (ed): *The Ciba Collection of Medical Illustrations*, vol I, *Nervous System*, ed 12. Summit, NJ, Ciba Pharmaceutical, 1977, p 25.)

the interspinous and supraspinous ligaments of other levels. Composed of fibroelastic tissue, it extends from the external occipital protuberance to the spine at the seventh cervical vertebrae and serves largely as a septum for muscular attachment (Fig. 7.42). In quadrupeds, it is much thicker and holds the grazing animal's head erect; muscular contraction is actually required for flexion. In humans, this ligament is of less importance and its strength is limited. The *supraspinous ligament* runs from the level of the spinous process of the seventh cervical vertebra to the sacrum, attaching each spinous process with a tough fibrous cord (Fig. 7.42). Above this level it is known as the ligamentum nuchae. It is continuous with the *interspinous ligament*, a thin membranous ligament spanning adjacent spinous processes and blending with the ligamenta flava. The interspinous ligament is not well developed in the cervical spine.

The *cruciform ligament* (so named because of its resemblance to a cross) consists of a thick strong band traversing and holding the

dens against the atlas. This portion is called the *transverse ligament of the atlas* (Fig. 7.43). Projecting cephalad from this ligament is the *upper vertical limb* of the cruciform ligament. This attaches the cruciform ligament to the occiput. Deep to this limb lies the *apical ligament of the dens* (Fig. 7.44). Running inferiorly from the cruciform ligament and inserting into the body of the axis is the *lower vertical limb* of the cruciform ligament.

The *alar ligaments* are strong fibrous bands that run from the medial sides of the condyles of the occiput around the posterior surface of the dens. These ligaments are also referred to as check ligaments, since they limit the amount of rotation that can occur upon the dens (Fig. 7.44).

The *intertransverse ligaments* (not illustrated) unite transverse processes. They are not well developed in the cervical spine and probably add little to its integrity. The fibrous capsules of the atlantoaxial joints are reinforced with the so-called *accessory ligament* which runs posteromedially from the atlas to the axis.

FASCIA

The term fascia is a general one used to described a sheet or layer of fibrous connective tissue. Fascia usually serves as a container or separator for muscular compartments or as a covering for an organ, but its definitive description is somewhat nebulous, in that all connective tissue is attached by definition to other connective tissue. The description and the understanding of this tissue, however, have real functional value.

Several forms of fascia exist in the body— *tela subcutanea* or the *superficial fascia* and *deep fascia*. The latter is a tough, thin, almost opalescent sheet of tissue that acts as a packaging material for muscles and muscle groups. From its undersurface emanate slips or septa of fascia down through individual muscles. Where it meets bone, it becomes continuous with the periosteum. In Figure 7.45 are illustrated the fascial layers in the cervical spine.

NEUROANATOMY

The central nervous system consists of the brain and spinal cord. The brain is covered with a three-layered substance known as the meninges. The *dura mater* is the tough outermost layer which forms a shell around the brain and a tube around the spinal cord. Just deep and adjacent to the dura lies the thinner *arachnoid membrane*. The *subarachnoid space* occupies the area between the arachnoid and the *pia mater*, the third layer of the meninges. The pia is closely adherent to the brain and spinal cord which are bathed and supported by the cerebrospinal fluid occupying the subarachnoid space (Fig. 7.46).

The *dentate* or *denticulate ligaments* arise from the pia mater of the cervical and thoracic spinal cord between the ventral and dorsal nerve roots. They consist of narrow, fibrous tooth-shaped projections (hence the name) that attach the cord to the dura and help to suspend it safely in the cerebrospinal fluid. Spaced between adjacent nerve roots, there are 20–21 of these ligaments (Fig. 7.47).

The neuroanatomy of the *cervical spinal cord* is illustrated in Figures 7.48 and 7.49.

From a clinical standpoint it is important to remember that the *spinal nerve* is composed not of discrete ventral and dorsal roots but of *root filaments* (Fig. 7.47) that emanate from the cord in a nearly continuous flow. In the cervical spine, the nerve roots exit the same foraminal level as that of their origin from the cord. This is in contrast to those in the lumbar spine that assume a more vertical course.

Both *parasympathetic* and *sympathetic nervous system* components may be found in the neck, although neither of these originate there. The *vagus nerve* of the parasympathetic system (or *craniosacral outflow*, as it is sometimes referred to) lies between the common carotid artery and the internal jugular vein as it traverses the cervical spine. It originates from a dorsal nucleus in the brain stem. The sympathetic nervous system (or *thoracolumbar outflow*) has its origin in the lateral column of gray matter from the first thoracic level to the upper two or three lumbar segments. These segments exit the spinal cord via the ventral roots and then, via the white rami communicates, join their sympathetic trunk ganglia or interganglionic parts.

The upper thoracic segments give rise to three or four cervical sympathetic ganglia which include the *superior cervical ganglion*, the *middle cervical ganglion*, the *intermediate cervical ganglion*, and the *inferior cervical ganglion*. From here they rise up into the neck, giving rise to several cervical ganglia which supply the head and neck. There are, therefore, no white rami communicantes in the neck. The inferior cervical ganglion is located at the level of the ventral aspect of the head of the first rib. When this ganglion is fused with the first thoracic ganglion, it is referred to as the *stellate* or *cervicothoracic ganglion*. It supplies gray rami communicantes to the seventh and eighth cervical and first thoracic nerves and, sometimes, to the sixth cervical nerve. The intermediate cervical ganglion is found at the level of the eighth cervical nerve. It joins the sixth and, sometimes, the seventh cervical nerve. The middle cervical ganglion is the smallest of the cervical ganglion and occasionally is absent. It is usually found at the level of the sixth cervical vertebra, anterior or superior to the inferior thyroid artery. It sends fibers to the fifth and sixth and, sometimes also, the fourth and seventh cervical nerves. The largest of the sympathetic trunk ganglia, the superior cervical ganglion, sends postganglionic (gray rami) to the first two and , sometimes, the third and even fourth cervical nerves.

The sympathetic innervation to the cranium is largely derived from the *internal carotid nerve* which is the cephalic continuation of the superior cervical ganglion. Other sources include the sympathetic plexuses that run with the common carotid and vertebral arteries.

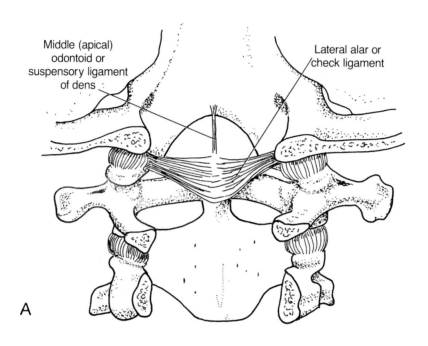

Middle (apical) odontoid or suspensory ligament of dens

Lateral alar or check ligament

A

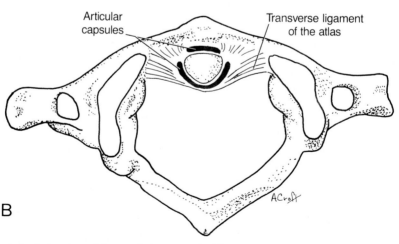

Articular capsules

Transverse ligament of the atlas

B

Figure 7.44.   A. Posterior view of the posterior aspect of the base of the skull, atlas, and axis deep to the cruciform ligament. **B.** Superior view of the atlas and dens. (Adapted from Kaplan A: The central nervous system. In Netter NH (ed): *The Ciba Collection of Medical Illustrations*, vol I, *Nervous System*, ed 12. Summit, NJ, Ciba Pharmaceutical, 1977, p 25.)

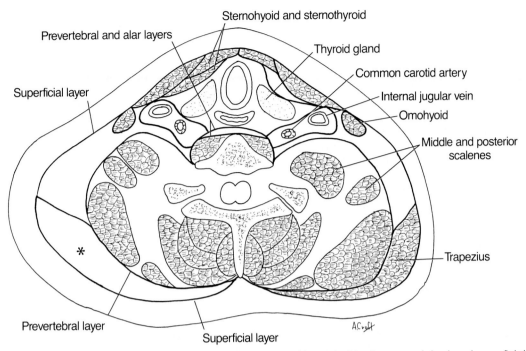

Figure 7.45. Fascial layers of the neck. One compartment bounded by the prevertebral and superficial layers (*asterisk*) is illustrated. (Adapted from Hollinshead WH: *Textbook of Anatomy*, ed 3. New York, Harper & Row, 1974, p 758.)

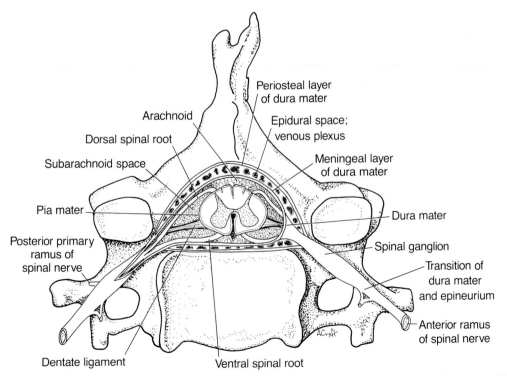

Figure 7.46. Neuroanatomy of the cervical spinal cord including meninges. (Adapted from Clemente CD: *Anatomy: A Regional Atlas of the Human Body*. Philadelphia, Lea & Febiger, 1975, fig 422.)

Physiologically, the autonomic nervous system is, in actuality, less "autonomous" than its name implies. For instance, it is greatly and rapidly affected by extrinsic stimulae, resulting in reflexes that are well known to us. It is also largely influenced by higher neurological levels of the central nervous system, including the brainstem reticular formation, the thalamic and hypothalamic nuclei, the limbic system, and the prefrontal lobe. The parasympathetic nervous system and the sympathetic nervous system serve to balance out each other in terms of their somatic effects. By way of review, the parasympathetic system acts to slow the heart rate and to increase the gut motility and glandular activity, whereas the sympathetic nervous system serves to increase the heart rate and to peripherally vasoconstrict, thereby increasing the return of blood to the heart. It also acts to inhibit gut peristalsis. Acetylcholine is released from parasympathetic terminals (hence the term "cholinergic"), whereas epinephrine (adrenaline) is released from the sympathetic terminals (hence the term "adrenergic"). The sympathetic supply to the upper extremities emanates from the cord levels T2–T6 or T7. The vasoconstrictor fibers supplying the arteries of the upper extremity are of the second and third thoracic nerves.

The average length of the adult human spinal cord is about 45 cm. It weights about

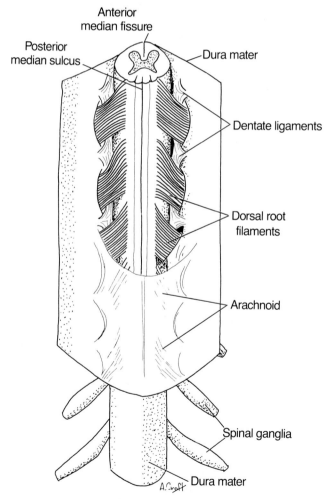

Figure 7.47. Spinal cord with dura mater dissected. (Adapted from Clemente CD: *Anatomy: A Regional Atlas of the Human Body.* Philadelphia, Lea & Febiger, 1975, fig 424.)

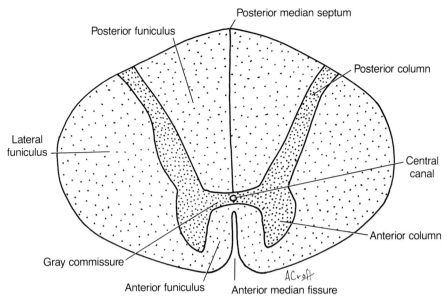

Figure 7.48. Schematic drawing of a section of spinal cord. In some segments of the spinal cord, a small lateral column is present (not illustrated). (Adapted from Warwick R, Williams PL: *Gray's Anatomy*, Br ed 35. Philadelphia, WB Saunders, 1973, p 808.)

30 gm. As the spinal cord descends, it generally tapers in its transverse diameter, with the exceptions of the *cervical* and the *lumbar enlargements* or *intumescentiae* that correspond to the neural connections and anterior horn cell collections associated with the upper and the lower extremities, respectively. At its widest point in the cervical spine, which is at about the level of C6, the transverse diameter of the cord is typically no more than 38 mm.

The spinal cord is divided into gray matter and white matter, with the former composed largely of cell bodies and terminal processes of axons and dendrites known as the *neuropil* and the latter composed largely

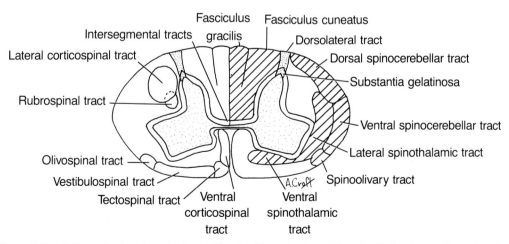

Figure 7.49. Schematic drawing of selected tracts of the spinal cord. The *shaded areas* are the ascending tracts; the *areas only outlined* are the descending tracts. (Adapted from Warwick R, Williams PL: *Gray's Anatomy*, Br ed 35. Philadelphia, WB Saunders, 1973, p 817.)

of myelinated nerve fibers. The gray component takes on the shape of an "H" and is composed of paired *posterior columns, lateral columns* (not seen in the cervical spine), and *anterior columns* which are joined together by the *gray commissure*. At the center of this structure lies the central canal (Fig. 7.48).

The posterior column or "horn," as it is sometimes referred to, contains the cell bodies of secondary sensory and other neu-

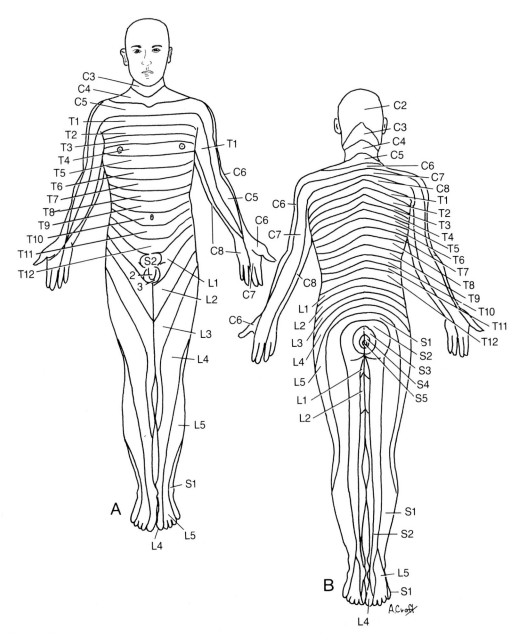

Figure 7.50. Segmental cutaneous innervation to the skin. Dermatome maps may vary somewhat. **A.** Anterior view. **B.** Posterior view. (Adapted from Kaplan A: The central nervous system. In Netter FH (ed): *The Ciba Collection of Medical Illustrations,* vol I, *Nervous System,* ed 12. Summit, NJ, Ciba Pharmaceutical, 1977, p 55.)

rons. The anterior column of horn contains the cell bodies of the spinal cord motor neurons. The lateral gray column is seen only in thoracic and upper lumbar levels and consists of relatively small cells that give rise to the sympathetic branch of the autonomic nervous system.

The white matter of the cervical spinal cord is divided into *posterior, lateral,* and *anterior funiculi* that contain bundles of fibers or tracts, both ascending and descending, carrying messages to and from the central nervous system. The more significant tracts are illustrated in Figure 7.49. Many other smaller tracts have been omitted from this figure for the sake of simplicity.

Major descending tracts of the cervical spinal cord include the lateral corticospinal, the anterior corticospinal, the tectospinal, the vestibulospinal, and the rubrospinal. The *lateral corticospinal tract,* also known as the *crossed* or *lateral pyramidal tract,* contains about 70–90% of the fibers of the pyramidal system, about 70% of which are myelinated. There are about 1 million fibers in this tract. In the *anterior corticospinal tract* or *uncrossed pyramidal tract,* these fibers do not decussate at the motor decussation but descend in the anterior funiculus and terminate at the anterior column in the cervical and thoracic levels, with most fibers crossing in the anterior white commissure. This tract is quite variable, in that it may (rarely) contain all corticospinal fibers or it may be absent entirely. Usually, however, it comprises 10–30% of the pyramidal system. The *tectospinal tract* that arises from the superior colliculus sends fibers that decussate in the dorsal tegmental decussation and reach the cervical spinal cord anterior horn cells that supply the neck muscles and upper extremities. This tract is presumed to mediate reflex postural movements in response to visual and perhaps auditory stimuli. The *vestibulospinal tract* mediates equilibrium and postural adjustment. Its fibers arise from the lateral vestibular nucleus and descend uncrossed to end on anterior horn cells throughout the cord, especially those associated with the lower extremities. The *rubrospinal tract* originates from the red nucleus of the midbrain and terminates in the spinal cord at the cervical levels. The most important function of this

tract is the control of muscle tone in flexor muscle groups.

The ascending tracts of the cervical spinal cord include the fasciculus gracilis, the fasciculus cuneatus, the dorsolateral fasciculus, the dorsal spinocerebellar, the ventral spinocerebellar, the spinoolivary, the lateral spinothalamic, and the ventral spinothalamic. The cervical *fasciculus gracilis tract* occupies half of each posterior funiculi. These fibers convey tactile and proprioceptive impulses from the lower half of the body primarily to the nucleus gracilis. The cell bodies are located in the dorsal root ganglia. The *fasciculus cuneatus tract* conveys tactile and proprioceptive impulses (primarily to the cuneate and lateral cuneate nuclei) from the upper half of the body. This tract lies lateral to the fasciculus gracilis. The *dorsolateral fasciculus tract* (of Lissauer) located at the tip of the posterior horn conveys pain and temperature to levels one or two segments above. The *dorsal spinocerebellar tract* carries proprioceptive and tactile impulses mainly from the lower extremities to the cerebellum. The *ventral spinocerebellar tract* relays information from neurotendinous and tactile endings to the cerebellum and also conveys tactile and proprioceptive information. The *spinoolivary tract* originates from neurons in the deep layers of cervical spinal cord gray matter and ascends to end on spinal regions of the dorsal and medial accessory olivary nuclei. This tract carries proprioceptive information from tendons and muscles as well as tactile sensation from cutaneous receptors. The *lateral spinothalamic tract* is composed of crossed fibers of secondary neurons carrying the sensation of pain and temperature to the thalamus. The *ventral spinothalamic tract* is composed of fibers of secondary neurons. This tract probably carries the general tactile sensations of crude touch and pressure.

The *fasciculus proprius* is composed of short fibers that interconnect adjacent spinal levels.

Segmental cutaneous innervation to the skin has been well mapped and described. Certainly from a neuroanatomical standpoint a slight variance from one individual to the next would be expected, but in fact there exists some minor variation from one reference source to the next. In Figure 7.50, an example of this dermal segmentation map is illustrated. Each segment constitutes a *dermatome*. These may not coincide perfectly with other anatomy texts and should be used as a general guide only.

It is also important to remember that there exists a fair amount of segmental overlap, especially in areas not related to the extremities, and that the sensations of pain and temperature overlap to a greater extent than does tactile sensation. Therefore, rhizotomy of a single spinal nerve root will generally only be perceived as hypesthesia rather than anesthesia or analgesia.

Conclusion

This chapter provides a brief review of the developmental and normal anatomy of the cervical spine and related structures. And although this textbook deals primarily with injuries of the neck resulting from whiplash, it would be incomplete without this overview of anatomy. In addition, this chapter provides a good foundation for understanding important concepts of pain presented in the following chapters. It

should also offer some understanding to those whose primary interest lies outside the field of chiropractic or medicine, and in this regard the glossary will lend additional support.

References

1. Warwick R, Williams PL: *Gray's Anatomy*, Br ed 35. Philadelphia, WB Saunders, 1973.
2. Langman J: *Medical Embryology*, ed 3. Baltimore, Williams & Wilkins, 1975.
3. Baily RW, Sherk HH, Dunn EJ, Fielding JW, Long DM, Ono K, Penning L, Stauffer ES: *The Cervical Spine*, The Cervical Spine Research Society. Philadelphia, JB Lippincott, 1983.

Suggested Readings

Carpenter MB: *Human Neuroanatomy*, ed 7. Baltimore, Williams & Wilkins, 1977.
Ham AW: *Histology*, ed 7. Philadelphia, JB Lippincott, 1974.
Harris JH Jr: *The Radiology of Acute Cervical Spine Trauma*. Baltimore, Williams & Wilkins, 1978.
Hollinshead WH: *Textbook of Anatomy*, ed 3. New York, Harper & Row, 1974.
Keats TE: The spine—cervical spine. In Keats TE (ed): *Atlas of Normal Roentgen Variants That May Simulate Disease*, ed 3. Chicago, Year Book, 1984, p 168.
McMinn RMH, Hutchings RT: *Color Atlas of Anatomy*. Chicago, Year Book, 1977.
Netter FH (ed): *The Ciba Collection of Medical Illustrations*, vol I, *Nervous System*, ed 12. New York, Ciba Pharmaceutical, 1977.
Rothman RH, Simeone FA (eds): *The Spine*, ed 2. Philadelphia, WB Saunders, 1982, vols I and II.

8

Soft Tissue Injury: Long- and Short-Term Effects

ARTHUR C. CROFT, DC, MS, DABCO

> "Physical pain is not a simple affair of an impulse, travelling at a fixed rate along a nerve. It is the result of a conflict between a stimulus and the whole individual."
>
> *Rene Leriche (1879–1955)*

The soft tissue injury, without question, remains one of the most baffling and enigmatic of all human afflictions. Nearly as ordinary as the common cold or headache, its definition, description, and cure seem to many physicians equally as elusive.

Since the invention of the automobile, humans have been continually plagued by the unique and yet consistent constellation of symptoms that Crowe first coined "whiplash" in 1928 (1). But motorists have not been the only ones to suffer the effects of the acceleration/deceleration injury. Injuries to the necks of military pilots that resulted from catapult-assisted takeoffs from aircraft carriers often caused permanent disability and early medical retirement. This inspired the construction of head restraints to prevent this type of whiplash.

In spite of the ultrasophisticated technology available today, we, as physicians, often find ourselves balancing on the horn of a dilemma as we approach the soft tissue injury case. Is this injury real or imagined? Are the subjective complaints consistent with the objective findings? What is the best way to treat the patient? What shall we say in our report? How, if asked do we describe the prognosis?

It is becoming increasingly tempting to rely on machines to solve our clinical puzzles. And these machines, be they magnetic resonance imagers, computed tomography scanners, scintillation cameras, electrodiagnostic equipment, x-ray units, or sequential multiple analyzers, may provide us with useful laboratory data, but it is only the human computer that is able to

271

take the history, give the detailed physical examination, and branch out from the diagnostic tree, sorting and re-sorting every bit of information until a final diagnosis is reached.

For reasons that will become obvious by the end of this chapter, a thorough work-up is important in each and every case no matter how trivial it may initially seem. The soft tissue injury must be approached rationally and with a good understanding of the underlying pathology. Haphazard and routine treatment directed merely at symptoms can not only delay the patient's recovery but can also unfavorably influence the long-range prognosis.

Experimental Studies

With the ever-increasing number of automobiles on the road, whiplash injuries have become more and more prevalent in our society. With an increase in this type of injury, of course, has come an increase in the number of personal injury liability suits. Those on the defense side in these suits generally have held that the plaintiff was fabricating or exaggerating his or her symptoms in order to attain a larger settlement, suggesting that once the case was over, the symptoms would miraculously clear up.

To many observers, however, it soon became clear that the constellation of symptoms complained of by these patients were relatively typical, consistent, and somewhat predictable. Such would not likely have been the case had these people truly been malingering. Several investigators began to experiment with anthropomorphic dummies, laboratory animals, cadavers, and human volunteers. The findings were sometimes surprising. Macnab (2) secured anesthetized animals to a chair mounted on vertical rails. The animals were dropped from heights ranging from 2 to 40 feet. At the end of the rail the chair would stop abruptly, thereby jerking the animal's head backward, simulating an acceleration injury. Depending on the height of the drop and hence the magnitude of hyperextension injury produced, various types and severities of lesions resulted. These ranged from minor tears in the sternocleidomas-

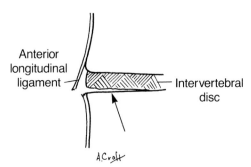

Figure 8.1. Tearing of the anterior longitudinal ligament and avulsion of the intervertebral disc from the vertebral body was seen in laboratory animals exposed to hyperextension injury.

toid muscle to tears of the longus colli muscle. This latter injury was usually associated with a retropharyngeal hematoma and occasionally with damage to the cervical sympathetic nervous system. Also noted were hemorrhages in the muscular coats of the esophagus. In some cases, the anterior longitudinal ligament was torn and the disc avulsed from the vertebra (Fig. 8.1). This was not detectable with standard x-ray procedures, however.

Although this experiment failed to reproduce the exact mechanism of injury as seen in a rear-end motor vehicle accident, some extrapolation of experimental results has been allowable. Macnab (2) states:

"[these injuries] suggest that lesions can vary from very minor injuries, such as a tear of muscle fibers, to serious lesions, such as separation of the disc or damage to the posterior joints. It is reasonable to presume that the same variation is seen clinically, with the majority of patients sustaining minor injuries only, but some suffering lesions of more serious significance."

Wickstrom et al. (3–5) have done extensive testing in this area, using Belgian hares initially and, later, primates. Three basic types of equipment were utilized in an effort to reproduce a more realistic acceleration injury. These included: (*a*) a pendulum-mounted hammer, (*b*) an air cylinder, and (*c*) an acceleration device (Fig. 8.2).

Their studies showed that these devices varied widely in the amount of G forces generated as well as in the duration of acceleration measured in milliseconds. The

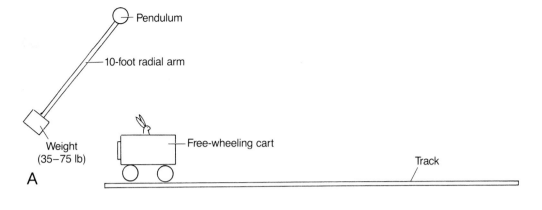

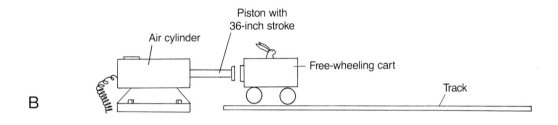

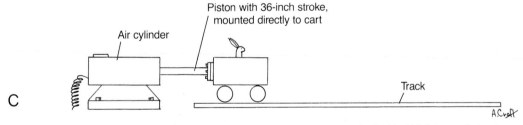

Figure 8.2. Experiments in hyperextension/hyperflexion injury were conducted by Wickstrom et al. using a free-wheeling cart that was struck from the rear by a pendulum-mounted weight (**A**), a free-wheeling cart that was struck from the rear by an air cylinder-powered piston (**B**), and a cart that had the air cylinder-powered piston directly fastened to it (**C**).

pendulum-mounted hammer, which varied in weight from 35 to 75 lb, produced a peak acceleration of 218 G within 1.5 msec. This weight, mounted on a 10-foot radial arm, was dropped from a fixed height and allowed to strike the test vehicle which could then run free on rails after impact. Surprisingly, none of the Belgian hares appeared to be injured in this type of apparatus, and this led to the adoption of the second device, the air cylinder. This device consisted of a cylinder with a piston stroke of 36 inches which directly accelerated the free-running vehicle to a force of 26 G in about 30–40 msec. As in the first case, the experimental animals seemed to tolerate these forces, and apart from being initially stunned, all recovered and appeared normal. Dissection in both cases failed to reveal any gross lesions in the soft tissues.

This failure to produce grossly visible lesions led to the development of the third acceleration device which again utilized the air cylinder, but this time the end of the piston rod was mounted directly to the vehicle, so that the cart could not run free following the acceleration. Peak acceleration forces of up to 70 G were obtained within 20–40 msec. This apparatus produced the most extreme forces, as the acceleration phase was quickly followed by a rapid deceleration force as high as 105 G. This deceleration force was consistently greater than the acceleration force by a factor of up to 3 and resulted in repeated hyperextension/hyperflexion movements of the head. Almost all of these animals were seriously injured or killed.

Upon close microscopic examination at necropsy, many animals in the pendulum and air cylinder group exhibited cerebral hemorrhage, and the majority in the piston-mounted device group sustained retroocular hemorrhage. Subsequent studies by Wickstrom et al. (3–5) and by Unterharnscheidt (6) using primates failed to produce retroocular lesions. It was noted in the case of the piston-mounted device group that with the animal facing forward the greatest force produced was hyperflexion, whereas with the animal facing backward the greatest force produced was hyperextension. In the hyperflexion/hyperextension injury, a higher proportion of injuries to the posterior elements (including the posterior ligamentous complex and nerve roots) occurred. Also, there were twice as many fractures, dislocations, and subluxations seen in this group. It was found that intracerebral hemorrhage occurred four times more often in the hyperextension injury than in the hyperflexion injury but that subdural, subarachnoid, and epidural hemorrhages were found with equal frequency in both groups.

Wickstrom et al. (3) biopsied muscle and other soft tissue from these animals and found inflammation or hemorrhage in the trapezius and splenius capitis muscles about 25% of the time. Several cases of retropharyngeal hemorrhage and intralaryngeal hemorrhage were discovered, and almost half of the thyroid glands biopsied showed evidence of inflammation or hemorrhage. These investigators also demonstrated brain damage in some animals as evidenced by electoencephalogram (EEG).

Katayama (7) studied the whiplash-type injury in rabbits and found ligamentous injury, capsular joint hematomas, circulatory changes in the venous component of the neuroforamen, and thrombosis. He found that with the rear-end acceleration, greater damage occurred in the upper cervical spine.

Unterharnscheidt (6) tested the effects of −Gx and +Gx acceleration forces on rhesus monkeys. These vectors are described in greater detail in Chapter 1, but for the sake of review, the −Gx force would produce hyperflexion or deceleration, whereas the +Gx force would produce hyperextension or acceleration. Although it is somewhat misleading, both are referred to as "acceleration" because the forces are initially applied by a horizontal accelerator and the force generated (i.e., −Gx or +Gx) depends upon which way the animal is facing at the time of acceleration (Fig. 8.3).

Unterharnscheidt (6) described these posttraumatic lesions in terms of central nervous system (CNS) lesions, vascular lesions, bony lesions, and muscular, ligamentous, and related structure lesions. His findings are summarized under the headings, "−Gx Vector Injuries" and "+Gx Vector Injuries."

−Gx VECTOR INJURIES

CNS Lesions

Rhesus monkeys were subjected to gradually increasing G forces up to the point where complete traumatic transections of the spinal cord occurred. Transections were generally observed above 127 G.

Incomplete traumatic transections occurred between 105 and 130 G. One animal who survived the 105 G sustained a thrombosis to the right vertebral and right posterior inferior cerebellar artery, producing a softening of the spinal cord at C1 and softening of the right cerebellar white matter (the Wallenberg syndrome).

The lowest force productive of tissue damage was 78.3 G. The lesion resulting from this force consisted of subarachnoid hemorrhage adjacent to the basilar and vertebral arteries. With peak sled accelerations ranging from 5.2 to 63.7 −Gx, Unterharnscheidt (6) was unable to detect any

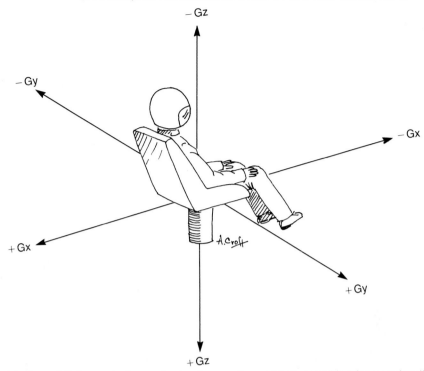

Figure 8.3. Vectors of G forces in the major body axes (x, y, and z) described for acceleration and vibration. + indicates a forward acceleration that results in a hyperextension injury, whereas − indicates an acceleration in a rearward direction, resulting in a hyperflexion injury (the term "acceleration" can describe both forces when qualified by the proper symbols). The *direction of the arrows* represents the direction of acceleration at the head; e.g., rear impact produces +Gx acceleration and hyperextension of the neck. (Adapted from Unterharnscheidt F: Pathological and neuropathological findings in rhesus monkeys subjected to −Gx and +Gx indirect impact acceleration. In Sances A Jr, Thomas DJ, Ewing CL, Larson SJ, Unterharnscheidt F (eds): *Mechanisms of Head and Spine Trauma.* Goshen, NY, Aloray, 1986, p 567.)

pathomorphological findings after extensive histological study of sections between the lower medulla oblongata and C2 with the light microscope. He noted, however, that Sances et al. (8), using slow application of axial forces to the vertebral column with forces that reduced the afferent or efferent evoked potential magnitude by 50%, produced a marked reduction in metabolic activity at the cervicomedullary junction and cervical spinal cord, as demonstrated by the ^{14}C-labeled deoxyglucose method of Sokoloff et al. (9–13). Light microscopic examination of tissue from these animals failed to reveal any significant lesions, but electron microscopic examination demonstrated shrinkage of the axoplasm and disruption of the myelin lamellae in the upper cervical cord. Direct impact of the odontoid process of the axis often produced a contusion to the cord.

Vascular Lesions

Thrombosis occurred in one animal previously described. Complete rupture of the vertebral arteries frequently accompanied complete traumatic transections. In some instances, the basilar artery was avulsed. No carotid artery ruptures were observed.

Bony Lesions

The bony lesions observed included atlantooccipital separations with massive dislocation of the segments and incomplete and complete C1-C2 separations. The only fractures to be observed were three cases of basilar skull fracture.

Muscular and Ligamentous Lesions

Unterharnscheidt found hemorrhages that were probably due to tears and ruptures of muscles near their origin. The tectorial membranes and posterior longitudinal ligaments were frequently observed to be disrupted, as were the transverse and cruciate ligaments.

+ Gx VECTOR INJURIES

CNS Lesions

CNS lesions similar to those resulting from − Gx vector acceleration were seen in this group of + Gx vector injuries. This included complete transections of the spinal cord that, in some cases, were identical to those seen with the − Gx vector acceleration (i.e., accompanied by rupture of both vertebral arteries). At this time, Unterharnscheidt had not yet finished compiling the neurohistopathological data on this group.

Vascular Lesions

As would be expected, the vascular lesions produced by the + Gx vector forces were somewhat different from those produced by the − Gx vector forces. Unterharnscheidt found extensive hemorrhages in the neck around the esophagus and aorta and extending into the upper as well as the posterior mediastinum with extensive retropleural and paravertebral hemorrhages around the lateral aspect of the spine. It was noted that in both − Gx and + Gx vector testing, no carotid artery ruptures were found. There were no cerebral subdural hemorrhages seen in the + Gx group, as were seen in the − Gx group, although spinal subdural hemorrhages were seen in both groups when transection of the cord occurred.

Bony Lesions

Bony lesions that resulted from these experiments included hairline fractures of the scapulae, fracture dislocations of the thoracic and the cervical spine, rib fractures, and spinous process fractures.

Muscular Ligamentous and Related Structure Lesions

Major alterations in the ligamentous structure were not described. Multiple hematomas and hemorrhages were found in the neck musculature, especially in the sternocleidomastoids.

Lin et al. (14) have shown with experimental animals that in addition to muscle fiber tears, muscular strains, and ligament injuries, damage to the brain can be produced by using acceleration injuries similar to those experienced by occupants of vehicles struck from the rear. Brain damage can sometimes be detected by EEG, but it is significant that in 24% of the 29 animals initially found to have "normal" EEG recordings, definite neurological lesions were found.

Bocchi and Orso (15) have reported on other studies in which monkeys subjected to + Gx vector accelerations suffered tearing of the sternocleidomastoid and other long muscles of the neck, fractures and dislocation, lesions of the meninges and brain, stretch of the anterior longitudinal ligament to the point of rupture of the disc, rupture of the posterior longitudinal ligament at the level of its attachment to the disc, and ruptures of the two alar ligaments or of the transverse and alar ligaments together.

In addition to the numerous forms of soft tissue injury described in animal experiments, similar lesions in humans who have been exposed to acceleration/deceleration injuries have been confirmed. Usually these are diagnosed from clinical examination or are presumed to exist from the patient's particular complaints and the nature of his or her presenting symptomatology. Other times, various laboratory and roentgenological studies may be used to define the nature and extent of damage. For example, some patients may present with marked muscle spasm in the cervical spine. Swelling may be grossly visible or may be discovered by serial circumferential measurements of the neck. Palpation of the cervical musculature may reveal marked tenderness, and active range of motion may be quite painful for the patient to perform. In severe cases, grossly visible ecchymosis may be present. These findings would strongly suggest moderate to severe muscle strain. When dysphagia is present, its cause is generally pharyngeal edema or retropharyngeal hematoma from extravasation of blood into the loose areolar prevertebral tissues from torn or ruptured paravertebral blood vessels or from fractures of the vertebrae and can be of serious prognostic significance (see Fig. 4.6). Hemorrhage and edema of the strap muscles may also cause hoarseness or dysphagia (16). Retropharyngeal hematoma will generally be visible on lateral plain films, as is described in Chapter 4. Damage to neural structures is first presumed from the history and physical examination and later confirmed by electromyography, nerve conduction velocity study, electroencephalography, or appropriate psychometric testing, as outlined in Chapter 3. Specialized radiological studies such as tomography, myelography, and cineradiography along with magnetic resonance imaging and computed tomography are also useful in evaluating various soft tissue lesions. These are described in greater detail in Chapters 3 and 5.

Muscular Injury. When a vehicle is struck from the rear, the occupant's torso is accelerated while his or her unrestrained head and neck are snapped backward. This is the so-called "pure" hyperextension injury. Some authorities debate whether this mechanism actually exists in a pure state,

i.e., uncomplicated by other movements. Their debate centers around whether a low-amplitude initial flexion phase actually precedes the hyperextension phase. For the sake of discussion, the existence of the pure hyperextension injury is assumed, since the alternate mechanism that has been proposed, most notably the "concertina effect" as described by Unterharnscheidt (6) (see Chapter 1), does consist primarily of hyperextension.

As the head rotates into hyperextension, the anterior cervical muscles are stretched, and when their tone is overcome, the brunt of the remaining force is taken up by the anterior longitudinal ligament and anterior fibers of the anulus fibrosus. If the rate of stretch of these muscles is rapid, individual muscle fibers may not have sufficient time to relax (17). This results in rupture of muscle. At or near the end of the acceleration phase, after hyperextension of the spine has occurred, the hyperflexion component of the injury takes place. This may be potentiated by a violent contraction of the flexors of the neck stimulated by a very powerful stretch reflex initiated by the preceding hyperextension phase (Fig. 8.4). If the victim's vehicle now strikes another ve-

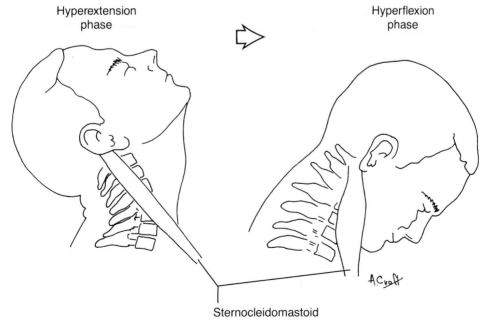

Hyperextension phase

Hyperflexion phase

Sternocleidomastoid

Figure 8.4. The hyperflexion phase of injury may be potentiated by violent contraction of the neck flexors as a result of a powerful stretch reflex initiated by the preceding hyperextension phase.

hicle or object in front, the resulting rapid deceleration further potentiates the hyperflexion injury. During the deceleration phase, when a shoulder harness is worn, a linear tractional injury occurs at or near the end of forward rotation of the cervical spine. Although McKenzie and Williams (18) have suggested that it is the hyperextension phase of whiplash that produces the greatest damage, it has been demonstrated by Wickstrom (3) and by Unterharnscheidt (6) under laboratory conditions that the deceleration of $-Gx$ vector acceleration that produces the hyperflexion injury is more injurious than the $+Gx$ vector acceleration. Unterharnscheidt (6) also pointed out that the upper cervical spine sustains the greatest injury, as it tends to be the biomechanical pivot point. I would agree with these findings and submit that it is because of this and the fact that the muscles in this region, i.e., suboccipital and occipitofrontalis muscles, are smaller and more specialized that they are so commonly traumatized to a greater degree than the larger paraspinal muscles. The concept of muscular rupture and tearing is well documented in the literature (15, 19–23).

Ligamentous Injury. In experimental studies conducted by Wickstrom et al. (24), ligamentous lesions involving the anterior longitudinal ligament were discovered.

These were sometimes so severe that they were accompanied by separation of the disc from its vertebral attachment (Fig. 8.1.) These lesions were not detectable by x-rays even after the passage of several months. Other reported injuries included facet joint capsule sprains and hemorrhages beneath the anterior and posterior longitudinal ligaments (Fig. 8.5).

Webb et al. (25) have described damage to the "posterior cervical complex" in traumatic flexion injuries to the neck. This complex is defined as the posterior articulations that are stabilized by the capsule, the interspinous ligament, and the ligamentum flavum. Disruption of these structures results in instability which may require surgical stabilization. In each operative case, ligamentous damage was confirmed.

Green et al. (26) studied the anterior subluxation of the cervical spine, a lesion resulting from hyperflexion trauma in which the posterior elements are disrupted. They noted that there was an approximately 20% incidence of delayed instability due to impaired ligamentous healing. Evans (27) has also described the traumatic ligamentous rupture seen at operation. Fielding et al. (28) studied the biomechanics of the transverse ligament of the atlas. They correlated the results of laboratory testing of cadaveric material with a

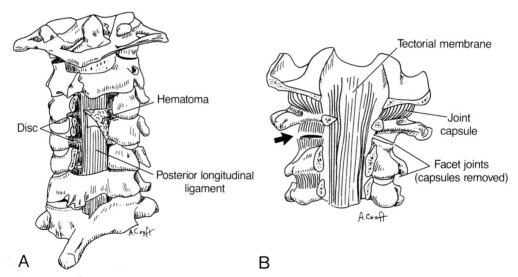

A

B

Figure 8.5.   A. A section of the posterior longitudinal ligament is reflected to illustrate a hematoma beneath it. **B.** Disruption of the facet joint capsule has occurred.

clinical series of 11 patients who had suffered traumatic transverse ligament ruptures from various traumas. The transverse ligament is the primary stabilizing component of the atlantoaxial ligament complex. When it is ruptured, the secondary stabilizing components—most notably, the alar ligaments—serve to protect against anterior displacement of the atlas and subsequent cord damage resulting from contact with the odontoid process of the axis (6, 28). Unterharnscheidt (6) has described cord contusions presumably from direct impact of the odontoid process against an area between the lower medulla oblongata and upper cervical spinal cord. In this case, two parts of the cruciform ligament—the transverse ligament and the vertical band—were ruptured along with the apical and alar ligaments. The concept of ligamentous injury is well documented in the literature (15, 19, 20, 22, 23, 27, 29, 30).

Several reports of vertebral injury resulting from the wearing of seat belts have been published (31–37). A spraining injury to the lumbar spine seems to be the most prevalent seat belt injury. This usually involves rupture of the supraspinous and interspinous ligaments. Other injuries include the so-called "fulcrum fracture" of the vertebral body which occurs as a result of severe forward flexion of the torso against the restraining seat belt. If the ligamentous structures remain intact, a horizontal fracture extends through the spinous process and usually through the pedicles and into the posterior aspect of the vertebral body. Occasionally, the fracture also runs through the transverse processes (36). This type of fracture was originally reported in the literature in 1948 by Chance (38). Smith and Kaufer (39) recognized this type of fracture occurring with certain seat belt injuries and named it the "Chance fracture." Other bony lesions include compression fractures, fracture dislocations, posterior arch fractures (40–42), pelvic fractures (34), rib fractures (43, 44), and flexion-compression fractures of the cervicodorsal junction (45).

Numerous reports of abdominal injury have been published, including injury to the small bowel, mesentery, omentum, kidney, liver, spleen, pregnant uterus, diaphragm, stomach, large bowel, and great

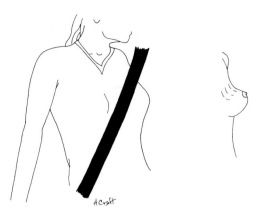

Figure 8.6. The female breast is commonly injured by the shoulder harness. In severe cases, traumatic fat necrosis has been reported.

vessels of the thorax (35, 46–48). Dawes et al. (49) have reported six cases of female breast trauma resulting from compression against a shoulder harness. In two cases, the soft tissues of the breast were actually separated. This left a transverse furrow in the breast (Fig. 8.6). Several cases were found to have suffered traumatic fat necrosis. Carcinoma was eventually diagnosed in three cases. Although studies (50) have shown some connection between trauma to the breast and the later development of carcinoma, the authors have thought that coincidence was the most likely explanation for their findings. Minor contusions to the breast from the transverse shoulder harness are fairly common and should be evaluated appropriately.

Intervertebral Disc Injury. As mentioned previously, Wickstrom et al. (3) produced a rupture of the anterior longitudinal ligament along with a tearing of the anulus fibrosus of the disc and a separation from its vertebral attachment. Green et al. (26) have described a tearing of the posterior anulus fibrosus following a hyperflexion injury. They noted anterior narrowing and posterior widening of the disc space along with anterior subluxation as subtle manifestations of this lesion (Fig. 8.7). Gotten (20) has also described this disc tearing and has suggested that it may result in fibrosis and abnormal motility of the vertebral joints.

Disc injury usually results in a posterior

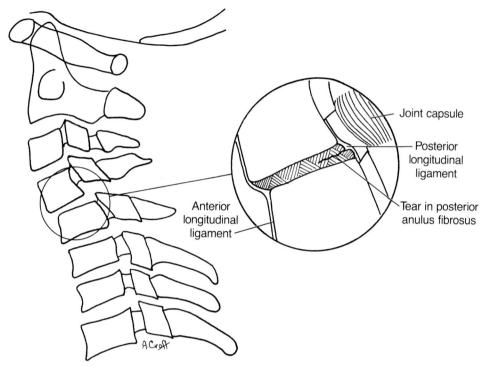

Figure 8.7. On the *left* is illustrated the x-ray appearance of anterior subluxation with the characteristic anterior narrowing and posterior widening of the disc space. These findings are subtle manifestations of annular tear. (Also see Chapter 1.)

tearing of the anulus fibrosus (51–53). This is seen on x-ray as a widening of the posterior disc space, a narrowing of the anterior disc space and, often, a concomitant anterior subluxation due to disruption of posterior elements (Fig. 8.7). Green et al. (26) described a 16% disc space narrowing in this condition and noted that the changes may be quite subtle. Loss of disc height in the acute time frame is probably the result of endplate fracture with extrusion of nuclear material into the body of the adjacent vertebrae or herniation or extrusion of nuclear material through the anulus fibrosus, which may or may not produce radiculopathy or myelopathy. Both conditions may be operant (Fig. 8.8). Swelling of the disc immediately following trauma has also been described as a subtle sign of disc injury.

Other Soft Tissue Injuries. Gotten (20) described direct trauma to nerve roots, occurring with the acceleration/deceleration injury. Symptoms of nerve root irritation include radiating pains into the shoulder and upper extremities, loss of deep tendon reflexes, muscular spasm or fasciculation, paresthesias, and decreased sensitivity to pinprick. These should not be confused with the brachialgias and paresthesias frequently seen in the aftermath of acceleration/deceleration trauma. These latter symptoms are usually caused by swelling and inflammation paravertebrally along with spasm of the scalene group and do not represent direct nerve root injury (54). They are most frequently seen in the ulnar distribution.

It is important to differentiate between neurovascular compression syndrome and nerve root compression syndrome. Both may arise out of trauma, and both may have had some chronic, although previously asymptomatic, etiology aggravated by the acceleration/deceleration injury.

The *neurovascular compression syndromes* include such entities as costoclavicular syndrome, supernumerary ribs or transverse bands from transverse processes, the knapsack syndrome of Falconer and Weddell, the thoracic outlet syndrome of Robb

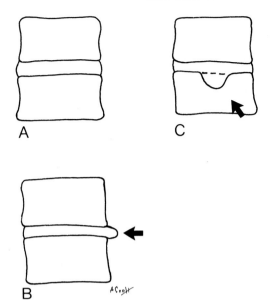

Figure 8.8. Loss of disc height in the acute time frame may result from annular bulge or herniation of nuclear material. **A.** Normal relationship. **B.** Annular bulge (with or without extrusion of nuclear material). **C.** Schmorl's herniation with endplate fracture.

and Standeven, the hyperabduction syndrome of Wright, and the scalenus anticus syndrome as described by Adson and Coffey. Symptoms of the neurovascular compression syndromes tend to be of an achy and diffuse nature and to be aggravated by movements or use of the arm or shoulder rather than the neck. Weakness is generally more a result of inhibition due to pain or clumsiness than to actual paralysis, and, the patient generally will have had some history of trouble in this area. A bruit can often be auscultated.

The reflex sympathetic dystrophies, which occasionally result from trauma to sympathetic plexuses, might also be included under the category of neurovascular compression syndromes. Symptoms of this disorder include pallor, redness, coldness, pulse loss, hyperhidrosis, and causalgia. None of these symptoms would be expected with a nerve root compression.

The *nerve root compression syndromes* may result from direct trauma to the nerve roots from the pincer-like action of the neuroforaminal architecture during an acute hyperextension trauma or from disc disease. This latter source may be a traumatic aggravation of chronic disc disease or an acute herniation or prolapse of disc material. Whatever the cause may be, the constellation of symptoms with nerve root compression syndrome are distinctly different from those with neurovascular compression syndrome or reflex sympathetic dystrophy and include proximal (root) pain and neck pain, distal paresthesias in dermatomal pattern, muscle weakness in one or several muscles supplied by a single root, loss of deep tendon reflexes, muscle fasciculations, and radiating pains aggravated by movements of the neck. The neck is generally held rigidly immobile by the patient. These points are summarized in Table 8.1.

The symptomatology of disc disease is remarkably variable, especially if both chronic disc degeneration, which may have been further aggravated by trauma, and acute disc herniation are considered together. Pain may be severe or subtle. Usually, in disc degeneration, pain will come and go and is frequently intensified by pressure over the spinous processes or deep cervical musculature. Sometimes, headaches will be the only symptom. These headaches generally follow the pattern of the greater and lesser occipital nerves, although retrobulbar pain can be produced with stimulation of the C2 nerve and this is also seen clinically in disc disease. Other confusing presentations such as pain in the shoulder, elbow, wrist, or hand—alone or in conjunction with paresthesias—may tend to divert attention away from the neuroforamina in the search for peripheral entrapment syndromes, especially in the absence of neck pain.

The *double crush syndrome* may be operant and serve to further confuse the clinician who orders electromyogram/nerve conduction velocity studies in the hope of finding the level of peripheral entrapment in such cases. In this phenomenon, the additive effects of distal compression and proximal impingement work synergistically to produce clinically recognizable symptomatology somewhere along the course of that nerve. A commonly seen example would be the middle-aged woman with a subclinical carpal tunnel compression who then sustains an acceleration/de-

Table 8.1.
Differentiation between Neurovascular Compression Syndrome and Nerve Root Compression Syndrome

Neurovascular Compression Syndrome	Nerve Root Compression Syndrome
Arm and axillary ache with feeling of swelling; ulnar paresthesias	Sharply radiating pain with generally discrete paresthesias of dermatomal genre
Pain aggravated by movements or use of arm or shoulder; not aggravated by movements of neck	Pain usually greatly aggravated by neck motions; not generally affected by use of shoulder or arm
Neck pain mild or absent	Neck pain is often major complaint
Muscle spasm in neck absent or mild	Muscle spasm in neck pronounced
Pain usually unaffected by soft cervical collar	Pain greatly relieved by soft cervical collar
Often, symptoms have occurred previously	Usually acute onset associated with known event or injury
No reflex changes present	May be reflex changes present
No fasciculations	May be fasciculations present
Can often locate lesion by ausculation of bruit	No bruits present
Weakness is generally diffuse and related more to inhibition from pain than to actual motor deficit	Discrete paresis usually associated with monoradiculopathy
Orthopaedic tests such as Wright's hyperabduction, costoclavicular, Adson's and Allen's are positive	Orthopaedic tests such as Bakody's, Jackson's, distraction and Spurling's are positive

celeration injury to the neck, which results in mild nerve root compression at a root level, which contributes to the median nerve. The proximal nerve root compression in itself is so mild that it would otherwise go unnoticed, and there are no proximal nerve root symptoms. Neck pain may be assumed to be of a strain or sprain variety only. However, the additive effects of the new proximal impingement and the preexisting, yet subclinical, carpal tunnel compression now result in a typical clinical manifestation of classic carpal tunnel syndrome. Very often this relatively common scenario results in an erroneous diagnosis of carpal tunnel syndrome secondary to spraining injury at the wrist from contact with the steering wheel or stick shift. In cases such as this, electrodiagnostic studies are often normal. Treatment should be directed not only to the wrist but also to the cervical spine.

Some patients with chronic radiculopathies may present only with atrophy. Others may have suffered neck pain for a short period of time only to be left with chronic shoulder or elbow pain. This again may result in an erroneous diagnosis of bursitis, tendonitis, or osteoarthritis. Neck movements are often painless.

Still other patients may present with numbness of one or more fingers and no pain. This numbness may persist indefinitely. Motor weakness is generally seen in association with paresthesias but occasionally may be seen in the absence of other symptoms.

Monoradiculopathies usually affect muscles that may be subserved by other healthy roots, so that total paralysis is not generally seen. These muscles also tend to function within a group of muscles that have a healthy nerve supply. This makes the discovery of discrete muscle paresis difficult in some cases. Careful comparative muscle testing of the deltoid, biceps, triceps, and intrinsic muscles of the hand, however, will uncover the majority of radiculopathies in which motor strength is affected. Symptoms of nerve root compression syndromes as seen at different cervical levels are summarized in Table 8.2, and the motor and reflex changes associated with these syndromes and seen at different levels are summarized in Table 8.3. Because a monoradiculopathy affects only one root, the patient may be able to compensate quite well for that weakness and may be quite surprised to find out just how weak an isolated muscle might be.

Table 8.2.
Symptoms Associated with the Nerve Root Compression Syndromes[a]

Nerve Root	Disc Level	Symptoms
C3	C2-C3	Pain and numbness in back of neck, especially at mastoid process and pinna of ear
C4	C3-C4	Pain and numbness in back of neck, radiating to levator scapulae and, occasionally, to anterior chest
C5	C4-C5	Pain radiating from side of neck to top of shoulder; numbness over deltoid muscle
C6	C5-C6	Pain radiating down arm and forearm, often into thumb and index fingers; numbness of tip of thumb and over first dorsal interosseous muscle
C7	C6-C7	Pain radiating down middle forearm, usually to index and ring finger
C8	C7-T1	Pain down medial aspect of forearm to ring and small finger; numbness in medial aspect of ring finger but rarely in forearm

[a]Adapted from Simeone FA, Rothman RH: Cervical disc disease. In Rothman RH, Simeone FA (eds): *The Spine*, ed 2. Philadelphia, WB Saunders, 1982, vol 1, p 454.

Occasionally, with severe acceleration/deceleration trauma, acute disc herniation is seen in association with myelopathy. This may be the result of posterior osteophyte formation and occasionally is due to chronic disc degeneration. The anterior spinal artery has also been implicated in this disorder. Myelopathic symptoms include the so-called long tract signs. With coexistent acute disc disease and radiculopathy, a combination of upper and lower motor neuron lesions is to be expected. Deep tendon reflexes are depressed at the level of the root lesions. Hyperreflexia at other levels and brisk Hoffmann's signs are usually present, whereas abdominal reflexes are usually absent. Spasticity and hyperreflexia in the lower extremities, often with clonus at the ankle, and downgoing plantar reflexes are common. In severe myelopathy, an extensor plantar response (Babinski) may be seen, and pain and temperature sensation may be blunted below the level of the lesion. The patient will not complain of numbness, however, as in the case of nerve root compression. This is because the touch sensation is preserved. Proprioceptive loss, which is most common in the lower extremities, may be responsible in part for the wide-based gait frequently observed in these individuals.

Macnab (55) has stated that pain radiating down the arm may also represent a referred pain from damaged tissues in the spine and may not indicate nerve root pressure. The mechanism of this referred pain is explored later in this chapter.

Vertebral artery insufficiency, whether permanent or transitory, has been implicated as an explanation for some of the symptomatology seen with hyperextension/hyperflexion injuries (15, 56). The course of the vertebral artery in the cervical spine is quite tortuous, and the artery passes through, over, and around structures that, following trauma, may become malaligned because of myospasm or ligamentous instability (Fig. 7.36). Abnormal pressures or tractional stresses may impede the circulation through these arteries. The

Table 8.3.
Motor and Reflex Changes Associated with Nerve Root Compression[a]

Nerve Root	Disc Level	Motor and Reflex Changes
C3	C2-C3	Weakness detectable only by electromyogram; no reflex change
C4	C3-C4	Weakness detectable only by electromyogram; no reflex change
C5	C4-C5	Weakness of extension of arm and shoulder, especially above 90°; atrophy and weakness of deltoid; diminished biceps reflex (biceps is innervated by C6 as well)
C6	C5-C6	Weakness of biceps muscle and wrist extension; diminished biceps reflex and brachioradialis reflex
C7	C6-C7	Weakness of triceps muscle; diminished triceps reflex
C8	C7-T1	Weakness of triceps and intrinsic muscles of hand; no reflex changes

[a]Adapted from Simeone FA, Rothman RH: Cervical disc disease. In Rothman RH, Simeone FA (eds): *The Spine*, ed 2. Philadelphia, WB Saunders, 1982, vol 1, p 154.

vertebral arteries may also be compressed as a result of chronic degenerative disease in the cervical spine. This may occur at any point along its usual course from C6 to C2. This condition may become symptomatic as a result of cervical spine trauma. Three mechanisms have been described, including (*a*) osteophytes from the lateral disc margin, (*b*) anteriorly extending osteo- phytes from the facet joint, and (*c*) compression from the inferior articulating facet from posterior subluxation and a scis- soring effect by the adjacent superior artic- ulating facet. On the other hand, increased tissue pressures from myospasm, edema, or hemorrhage may also compromise the flow of blood through the vertebral artery, especially when patency is already com-

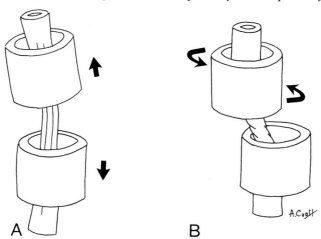

Figure 8.9.   Schematic drawing of two causes of impedance to blood flow through the vertebral arteries. **A.** Tractional force. **B.** Combined rotational and shear force exerted by adjacent vertebral structures.

promised because of atherosclerosis or congenital underdevelopment. Arterial spasm may also occur (Fig. 8.9). As noted earlier, animal experiments have shown that the occipitocervical region is commonly the most severely traumatized, as this serves as a mechanical pivot point in rotational injuries (6). All of the structures adjacent to the vertebral artery have been shown to be injured, and as previously mentioned, the arteries themselves may be traumatized—to the point of rupture—by increasing G forces. With moderate degrees of trauma, intimal disruption occurs. This may result in complete thrombotic occlusion or in subintimal hematoma formation. Pseudoaneurysm or complete dissection of the artery may also result. Milder mechanical trauma may induce a nonspecific arteritis characterized by edema, fibrin precipitation, and leukocytic infiltration in the affected arterial wall. If the inflammatory involvement is prolonged, fibroblastic proliferation may eventually result in narrowing of the lumen (57).

Three areas in which the vertebral artery is most susceptible to trauma include: (*a*) the posterior atlantooccipital membrane, which is dense and relatively inelastic and may become calcified (it is firmly attached to the artery); (*b*) the space between the occiput and posterior arch of the atlas, especially during extension; and (*c*) between the lateral mass of the atlas and the transverse process of the axis, especially with extension and rotation. Macnab (56) has noted that older patients with preexisting atherosclerotic disease are at greater risk of injury, resulting in *vertebral artery syndrome* which may be assumed to be synonymous with vertebrobasilar insufficiency. The vertebrobasilar syndrome is usually the result of thrombosis and generally results from extreme extension and rotation of the neck. Symptoms include vertigo, nausea, vomiting, dysarthria, nystagmus, and partial facial paralysis. If a thrombus or plaque is released, it could occlude the posterior inferior cerebellar artery, resulting in the *lateral medullary* or *Wallenberg's syndrome*, a common sequela to vertebrobasilar syndrome. Wallenberg's syndrome consists of an ipsilateral loss of cranial nerves V, IX, X, and XI, cerebellar ataxia, Horner's syndrome, and a contralateral loss of pain and

temperature sensation. In more severe cases, the basilar, superior cerebellar and posterior cerebellar arteries may be affected. This may result in death or in the *locked-in syndrome*, which includes quadriplegia and loss of the lower cranial nerves, allowing only blinking. To date, I have been unable to find any reports of experimental studies in which the hemodynamics of the cervical and cerebral structures was studied pretrauma and posttrauma. Further research in this area is needed.

Pollock et al. (58) presented four cases of esophageal and hypopharyngeal perforations occurring in patients subjected to hyperflexion injuries. Two of these injuries were from motor vehicle accidents. Results of previous reports have generally indicated that the hyperextension injury is responsible (59). Lesser trauma may produce hemorrhage into the musculature of the esophagus. Pollock et al. (58) have indicated the posterior sling formation of the cricopharyngeal muscle as the inherent weak spot that renders the esophagus susceptible to trauma from bone fragments or osteophytic spurs. Others have proposed alternate mechanisms. Stringer et al. (60) have suggested that after the hyperextension phase of an injury, when the anterior longitudinal ligament has been ruptured and the disc has been torn such that the vertebral bodies separate, the esophagus is caught between the gap in the vertebral disc defect during the hyperflexion phase. This has been seen at autopsy (61). Some authors (61, 62) have implicated impalement on the sharp edge of the vertebra as a likely mechanism. All are likely to be causative, depending on the individual case. Certainly the elderly or those with advanced spondylosis of the cervical segments are at greater risk. Esophageal perforation carries a relatively high mortality rate because of the multitude of complications that can occur, such as bronchopneumonia, mediastinitis, and meningitis. Any unexplained fever, neck swelling, dysphagia, leukocytosis, hematemesis, hemoptysis, or wide mediastinum or subcutaneous emphysema seen on x-ray in a patient after acute cervical spine injury should be considered cause for a thorough workup. According to Love and Berkon (63), plain films of the cervical spine show pre-

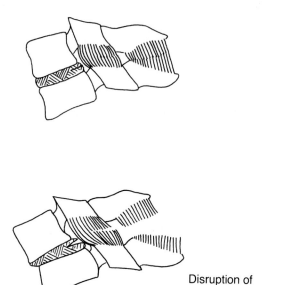

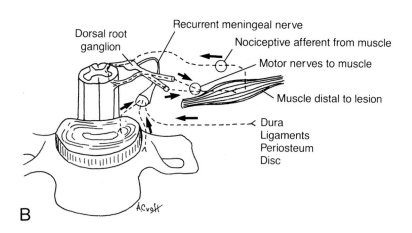

A   Acroff   Disruption of posterior elements

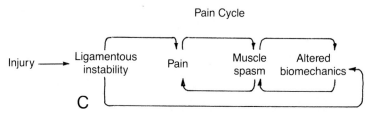

B

Dorsal root ganglion
Recurrent meningeal nerve
Nociceptive afferent from muscle
Motor nerves to muscle
Muscle distal to lesion
Dura
Ligaments
Periosteum
Disc

Pain Cycle

Injury ⟶ Ligamentous instability → Pain → Muscle spasm → Altered biomechanics

C

Figure 8.10. Rupture of stabilizing soft tissues in the cervical spine results in biomechanical instability and a consequent positive feedback loop or vicious circle of pain. **A.** Ligamentous instability. **B.** Afferent noxious stimuli from injured paraspinal tissues are transmitted via the recurrent meningeal (sinuvertebral) nerve, which via segmental cord reflexes, results in muscle spasm and pain in healthy muscles distal to the lesion. (Adapted from Cloward RB: *J Neurol Neurosurg Psychiatry* 23:321, 1960.) **C.** Schematic drawing illustrating the multiple mechanisms of the pain cycle.

vertebral air in all cases of perforation. Chest films show mediastinal air, air/fluid levels in the mediastinum, wide mediastinum, subcutaneous emphysema, pneumothorax, and pleural effusion. Esophagography with contrast media may be diagnostic in only 50% of cervical level perforations (64) and in 75–86% of thoracic perforations (64–66). Esophagoscopy with a flexible fiberoptic endoscope may also be useful, but Pollock et al. (58) have reported studies in which successful diagnosis with this method did not exceed 30%.

Injuries to the temporomandibular joint occur when the patient's head is abruptly hyperextended and the force generated by it overcomes the tone of the anterior cervical and masticatory muscles. When this occurs at the temporomandibular joint, as is the case with the cervical spine, the ligaments that support the joint may become stretched or torn. This may result in subluxation of one or both joints along with displacement of the meniscus. In severe cases, luxation is possible. It is likely that the muscles of mastication will also be strained, which may further complicate the picture. The temporomandibular joint is discussed in further detail in Chapter 10.

Symptoms

NECK PAIN

Neck pain is the most commonly reported symptom following acceleration/deceleration trauma. It may be immediate, but it is generally delayed in its onset, occurring usually within several hours. Symptoms may commonly be delayed up to 24 (55) to 48 hours (51). This has undoubtedly served to skew certain statistics regarding this form of injury, especially when there is reliance on data derived from emergency room notes that often describe the patient's condition only minutes to hours posttrauma. It is not uncommon for pain to appear several days (20) and, occasionally, weeks after the injury (15, 67, 68). Braaf and Rosner (68) have strongly emphasized that symptoms may be delayed months or even years.

The timing of onset of symptomatology is largely dependent upon the nature and extent of the soft tissue lesion. Neck pain is generally followed by a general myospasm of the cervical paraspinal musculature, either from reflex or from muscular rupture or tear. Range of motion is quite limited, and passive movements are generally painful. On palpation, tenderness is usually noted over strained muscles anteriorly or posteriorly. Occasionally, the patient may present holding his or her head. This generally indicates that significant soft tissue injury has occurred and ligamentous damage may be severe.

The incidence of neck pain following acceleration/deceleration injury has been variously reported as 62% (69) and as more than 98% (67, 70, 71).

Several authors have reported a higher incidence of injury in women than in men (15, 67, 70). One possible explanation may be that men generally have a heavier musculature in the cervical and thoracic spine and so are more resistant to injury.

Neck pain is often protracted. There may be numerous factors that contribute to this phenomenon. Stretched and torn ligaments can allow abnormal range of motion at the intervertebral joints, zygapophyseal joints, atlantoaxial joints, and atlantooccipital joints. Both stretched and torn ligaments, by direct inflammation, and hypermobile joints, by overstretching of joint capsules, can elicit pain. This latter condition results in an increased tone in the supporting musculature of the cervical spine which then attempts to stabilize and splint this aberrant motion. This muscular hypertonicity begins with the shunt muscles that stabilize the joints and act to coordinate fine intersegmental movements (Fig. 8.10). Clinically, this condition is seen as myospasm of the larger muscle groups that act as postural muscles and coordinators of gross movements of the neck.

Damage to the muscles themselves can also serve as a potent source of continued neck pain. Healing of muscle and tendon is a slow process, and healing of ligaments is even slower and, owing to their poor blood supply, is often incomplete (26).

As is discussed later in this chapter, long-term changes may result in cervical disc disease and spondylosis. Proliferative changes of the bone result in osteophytic spurs that may encroach upon the neuroforamen. Initially, the cervical nerve root

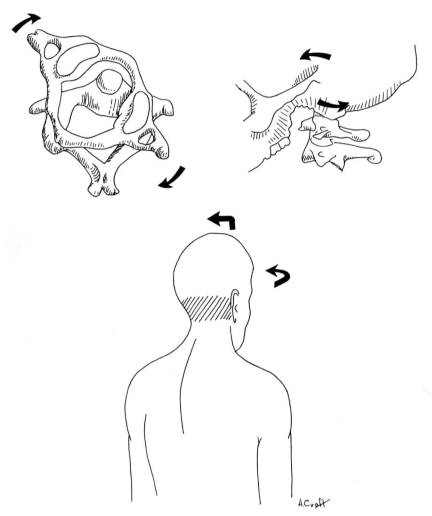

Figure 8.11.   Atlantoaxial arthrosis produces characteristic patterns of pain in the suboccipital (*shaded*) area with rotation of the head. Nodding motions occur between the occiput and the atlas and do not generally produce this effect. (Adapted from Hoppenfeld S: *Orthopaedic Neurology*. Philadelphia, JB Lippincott, 1977, p 29.)

may be able to migrate away from this osteophyte, but with gradual bony extension, or with sudden increased motion or injury the nerve root may become entrapped, resulting in the characteristic nerve root compression syndrome.

Somewhat less recognized are the syndromes that result from arthrosis of the diarthrodial joints of the upper cervical spine. Nerve roots in these areas are less vulnerable to exuberant osteophytic reaction and, even when directly irritated, may not be productive of commonly known symptoms. Atlantoaxial arthrosis may be

evidenced by well-localized suboccipital pain with rotation of the head (72) (Fig. 8.11).

HEADACHE

Headache is the second most frequently reported symptom in the acceleration/deceleration injury. It is almost invariably present with moderate to severe trauma to the cervical spine. In the series reported by Schutt and Dohan (67), 70% of patients presented with headache. Hohl (70) noted headache complaints in 66% of the patients

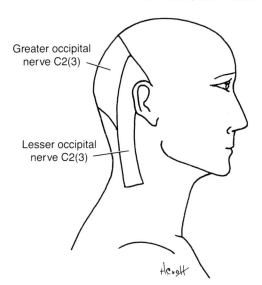

Greater occipital
nerve C2(3)

Lesser occipital
nerve C2(3)

Hevott

Figure 8.12. Areas on the scalp supplied by the greater and lesser occipital nerves.

in his study. Braaf and Rosner (68) have stated that headache occurs in 92% of trauma cases, while Norris and Watt (71) have noted complaints of headache in virtually all of the patients in their study (Table 8.4).

The pain may be unilateral or bilateral, intermittent or constant, localized or general. It may recur in a consistent pattern or vary greatly in its presentation from day to day. The occipital and frontal areas are most commonly affected, although parietal and temporal areas may also be involved, especially if there is injury to the temporomandibular joint.

Headaches may be of several types. Perhaps the most common is the muscle contraction headache or the so-called "tension headache." These are generally associated with occipital or frontal pain and are often

felt behind the eyes. They may also be neuropathic or vascular in origin.

A number of mechanisms may be responsible for this annoying and often debilitating complaint. The injury may have aggravated a previously quiescent condition that has become symptomatic posttraumatically. The most common example of this is spondylosis. Cailliet (73) has stated that a headache is the single most common presenting symptom of cervical spondylosis. Another mechanism described by Cailliet (73) is that of spasm, injury, or inflammation to the muscles of the cervical spine or myofascial connection to cranial periosteum such that the greater and lesser occipital nerves may become trapped and irritated within these structures, resulting in pain along the distribution of the nerves (Fig. 8.12). Headaches occurring in the areas supplied by the greater and lesser occipital nerves may also be caused by cervical disc degeneration at the upper and lower levels of the cervical spine. The mechanism of referred or sclerotomal pain as described later in this chapter is also operant in cases of cervical spine trauma in which ligamentous and/or deep muscular damage has occurred.

Muscular, myofascial, or ligamentous tear or rupture may produce a chronic local inflammation with its attendant release of irritating substances such as substance P, bradykinin, and other pain-producing polypeptides as well as proteolytic enzymes that are released from damaged tissues. Ischemia from muscle spasm also produces pain. In the presence of these compounds, afferent nerve endings are stimulated and send messages to the cord, which reflexly increases the contraction via

Table 8.4.
Incidence of Headache and Other Common Symptoms after Acceleration/Deceleration Injuries to the Neck That Were Sustained in Motor Vehicle Accidents[a]

Symptoms	Schutt and Dohan (67) (n = 74)	Braaf and Rosner (68) (n = 101)	Hohl (70) (n = 146)	Norris and Watt (71) (n = 61)
Neck pain	100	100	98	100
Headache	70	92	72	48–80
Pain or paresthesia in upper extremity	7	75	12	33–100[b]

[a]n equals number of patients.
[b]See Table 8.7.

internuncial and intraspinal neurons acting on anterior motor neurons, creating in effect a positive feedback loop. The increased ischemia that results tends to perpetuate the cycle and probably also impedes the cellular repair process by altering the tissue hemodynamics and local pH.

Vascular causes have also been implicated in many cases of headache following trauma (74–77). Patten (78) has stated that migraine headache may occur in patients after quite trivial head injury. This may occur in those with no previous history of migraine. That some headaches are vascular in nature can be demonstrated by the patient's favorable response to vasoconstrictors such as ergotamine tartrate. This type of headache tends to be of a throbbing and unilateral nature but represents only a small fraction of those seen posttraumatically (79).

An air of controversy continues to surround the subject of *posttraumatic* or *postconcussion headache*. The symptoms frequently encountered with this type of headache are fairly consistent, so it may be more appropriate to refer to this as *posttraumatic* or *postconcussion syndrome*. The difference between the terms posttraumatic and postconcussion is really one of semantics. By classic definition, concussion implies a loss of consciousness, although I agree with some authors who believe that this is not a prerequisite. Patten (80) has stated that the syndrome is usually not preceded by a loss of consciousness.

Symptoms associated with this disorder include headache, neck pain, dizziness, difficulty concentrating, memory loss, insomnia, irritability, depression, anxiety, intolerance to alcohol and, in some cases,

Table 8.5.
Signs and Symptoms Associated with Posttraumatic Headache Syndrome

Headache	Irritability
Neck pain	Depression
Dizziness	Anxiety
Difficulty concentrating	Intolerance to alcohol
Memory loss	Personality changes
Insomnia	

personality changes (Table 8.5). Rutherford et al. (81) found women experienced significantly more symptoms than did men.

The finding that brain damage can occur from whiplash injury without loss of consciousness has been documented by several researchers using both animal experimentation with primates (3, 82, 83) and clinical studies (52, 74, 84–90). Wickstrom et al. (3) and Ommaya (82) have found EEG changes in experimental primates subjected to whiplash injury. These changes are similar to those seen after blunt, closed head injury and concussion. In these and other studies, loss of consciousness does not seem to be a requisite condition for organic brain damage (52, 84–92), although it may be significant in terms of long-term prognosis; i.e., loss of consciousness is associated with a less favorable prognosis. Torres and Shapiro (89) compared 45 cases of whiplash injury without head injury and 45 cases of closed head trauma. They found EEG abnormalities of moderate or marked degree in 46% of the cases of whiplash and in 44% of the cases of closed head trauma and concluded that both injuries present a similar clinical picture. Gibbs (52), in describing this phenomenon, has recommended evaluation by EEG beginning as soon as practicable after the injury. If it is abnormal, he recommends repeating the study every 3–6 months and, if it is still abnormal, yearly thereafter.

Jacome and Risko (74) studied patients suffering from posttraumatic syndrome. These patients had sustained either closed head injury or whiplash. Their testing failed to demonstrate EEG changes in the seven cases of whiplash injury without accompanying head injury.

Simons and Wolff (93) have characterized three types of posttraumatic headache: generalized, focal, and unilateral (Table 8.6). The generalized headache is the most frequently seen and probably represents a muscle contraction headache (79). The focal headache may represent local scar formation, fibrositis, or periostitis and is usually described by the patient as sharp and stabbing. The clinician must always be alert to symptomatology suggestive of late-occurring chronic subdural hematoma (79, 94). Mild confusional states or progressive

Table 8.6.
Characteristics of Three Types of Posttraumatic Headache[a]

Type of Headache	Possible Causes	Signs and Symptoms
Generalized headache	Ligamentous and muscular injury to head and neck	Intermittent or constant pain increasing with exertion; sensations of heaviness, pressure, dizziness
Focal headache	Local scar formation, fibrositis, periostitis, intracranial injury	Sharp, jabbing, or stinging pain
Unilateral headache (similar to vascular headache)	Localized sympathetic overactivity	Throbbing, episodic pain, nausea, vomiting

[a]After Simmons and Wolff (93) and adapted from Ford JS: Posttraumatic headache. *Med Recertification Associates* 4(1):3–11, 1985.

intellectual impairment, an increase in severity or frequency of headaches, double vision, changes in gait, vomiting, or hemiparesis should be thoroughly investigated. The exact nature of this syndrome remains, for the most part, a mystery. Some authors deny that the syndrome exists at all. Other authors contend that nonorganic forces are operant (94–96). Hodge (53) has suggested that some patients may delay their recovery because of emotional instability and a desire for compensation. Abbott (97) has considered emotional tension to be a major factor in delayed recovery. And Threadgill (98) has concluded that self-delusion and malingering may be the correct diagnosis in many cases.

Ebbs et al. (69) sent out follow-up questionnaires to patients who had been injured in motor vehicle accidents and had been seen shortly thereafter in the emergency room of the local hospital. In their study of 137 patients who had been seen and then released, 85 (62%) complained of neck pain. In 15 of these, the pain lasted only 1 week. In 48, the pain had subsided within 6 months. Thirty-six had pain that lasted more than a year. These investigators found that at 6 months, 35% continued to complain of neck pain. Schutt and Dohan (67), in their study of women only, found that at 6 months, 75% continued to experience neck pain. This high number may reflect certain anatomical, physiological, or psychological differences between men and women.

Norris and Watt (71) studied a series of 61 patients whose vehicles had been struck from the rear, resulting in acceleration/deceleration injuries. These patients were

Table 8.7.
Symptoms, after Acceleration/Deceleration Injuries to the Neck That Were Sustained in Motor Vehicle Accidents, at Initial Presentation and at Final Follow-up, Indicated in Percentages[a]

	Percentages of Patients					
	Group 1		Group 2		Group 3	
Symptoms	At Presentation	At Final Follow-up	At Presentation	At Final Follow-up	At Presentation	At Final Follow-up
Neck Pain	100	44	100	81	100	90
Headache	48	37	78	37	80	70
Dysphagia	18.5	0	9.5	0	30	0
Paresthesias	33	37	43	29	100	60
Weakness	15	0	9.5	0	50	0
Visual symptoms	7.5	18.5	0	9.5	30	10
Auditory symptoms	7.5	11	0	14	30	20

[a]Adapted from Norris SH, Watt I: The prognosis of neck injuries resulting from rear-end vehicle collisions. *J Bone Joint Surg* 65B(5):608–611, 1983.

separated into three groups. Group 1 comprised patients who complained of symptoms associated with their injuries, although there was no gross abnormality found on physical examination. Group 2 comprised patients who, in addition to symptoms, had a reduced range of motion in the cervical spine but had no abnormal neurological signs. Group 3 comprised patients with symptoms, a reduced range of motion in the cervical spine, and evidence of objective neurological loss. These patients were followed for 6 months. The incidence of neck pain at 6 months in this study falls between that reported by Schutt and Dohan (67) and that reported by Ebbs et al. (69). It is surprising that at 6 months follow-up, 81% of the patients in group 2 and 90% of the patients in group 3 continued to complain of neck pain (Table 8.7).

Neck and muscle contraction headache symptoms following whiplash injury are known to persist for long periods of time despite conservative care. As mentioned previously, Norris and Watt (71) found residual neck pain in 44–90% of cases 6 months after injury. They also found that occipital headache may have particular significance, since 80% of patients with this complaint were involved in litigation. Schutt and Dohan (67) found similar statistics. Some patients were still under treatment 26 months after injury. Ebbs et al. (69) found persistent neck pain in about 35% of their patients at 6 months and in 26% at 1 year. Gotten (20) studied 100 cases of whiplash trauma that had gone to litigation. He found that 12% of these patients suffered severe residuals, another 34% suffered minor residuals, and the greatest percentage of recovery occurred in the first year.

Macnab (16) followed 575 cases of whiplash trauma. Of these, 266 had gone to litigation and been settled 2 or more years previously. He attempted to contact this latter group for follow-up, but only 145 patients responded. Of this 145 patients, 121 had residual symptoms. It was theorized that most of the 266 patients who were asymptomatic may have considered this study purposeless and a waste of their time and that it was more likely that only those who remained symptomatic would respond. If this were the case, and only 121

of the 266 were to be considered symptomatic, 45% had residual symptoms 2 years after litigation had been concluded. It is also conceivable, however, that those who had undergone endless diagnostic and treatment approaches and still suffered from neck pain or other symptoms might be somewhat disillusioned, disappointed, or perhaps even bitter toward the medical establishment. This group might also be unlikely to respond to this type of study, and so 45% is probably a conservative figure.

As mentioned previously, posttraumatic headache symptoms such as neck pain may also persist for months or years. Brenner et al. (99) reported that 40–60% of cases in his study persisted longer than 2 months. Russell (84) described persistence of headache longer than 6 months in 60% of 141 patients. Denker and Perry (91) found headache symptoms lasting longer than 1 year in 33% of patients and those lasting longer than 3 years in 15–20% of patients. Glaser and Shafer (84), in a review of 255 cases of posttraumatic headache, reported that 31% of patients continued to complain of headache after 5 years.

OTHER SYMPTOMS

Many other symptoms are commonly seen following the acceleration/deceleration injury. *Shoulder pain* is frequently described by patients and subsequently by clinicians. Although glenohumeral joint pain is uncommon in the absence of direct trauma, what is generally meant by "shoulder pain" is pain originating from the trapezius muscles. These are frequently strained and often found to be in spasm. The patient commonly will complain of pain radiating down the back of the neck and upper back into the midscapular region. This pain may represent one of three different conditions: muscle strain, herniated cervical disc, or sclerotomal pain.

In the case of muscle strain, the pain will be aggravated by passive stretching or active contraction of the muscle group, and edema may be present. In the case of herniated disc, the pain will be accentuated by movements of the neck and by orthopaedic tests such as Jackson's compression test and Spurling's test. Pain may be relieved temporarily by gentle manual cervical traction, and the patient may find that holding the arm in abduction with the hand and forearm above the head reduces the pain (Bakody's maneuver). This may serve to reduce the traction of a cervical nerve root against protruding disc material. Sclerotomal pain represents referred pain from deeper ligamentous, muscular, and osseous structures of the cervical spine which share a common embryologic derivation with the distal structures from which the patient perceives the pain emanating. This distal pain may be aggravated by movements of injured tissues but is of a referred variety and reacts very slowly to mechanical changes, unlike that seen in a case of disc herniation in which even slight movements of the neck result in immediate lancinating pain.

The character of pain may be of some diagnostic importance. Muscle tears or strains are generally described as burning pain and often can be localized to relatively discrete areas. Radicular pain is generally sharper and often described as shooting or electric shock-like pain. It is often associated with paresthesias more distally in the affected extremity along with changes in deep tendon reflexes and cutaneous sensitivity. Fasciculations of the muscles innervated by the affected root may be present. Sclerotomal pain is often difficult for the patient to describe in terms of both quality and distribution. It is generally described as a deep aching pain and may be affected by stretching of the injured referring structures; i.e., pain felt in the midscapular area may be increased by rotation of the neck with consequent stretching of damaged spinal ligaments. This finding, however, is not consistent.

Tenderness to palpation may be present in all cases and is not particularly reliable from a diagnostic standpoint. Paresthesias and brachialgias are relatively common following a hyperextension/hyperflexion injury and usually represent muscle spasm in the scalene group. The most common distribution of pain and paresthesia in this case is the ulnar nerve.

Chest pain and pain over the female breast may result from contact with the shoulder harness. *Low back pain* is a very common complaint following acceleration/deceleration trauma and has been reported by Braaf and Rosner (68) as occurring in 42% of their patients, with sciatica occurring in 15%. Croft and Foreman (unpublished observations) have described low back pain occurring in 57% of cases of moderate to severe injury resulting from rear-end collision and in 71% of those resulting from side-to-side impact, such as when the victim's vehicle is struck broadside. The lumbar spine is much more vulnerable to lateral flexion trauma than to flexion/extension in the sagittal plane. As with cervical spine injury, chronic pain syndromes may result.

Symptoms associated with the eyes, ears, nose, and throat are common but often difficult to explain. *Dysphagia*, as noted earlier, may be of grave prognostic significance and often is indicative of esophageal injury, pharyngeal hemorrhage or edema, or retropharyngeal hemorrhage. It may also result from severe muscle spasm. Visual disturbances generally take the form of *blurred vision* and may be associated with retrobulbar pain. Although these may be psychoneurotic in origin, they may indicate (*a*) transient disturbances in blood flow to the brain via the vertebral arteries or (*b*) injury to the sympathetic nervous system (15, 56, 71, 79). In some cases, a Horner's syndrome may be present. Other visual disturbances may include photophobia, dry eye, nystagmus, or temporary visual loss. Auditory disturbances, such as loss of hearing in the upper ranges, may be present (56). These are often associated with *tinnitus*. The precise cause of tinnitus is unknown in most cases, but it has been suggested that the aftereffects of CNS injury, (100) as well as sympathetic nervous system injury, vascular impairment (21), or temporomandibular joint dysfunction (56) may be to blame.

Another commonly described subjective complaint is *dizziness*. This symptom may also be caused by injury to the sympathetic nervous system, by vascular injury, by impairment (vertebrobasilar syndrome), or by injury to the CNS, as in posttraumatic headache syndrome. Dizziness, which is a subjective feeling of disorientation with one's surroundings or of simple light-headedness, should be distinguished from *vertigo*, which is a sensation of rotation of one's self (subjective vertigo) or of one's surroundings (objective vertigo) in any

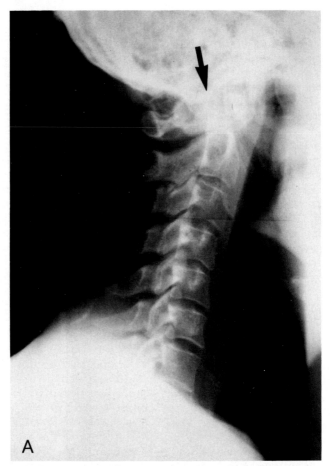

Figure 8.13. **A.** IR is a 27-year-old man who sustained a severe hyperextension injury when his pickup truck was struck from the rear by a semi-tractor trailer. The impact propelled his head into the back window, resulting in multiple stable fractures in the cervical spine (not well visualized here). Soft tissue hemorrhages around the vertebral artery produced vertigo first noticed in the hospital with rotation of the head. Later, this organized into fibrous scar tissue around the vertebral artery (*arrow*). After several months, this patient, who is a tree surgeon, continued to experience vertigo upon extension of the neck. This was resolved with physical therapy and manual manipulation. **B.** Illustrations *1–6* represent a digital run on a patient who sustained a severe lateral flexion injury to the cervical spine. The catheter was placed just proximal to the beginning of the vertebral artery in the aortic arch (*arrows*). A traumatic dissection was present at this level, preventing filling of the artery which is then seen to fill in subsequent pictures by backflow from collaterals (*arrowheads*). **C.** Schematic drawing.

plane. The latter generally represents a more severe injury or compromise of the vertebral artery and may be caused by extension and/or rotation of the head. Loss of consciousness may also occur. Examples of trauma to the vertebral arteries are illustrated in Figure 8.13.

Of the psychosomatic symptoms, *fatigue* and *general irritability* are present about 90% of the time (68). Fatigue may vary from a sense of mild tiredness to extremes of ex-

haustion and may be associated with restless sleep or insomnia. Quite often the patient will require more hours of sleep per night than he or she usually got and will still complain of fatigue. Other complaints may include mood changes, dysphasia, poor concentration, mental sluggishness, depression, anxiety, and ruminations about the accident. Many of these complaints have been considered to be exaggerations or fabrications on the part of the patient in order

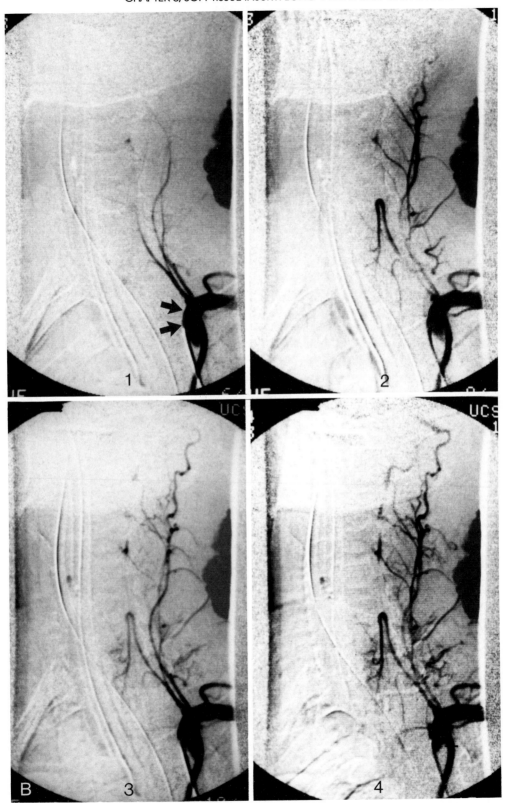

Figure 8.13.B *(1-4)*.

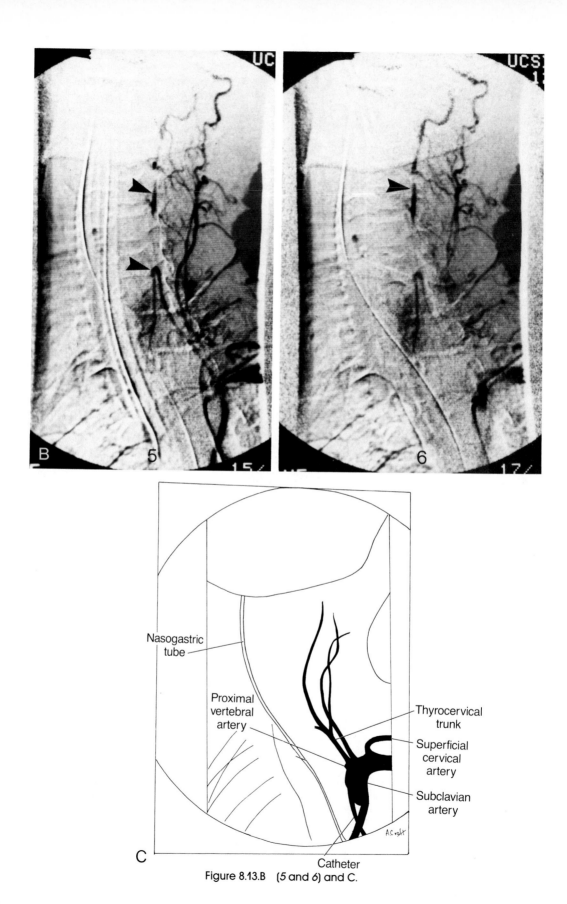

Figure 8.13.B (5 and 6) and C.

to secure a higher award in litigated cases, especially when no objective evidence of injury can be found. This constellation of symptoms, which are sometimes bizarre and certainly difficult to explain, are remarkably consistent, however, and the physician should realize that these symptoms are seen just as often in nonlitigated cases as in litigated ones and an organic basis for their presence should be sought. All too often in this type of trauma, after the examination is completed and x-rays are taken and found to be normal, the well-meaning physician will say to the patient, "There is nothing wrong with you." In actuality this may sometimes be the case, but often this statement represents the examiner's lack of knowledge or clinical acumen in this specialized area. The patient, if truly suffering, is looking for support, understanding, and relief; this type of statement, which is tantamount to accusing the patient of malingering or of being neurotic, serves no useful purpose and will generally send the patient looking for someone who can explain his or her symptoms.

Gross Tissue Changes

MUSCLE

Many researchers have produced grossly visible tears and ruptures in muscles of primates that were subjected to acceleration/deceleration forces. The degree of strain is often quoted as grade I, II, or III, depending upon severity. Grade I describes a condition in which the muscle remains grossly intact and functional and only some muscle fibers have been damaged (usually from overuse or overstretching). Grade II describes a more severe condition in which a part of the muscle has been damaged, although it still remains functionally intact. Grade III, the most severe form of injury, describes complete rupture of the muscle belly or tendon. This grading system, however, is more useful for describing the appendicular than the axial muscles. Unless the initial trauma is severe, most cases will be grades I and II, although it is generally not useful to describe them in this manner. Marked ecchymosis appearing under the skin may be seen with grade II strains of the larger and more superficial muscle groups. Injury can also occur at the musculotendinous junction or at the tenoperiosteal junction.

LIGAMENT

Ligaments and related structures such as the fascia and discs have also been shown to be damaged or disrupted in hyperextension/hyperflexion trauma. Both the anterior longitudinal ligament and the posterior ligamentous complex (intervertebral disc, zygapophyseal joint capsules, posterior longitudinal ligament, ligamentum flavum, interspinous ligament, and the ligamentum nuchae) have been shown experimentally (on primates subjected to +Gx

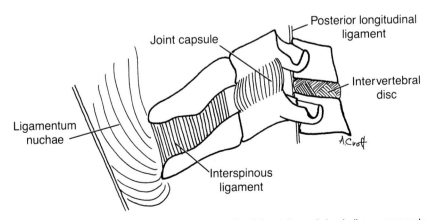

Figure 8.14. The posterior ligamentous complex consists of the intervertebral disc, zygapophyseal joint capsule, posterior longitudinal ligament, ligamentum flavum (not illustrated), interspinous ligament, and ligamentum nuchae.

and −Gx vector acceleration) to rupture either partially or completely (Fig. 8.14). Ligaments of the upper cervical spine, such as the cruciform ligament, the suspensory or apical ligament of the dens, and the alar ligaments, have also been found to be ruptured or disrupted (3, 6).

NERVES

Trauma to the cervical spine may injure the nervous tissue and related structures in several ways. During the hyperextension phase of the injury, nerve roots may suffer a compression injury at the point of exit

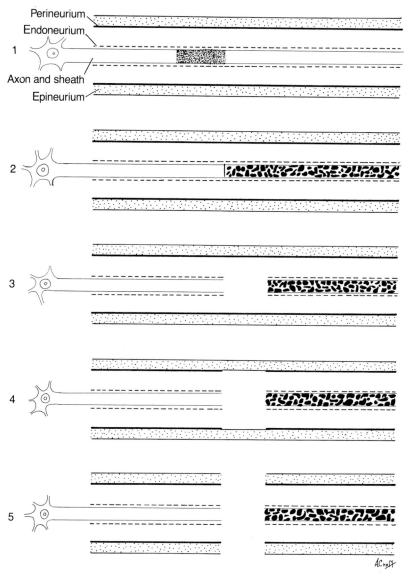

Figure 8.15. The histological structure of the nerve trunk in the five stages of nerve injury. *Stage 1* represents a simple conduction block or *neuropraxia*. Recovery is spontaneous and complete within several days or weeks. In *stage 2*, the axons are damaged such that wallerian degeneration takes place. Recovery is complete following regeneration. This may be described as *axonotmesis*. In *stage 3*, regeneration is incomplete and imperfect. In *stage 4*, the obstacles to establishment of good continuity are great and recovery is not expected. In *stage 5*, the nerve is completely severed and the chances of reestablishing useful connections are quite minimal. This is described as *neurotmesis*. (Adapted from Sunderland S: *Nerves and Nerve Injuries*, ed 2. Edinburgh, Churchill Livingstone, 1978, p 3.)

from their neural foramina. The nerve root may become contused severely enough to produce actual disruption of axons and resulting axonotmesis. Because the internal structure is fairly well preserved, however, recovery is generally spontaneous. Neuropraxic injury is more common and is clinically manifested as the transient paresthesias seen most often during the week or several days after the trauma (Fig. 8.15).

Spinal cord, dura, and arachnoid may also be contused. Subarachnoid hemorrhage has been demonstrated in experimental animals by Unterharnscheidt (6) and others.

During the hyperflexion phase, tractional injury may occur. These injuries are described in greater detail in Chapter 9.

FAT

Traumatic fat necrosis has been described in several cases in which the female breast had been contused by the shoulder harness (49). This lesion can be seen as a focal area of necrotic liquefied fat cells surrounded by an acute inflammatory area. This nodule gradually becomes more firm and less tender and generally is accompanied by a retraction of skin over a dense fibrous scar, not unlike certain forms of cancer that, of course, must be included in the differential diagnosis. Dawes et al. (49) reported on six cases in which shoulder harness trauma resulted in traumatic fat necrosis. As mentioned previously, a connection has been made between shoulder harness trauma and carcinoma of the breast (49). Some cases have even gone to litigation on this assumption (101). Mammography will almost invariably make the distinction between carcinoma and traumatic fat necrosis.

Repair Process

ACUTE STAGE

When the trauma of hyperextension/hyperflexion is great enough to produce tissue damage, the initial reaction is one of inflammation. This process is controlled largely by several chemical mediators (102) which can be categorized as follows:

Amines
  Histamine
    Inactivation of epinephrine and norepinephrine
Kinins
  Bradykinin (9 amino acids)
  Lysyl-bradykinin (10 amino acids)
Protein and tissue extracts
  Globulin permeability factor of Miles
  Cleavage fragments of complement
  Lymph node permeability factory
Miscellaneous
  Slow-reacting substance
  Lysolecithin
  Esterases of complement

Histamine is the major mediator of the acute inflammatory response, producing dilation of arterioles and venules, constriction of veins, and increased permeability primarily in the venules. Robbins (103) has stated that "contrary to earlier beliefs, the venules are the principal actors in the early phases of acute inflammatory drama. Capillaries play a larger role in the later phases of more severe injury."

Epinephrine and *norepinephrine* may play a small, rather indirect part in the inflammatory response. Normally, these substances produce vasoconstriction. At the site of injury, however, they may be degraded by monoamine oxidase, with the net effect being vasodilatation and increased permeability.

Kinins, which are a group of polypeptides, are major mediators of inflammation. They have been shown to produce pain, dilate arterioles, increase vascular permeability, and cause margination of leukocytes in vessel walls (104).

Globulin permeability factor causes increased vascular permeability. This agent may be related to and may activate the kinins.

Cleavage fractions of complement (C3 and C5) indirectly contribute to the overall process of inflammation by inducing mast cells to release histamine. Lysosomal enzymes and proteases released from injured cells as well as from neutrophils participate by activating kinins and probably also by direct enzymatic catabolic damage to healthy tissues.

Lymph node permeability factor has been suggested by some (105) to contribute to a delayed increased vascular permeability while *slow-reacting substance* and *lysolecithin* have also been shown experimentally to produce this effect. Many of these chemical mediators may not be directly involved with mechanical trauma and may only be operant in cases of immunological inflammatory responses.

Other mediators undoubtedly play greater or lesser roles in the acute inflammatory response, and although much research has been carried out in this area, much is still needed, since, as Robbins (106) puts it, "no single unifying concept fits all of the collected observations."

The cardinal signs of inflammation are calor (heat), rubor (redness), dolor (pain), and tumor (edema). Heat and redness result from the opening up of the local tissue microcirculation. This response may be delayed by several hours. Pain may be associated with a number of phenomena: actual tissue damage, such as torn or ruptured soft tissue; ischemia resulting from a disruption in vascular supply, which in turn may result from rupture of small blood vessels, vascular thrombosis, or vascular compromise due to swelling or muscle spasm; changes in the microcirculation which produce pH changes which, in turn, have an irritating effect on free nerve endings; some of the chemical mediators already mentioned which are also known to produce local pain; and, finally, swelling itself which produces an increased hydrostatic pressure within the tissues, which can be pain producing.

Swelling usually takes several hours to develop. When it is immediate, it often indicates that substantial bleeding has occurred. Less bleeding will occur when muscle fibers, fibrous tissue (collagen), elastic fibers, and other soft tissue elements are disrupted. The red cells released into the tissues break down into cellular debris and release hemoglobin. Platelets release thrombin which converts fibrinogen to fibrin. In a large inflammatory exudate, large quantities of fibrin are released and this ultimately organizes into collagenous scar tissue. Swelling may continue to increase for several days.

Regeneration of damaged tissues in humans generally leaves a new tissue that is somewhat less than perfect. Several factors that influence the eventual outcome of new tissue architecture are briefly discussed.

The cells of the body, as they relate to regenerative capacity, can be divided into three main categories. These are *labile, stable*, and *permanent*.

Labile cells possess the greatest regenerative capacity. This group includes the epithelial cells such as those lining the oral and vaginal cavities, the gastrointestinal tract, and the uterus.

Stable cells are those that are not normally engaged in regular mitotic activity. Their reproductive program is usually switched off. It has been suggested that injury to these cells suppresses the genetic message that maintains them in this genetically dormant state so that regeneration again becomes possible (107). These cells include all glandular parenchymal cells and mesenchymal derivatives, such as fibroblasts, osteoblasts, and chondroblasts.

Permanent cells are those that cannot, under any circumstance, be regenerated. The genetic message that represses their mitosis is unalterable. Nerve cells of the CNS constitute this group. When they are destroyed, whatever specialized function they were responsible for is lost forever, although other processes of adaptation may compensate to some degree, depending on the severity of injury. Peripheral nerves can regenerate if the cell body is spared. Degeneration of the distal portion is complete. Proximal to an injury, degeneration occurs only to the closest node of Ranvier. If the proximal stump remains in contact with the original channel, regeneration will usually take place.

Most injuries of the acceleration/deceleration type involve damage to stable cells. Fibroblasts are the major players involved in the repair process, and although unanimous agreement as to the origin of these cells does not exist, the general consensus is that they are derived from tissue adjacent to that which is injured. They are multipotential, being capable of differentiating into any other type of supporting cell.

It is now generally accepted that skeletal muscle fibers can regenerate (52), and evidence supports the contention that cardiac and smooth muscle also can regenerate (108, 109). This regeneration process may begin as early as the second day after trauma and become intensive between the fifth and twenty-first days, decreasing markedly during the next 3 weeks (110). Allbrook et al. (111), studying skeletal muscle injury in vervet monkeys, found healing to be complete in 21 days.

Severely damaged fibers do not recover but instead are phagocytized. They may regenerate later. Sarcolemmal tubes that are cleared of all cellular debris become lined with columns of myoblasts. It is a coalescence of individual myoblasts that ultimately forms individual muscle fibers. The source of these myoblasts is said to be the satellite cells of Mauro (112).

In the tissue spaces, muscle fibers attempt to grow by essentially the same process as that of the surviving sarcolemmal tubes. Unless these new fibers are accompanied by a nerve supply, however, they fail to mature and remain at the myotube stage, eventually atrophying (113).

Concomitant with this muscle regeneration is the proliferation of fibroblasts. The resulting collagen deposition often impedes the longitudinal growth of regenerating muscle fibers (114). This same process also may interfere with the ingrowth of nerve axons and result in noninnervated and, therefore, useless muscle tissue (115).

The proliferation of collagenous scar tissue is seen in virtually all soft tissue injuries (116) and may be influenced in several ways. Initially, the greater the amount of exudate released during the posttraumatic inflammatory period, the greater the amount of fibrin released to the tissues. As inflammation may persist for several days, it is important to minimize this exudative process for some time.

The question of mobilization versus immobilization in muscle injury has been disputed over the years. Allbrook et al. (111) described persistent tissue space edema and excess collagen deposition to be closely or perhaps causally associated with each other.

Lehto et al. (110) studied the effects of physical activity on granulation tissue production, scar formation, and muscle regeneration at various stages of healing in rats after skeletal muscle injury. These investigators found that immobilization after injury accelerated production of granulation tissue but that prolonged immobilization resulted in a poorly organized scar and regenerated muscle that was of inadequate tensile strength to withstand subsequent mobilization. They concluded that mobilization at the correct interval was essential for the quicker resorption of scar tissue and the better organization of muscle. This contention is now generally accepted (111, 117).

Jarvinen (117) also studied skeletal muscle healing in rats, comparing mobilization and immobilization, and found that hematoma, inflammatory cells, necrotic tissue, and degenerative changes disappear more rapidly in muscles treated by mobilization than in those kept immobilized. Denny-Brown (118) observed that normal muscle tension in healing skeletal muscle increased the speed of repair, while decreased tension resulted in randomly organized regenerated muscle and connective tissue fibers.

The general consensus is to immobilize for 1–5 days, depending on the severity of injury. Mobilization should follow this period.

As stated before, ligaments heal slowly and incompletely, if at all. Their blood supply is generally superficial and rather limited.

CHRONIC STAGE

Other connective tissue heals by proliferation of neighboring fibroblasts; scar tissue is the usual result. Scar tissue is less elastic, less resilient, less pliable, and less resistant to shear and tensile forces than is the original tissue. It can adversely affect mobility and extensibility and, therefore, may play a part in altered biomechanics. An example of this would be the thickened fibrous scar of the zygapophyseal joint, which is less elastic than the original tissue and functionally restricts local intervertebral kinetics (Fig. 8.16). The lack of motion at one level will be compensated for by hypermobility at adjacent levels, which in turn will usually result in degenerative disc disease and osteoarthritis some time in the future.

The concept that cervical spondylosis and cervical disc degeneration are causally associated with trauma is not a new one (72, 119, 120). Jackson (119) has stated that degenerative joint changes are, for the most part, the result of traumatic experiences, either single or multiple, or may have re-

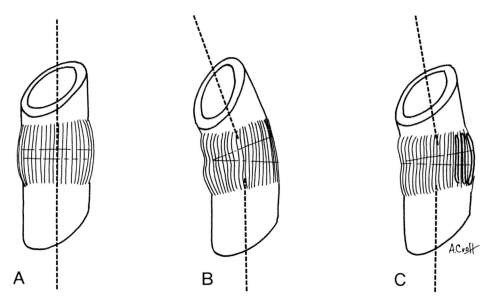

Figure 8.16. Schematic drawing of the kinematics of the zygapophyseal joint. **A.** Normal nonstressed joint and joint capsule. **B.** Normal joint in flexion. **C.** Restricted range of motion imposed by nonelastic scar tissue.

sulted from a mechanical imbalance of the motor units involved. Ehni (72) has associated trauma and changes described as "traumatic arthritis":

"Acute injury (sprain) of a joint produces synovial effusion, histamine release, capsular or ligamentous stretch or tear, bleeding, and associated clinical disabilities. Some of this is visible and palpable in joints in the extremities, such as the ankle and knee, but not in those of the spine. With repetition of the traumatic process or with chronic stress in the joint from shearing and other forces, as the disc thins and the superior facet moves cephalad under the inferior facet of the vertebra above, a chronic synovial reaction becomes established, which extends to the underlying articular cartilage. The cartilage undergoes fibrillar change, softens,

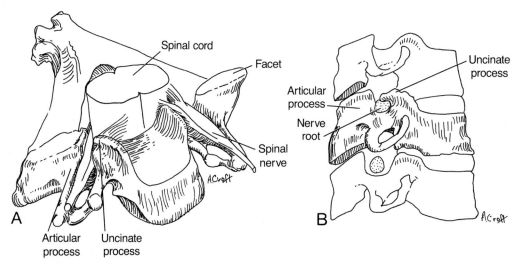

Figure 8.17. Hypertrophy of facet joints, articular processes, and uncovertebral joints or joints of Luschka may impinge upon spinal nerve roots. (Adapted from Hoppenfeld S: *Orthopaedic Neurosurgery.* Philadelphia, JB Lippincott, 1977, pp 40 and 41.)

and becomes rough and eroded. Stresses in the capsule and periosteum result in marginal osteophytosis, which may encroach on the underlying nerve root [Fig. 8.17]. A loose body may develop in the joint cavity, or an osteophytic process may fracture and lie free or loosely attached in or near the foramen. The facetal bone may thicken or hypertrophy, and the laminae may do so as well, but not to the same degree as seen in the lumbar spine. Degenerative enlargement of facets with irritative compression of one or more cervical roots may occur...."

In the spine, the term *osteoarthritis* is most appropriately applied to the diarthrodial apophyseal joints, while *spondylosis* may describe the amphiarthroidial intervertebral joints (121). Another term used to describe osteoarthritis of the posterior joints is *facet arthrosis*. Such other terms as *degenerative joint disease*, *osteoarthrosis*, and *hypertrophic arthritis* have also been used to describe this degenerative condition (122), but they are unsuitable. Degenerative joint disease implies a catabolic or running-down process, which is certainly not the case. Osteoarthrosis implies the condition is not inflammatory, and hypertrophic arthritis is an older term generally not used today. It implies hypertrophy of joint tissue. Osteoarthritis is, therefore, the most descriptive and suitable term used to describe this condition.

Some have suggested a mechanical origin in the development of osteoarthritis (123, 124), although this etiology is debated (122, 125). Huskisson et al. (126) has suggested an active metabolic abnormality as the underlying etiological factor. It is probable that a multiplicity of factors may be responsible for the development and progression of this condition. These may include hormonal influences such as insulin, estradiol, and human skeletal growth factor, which intensify osteoarthritis. Hypothyroidism is associated with a higher incidence of osteoarthritis. Virtually all hormones act either directly or indirectly on the fibroblast, osteoblast, and chondroblast (127).

Trauma may be one of the most common agents in the development of this disorder. This trauma, however, must be distinguished from that purported to occur according to the so-called "wear and tear"

theory. According to this theory, which is in such common use today and yet is truly untenable by strict definition, osteoarthritis and spondylitis result from the normal use of the joints over a long period of time. The normal human synovial joint simply will not wear out with normal use and under normal loads as suggested by this theory. Shear force is almost nonexistent, and the coefficient of friction is roughly equal to that of ice on ice (128, 129). In short, this joint is highly efficient and should last at least as long as the rest of the body.

The high incidence of cervical osteoarthritis and spondylosis observed in those presenting with symptoms years after an acceleration/deceleration injury suggests a very strong causal relationship, especially when the disease is localized to one or two levels. This has been recently investigated by Hohl (21) who found a high percentage of degenerative changes at long-term follow-up in patients who had been involved in motor vehicle accidents and in whom there was no prior history of degenerative disease.

All of these degenerative changes are permanent, and most ultimately affect function to one degree or another, often leaving the victim with years or perhaps a lifetime of residual pain or disability. "To add salt to the wound," often the injured patient is accused of hysterics, neurosis, or outright malingering.

Sources of Pain

Pain may result from numerous sources. Fractures and avulsion injuries involve pain-sensitive periosteal tissue and usually result in hemorrhage. Microfractures of bone that may not be visible on x-ray can also produce pain. Sudden deceleration may produce cervical disc herniation and annular tearing as well as fracture of the cartilaginous endplate with disc herniation into the body of the vertebra. These are usually seen on the superior endplate. The resulting increase in venous pressure within the vertebral body is thought to be a source of pain.

Herniation or extrusion of disc material

Table 8.8.
Sources of Pain Associated with Acceleration/
Deceleration Injury

Primary Sources of Pain

Fracture including avulsion injury, microfracture
and infraction

Dislocation

Subluxation

Periosteal tear

Ligamentous tear

Tendinous tear

Muscular tear

Fascial tear

Disc injury including annular tear and herniation of
nucleus

Hemorrhage

Edema

Ischemia

Spasm

Local changes in tissue metabolism including pH
changes and release of chemical mediators of
the inflammatory response

Adhesions

Altered vertebral kinetics including subluxation,
static fixation of diarthrodial joints, and hypermobility or instability

Secondary Sources of Pain

Chronic pain cycles associated with alterations
in vertebral kinetics

Myofascial disorders

Osteoarthritis

Congenital anomaly

may produce cord pressure or nerve root irritation, the symptoms of which have been described. Tearing of ligaments, muscles, tendons, and fascia, whether complete or partial, is productive of characteristic pain, while overstretch of these tissues may produce similar but milder symptoms. Changes that occur following these injuries result in inflammatory responses (e.g., ischemia, edema, direct irritation of local tissue, free nerve endings by chemical mediators of inflammation) that, in turn, produce pain as described previously.

When ligamentous stability has been compromised, as in the case of disruption of the posterior joint complex, anterior sub-luxation often is the end product. The resulting instability can produce constant muscle spasm and a chronic pain syndrome. This condition often requires surgical stabilization (see Fig. 6.16). Other sources of pain include preexisting conditions such as osteoarthritis and spondylosis, congenital anomalies, osteoporosis, and metabolic diseases of bone that may have been previously quiescent and now have become symptomatic or that, following trauma, have been markedly exacerbated (Table 8.8).

Several authors (54, 130–132) have described a kind of pain that is thought to be referred from injury to deep skeletal and soft tissue structures. Inman and Saunders (131) in 1944 coined the term *sclerotomal pain* to describe this type of pain.

In an attempt to understand the similar quality of referred pain resulting from such unrelated lesions and disorders as ligamentous and tendinous trauma, subdeltoid bursitis, calcific tendonitis, scalenus anticus syndrome, bone cysts, osteoid osteoma, and metastatic carcinoma of bone, these same investigators (131) stimulated the deep tissues of a group of human volunteers (consisting mostly of doctors, nurses, and medical students) by injecting various compounds, such as Ringer's solution, 6% saline solution, and a 1:3000 solution of formic acid, through small-caliber needles into various deep tissues (i.e., muscles, tendons, periosteum, fascia, tendon, and joint capsules) and observing the results. They also tested mechanical stimulation of these tissues by using a Mathews

Table 8.9.
Thresholds of Pain for Various Tissues, Listed in
Order from the Lowest Threshold (Periosteum) to
the Highest (Muscle)[a]

Periosteum

Ligament, especially near bony attachments

Fibrous joint capsule, especially near bony
attachments

Tendon

Fascia

Muscle

[a]After Inman VT, Saunders JB de CM: Referred pain from skeletal structures. *J Nerv Ment Dis* 99:667–1944.

wire and scratching or drilling the tissues with it.

Several interesting observations were made from these experiments: (a) the experimental subjects had great difficulty localizing the stimulus—the deeper the stimulus, the poorer the ability to localize; (b) there was a notable lag between the time of injection or stimulation and the time that pain was felt (up to one minute for full intensity); (c) different pain thresholds were noted for different tissues (Table 8.9); (d) stimulation of the periosteum or the tendinous attachments of ligaments and tendons was accompanied by an extensive radiation of pain; (e) the radiation of pain was associated with soreness of muscles and tenderness over bony prominences; (f) vasomotor disturbances such as sweating and blanching sometimes occurred; (g) the peripheral radiation of pain, although similar to that of the local experimental lesion (injection point), sometimes appeared only after several minutes or even several hours; (h) the pain sometimes occurred for several days even when the lesion was quite small; and (i) the characteristic pain was so reproducible that pain charts could be made that demonstrated consistent patterns of pain.

Feinstein et al. (130) reproduced this study some 10 years later. They also used 6% saline solution. The experimental subjects included the authors, 75 medical students, and three laboratory assistants. Their findings were consistent with those of Inman and Saunders (131), but they made several additional observations: (a) upon stimulation of the first cervical level, pain was often evoked in the occipital region, and in one case, it radiated to the forehead; (b) upon injection, stimulation of a group of muscles innervated by the same roots of the brachial plexus referred pain to the identical areas; e.g., injection of the latissimus dorsi innervated by cervical roots 6, 7, and 8 produced a referred pain pattern consistent with that produced by the injection of individual muscles from each of these three root levels, i.e., flexor carpi radialis longus (sixth root level), abductor pollicis longus (seventh root level), and the first dorsal interosseus (eighth root level); (c) deep tenderness and muscle spasm were noted in most cases; (d) hypoalgesia rather than hyperalgesia was usually noted on the skin overlying areas of referred pain; (e) autonomic reactions such as pallor, sweating (which was usually generalized), bradycardia, hypotension, a "faint" feeling, and nausea were most common with thoracic injections and were not found to be proportional to the severity of pain; i.e., relatively minor pain was occasionally accompanied by overwhelming autonomic symptoms; (f) that sympathetic nervous system was not responsible for pain referral (this was demonstrated by performing a sympathetic block with 10 ml of 2% procaine (which produced a Horner's syndrome), but rather than abolishing the pain, it often intensified it;) and (g) peripheral nerve function or axonal reflex was not responsible for referred pain (this was demonstrated by complete anesthetic block of the branchial plexus). Axial injection, as noted previously, readily produced sclerotomal pain distally in the anesthetic area. The concept that the peripheral nervous system was not involved in the propagation of referred pain was further dramatically demonstrated by injecting interspinous areas and producing the characteristic "phantom pain" reported in amputees (132). The pain elicited in these experiments was always remarkably reproducible (130–132) and was described as "gripping," "heavy," "cramp-like," "aching," and "burning."

These experiments suggest a segmental origin of pain. This concept is consistent with the development of the human embryo, in that muscles and other tissues to which pain is referred derive their nerve supply from the same segments that are injured. As the ontogeny of the embryo and fetus proceeds with the accompanying limb rotations and varying tissue migrations, these structures maintain their primordial segmental connection with each other via nerve fibers from individual nerve roots. (For a review of developmental anatomy, see Chapter 7.)

Another concept that is well known to those experienced in working with musculoskeletal disorders is that of the "vicious circle" that often results from an injury to a particular tissue, which then produces muscle spasm in another segmentally re-

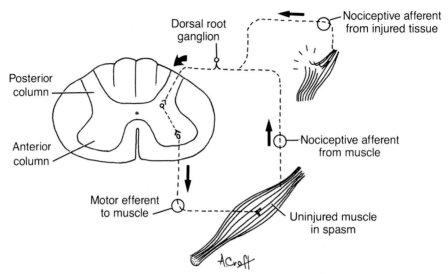

Figure 8.18. The vicious circle of pain originates in injured tissue such as ligament or muscle and is perpetuated by reflex arc via segmental spinal cord connections, resulting in muscle spasm in segmentally related yet uninjured muscle distal to the lesion.

lated (albeit uninjured) tissue. (This is akin to the well-known concept of viscerally referred pain as is seen in myocardial infarction.) The secondary muscle spasm is another source of pain (sometimes more intense than that of the original injury) and, via sensory reflex arc and segmental spinal cord connections, perpetuates the firing of anterior horn cells and thus the muscle spasm (Fig. 8.18). This condition, if left untreated, ultimately results in chronic, painful myofascial disorders. Treatment must

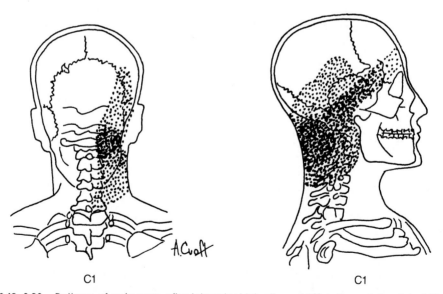

Figures 8.19–8.28. Patterns of pain seen after interspinal injection of 6% saline solution into 140 normal volunteers as described by Feinstein. *More darkly shaded areas* represent the more frequently localized areas of pain. For example, in Figure 8.19 the C1 interspinal space was injected, and the characteristic pattern of referred pain is shown from the rear and from the front. (Adapted from Feinstein B: Referred pain from paravertebral structures. In Buerger AA, Tobias JS (eds): *Approaches to the Validation of Manipulation Therapy.* Springfield, IL, Charles C Thomas, 1977, pp 155–160.)

be aimed at the original focus of injury if resolution of secondary symptoms is to be permanent. This often presents a diagnostic dilemma, especially to those unfamiliar with this concept.

The studies of Inman and Saunders (131) and Feinstein et al. (130) have shed much light on the etiology of these self-propogating myofascial syndromes and should be borne in mind when evaluating cases of acceleration/deceleration trauma in which the symptomatic complaints include radiating pain patterns to the head, back, and extremities. Many times, a direct correlation will be found between these pain patterns and injured spinal segments. The segmental referred pain patterns observed by Feinstein et al. (130) are illustrated in Figures 8.19–8.28. These figures represent the cumulative overlap of 140 individual observations of pain occurring after experimental injections of 6% saline solution at various interspinal levels. The segmental patterns described by Inman and Saunders (131) are illustrated in Figures 8.29 and 8.30.

Rationale for Treatment

Appropriate treatment depends upon an accurate diagnosis, for it is only with a clear understanding of the underlying pathology and its extent that the clinician can effectively prescribe a course of treatment that will not only help to alleviate the patient's initial pain but will also gradually lead the patient along a sensible course of rehabilitation. It must, therefore, be recognized that the course of treatment will encompass multiple phases of healing and the appropriate therapy must be geared not only to the nature and extent of the injury but also to whatever phase of healing the patient demonstrates. The patient may initially present at any stage in this process, from the early acute stage to the more chronic long-term stage, at which point the patient may have received no care, inadequate care, or improper care.

The popular acronym RICE (rest, ice, compression, and elevation) provides an easily remembered and generally useful and applicable rationale for proceeding with most injuries in the acute stage. As described earlier in this chapter, it is recommended that injured soft tissues be rested for 1–5 days. This has been shown to be associated with the most favorable outcome. More severe injuries may require slightly longer periods of rest and immobilization. When the spine has been injured, the most effective form of rest is bed rest. In most cases, however, this may not be necessary. Generally, if the patient is kept at home and quiet, he or she will find the proper atmosphere to begin the healing process.

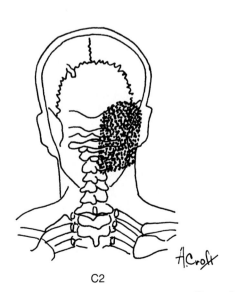

C2

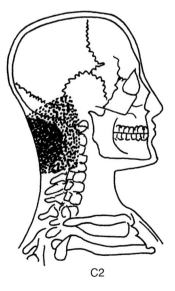

C2

Figure 8.20.

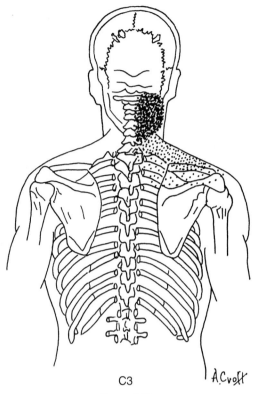

C3

Figure 8.21.

During the initial stages it is recommended that the patient wear a soft cervical collar which should be snug but not tight. The collar should also be tall enough to provide slight traction. Before putting the patient in the collar, however, the clinician should apply a slight amount of manual traction to the neck. This should provide some temporary relief of pain. If it aggravates the patient's pain, the cervical collar is contraindicated.

Some clinicians have recommended bracing in slight flexion or slight extension, depending on the major force of injury. I fail to see the wisdom of bracing an injured spine in a nonphysiologic position, regardless of the major vector of injury or type of presumed soft tissue damage, and, conventional wisdom not withstanding, have many times taken one of these rigid contraptions off a patient and replaced it with a soft collar, much to the relief of the patient. These flexible collars usually provide a surprising amount of support and comfort. Some patients even find that sleeping

in the collar initially provides them some relief. During the initial 48 hours, however, the patient should be icing the neck at regular intervals, which is another reason for having the patient at home.

When soft tissue injuries are severe or when stability is a problem, a more secure or restricting orthosis may be used. The most rigid of these devices is the adjustable four-poster brace with back and chest plates. These are usually only used in cases of fracture or after some types of surgery (Fig. 8.31).

Contrary to popular belief, the soft cervical collar does not promote muscle atrophy, although its use should be limited so that the patient does not develop a psychological dependency.

The use of ice during this acute inflammatory stage provides mild sedation and analgesia as well as limiting exudation and reducing muscle spasm. Gentle massage is useful to help relieve muscle spasm and promote drainage.

To aid in phagocytosis, it is recom-

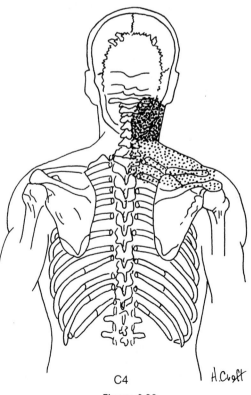

C4

Figure 8.22.

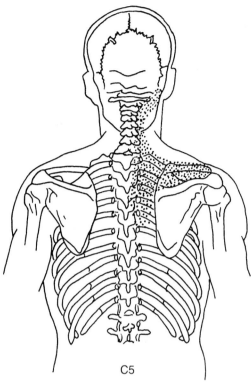

C5

Figure 8.23.

mended that modalities of physical medicine that agitate the tissue be employed. These might include gentle massage and low-intensity pulse muscle stimulation or ultrasound along with low-level muscular movements (133). Ultrasound is also said to "possess" mild analgesic properties and aid in dispersal of tissue fluids. It is also thought to improve fibroblastic repair (134) and is invaluable in the acute stages of soft tissue injury.

Other forms of physical therapy have been shown to be effective in the acute stage of injury. These may include high voltage galvanism, transcutaneous electrical neural stimulation, and electroacupuncture (which may also be referred to as hyperstimulation analgesia).

Several researchers (110, 111, 117, 118, 131) have shown that early mobilization of injured muscle tissue provides the most favorable outcome. Initially, the patient should be given isometric exercises to do at home. As an alternative, it may be advisable to have a therapist assist the patient in this exercise, especially if the patient is very old or very young or if the injuries are severe or multiple. I myself prefer to instruct all patients in specific exercise programs. Our therapists perform deep tissue massage and physical medicine procedures only. Later on, as the patients's recovery proceeds, active resistive exercises can be added. This should be encourage at every meeting with the patient, and their importance in the overall rehabilitation cannot be overemphasized, for in this type of injury it is almost axiomatic that poor muscle tone retards and, in some cases, may prevent the healing process. The patient must take an active part in his or her treatment from an early stage.

After the acute phase of inflammation has subsided, cervical traction may be instituted. Some authors advocate its use in the inflammatory stage to help reduce muscle spasm. The amount of traction applied at this early stage, however, should be light—perhaps 10–20 lb. At this stage, the traction should be continuous rather than intermittent. I do not recommend its use at this very early stage, however, as it may serve to intensify rather than relieve the patients's symptoms.

Most authorities (15, 68, 135, 136) recommend the use of cervical traction in the subacute and chronic phases of injury. As described previously, Denny-Brown (118) has shown that tension applied to the long axis of healing muscle provides for rapid healing with the strongest scar formation. Scar tissue, however, will also form in areas where it is not desirable, such as the fibrous joint capsules. Traction applied at regular intervals will help to prevent fibrous adhesions from occurring in these areas, thereby reducing the likelihood of delayed symptomatology resulting from secondary biomechanical changes (68, 137).

Although some clinicians (68, 137) have stated that traction should be considered palliative only, others (15, 135, 139) have recommended its use emphatically. I agree with Jackson when she states, "Anyone who treats cervical spine disorders should utilize motorized intermittent traction."

Jackson, using cineradiology, has shown that separation of the intervertebral foramen does occur when cervical traction of

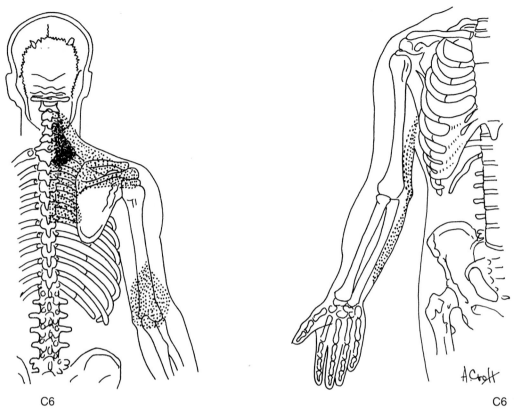

C6   C6

Figure 8.24.

more than 15–20 lb is applied (135). Depending upon the condition and size of the patient, she has recommended as much as 40 lb of traction in chronic disorders and up to 50 lb in those with thick muscular necks. Wickstrom and La Rocca (138) have suggested at least 20–25 lb of cervical traction for 20 minutes. They have also recommended that prior to traction, the patient should be given heat over the area and that in some cases in which mobility of the neck has not returned to normal, traction should be followed by rotary manipulation. Moist heat should precede cervical traction in the acute and subacute phases and is also useful in the chronic phase. Muscle stimulation with either a pulse or a surging current is useful in combination with heat preparatory to traction.

In general, it is advisable to initiate traction with very light forces and relatively short treatment times. This treatment should be observed closely for patient tolerance and discontinued if headache, occipital nerve irritation, or pain is observed. Before the patient is placed on traction, the clinician or therapist should apply firm manual traction to this patient. If the patient experiences some relief of symptoms, he or she is a good candidate for this modality. If symptoms are intensified, however, motorized traction should not be attempted.

Modern motorized traction equipment will usually have the following features: (*a*) a digital real-time display of pounds of traction applied, (*b*) a control that varies the mode of traction, i.e., progressive intermittent, intermittent, static, and progressive static, (*c*) settings to control the length of the "on" phase and "off" phase, (*d*) a setting for the number "steps" when used in the progressive mode, (*e*) a timer, and (*f*) a panic button or kill switch with which the patient can instantly turn the machine off and release the traction (Fig. 8.32). In addition, the halter harness that fits beneath the mandible and occiput should not be used, as it may irritate or injure the temporomandibular joint. Instead, newer equipment that pulls only from the mastoid area, thereby eliminating any pressure whatsoever on the temporomandibular joint, is available. This device also has the ability to be rotated several degrees in the coronal plane, so that a slight lateral flexion component can be added (Fig. 8.33).

When traction is being applied to the cervical region, the spine should be flexed approximately 10–15° in the sagittal plane. This provides the proper physiological and biomechanical advantage. The focal point

of traction can be somewhat controlled by varying this parameter. The upper cervical segments receive the greatest distractive force when the amount of flexion is the least. The lower cervical and upper thoracic segments are distracted with both increasing force and increasing forward flexion (Fig. 8.34).

When traction has proved efficacious for the patient, it may be augmented with home traction. These units are simple, effective, easy to use, and inexpensive. They consist of a water bag (which is filled to varying levels, depending on the amount of traction force desired) connected to a rope that runs up and over a pulley device that mounts on a door. The rope then runs down to attach to a halter that is worn by the

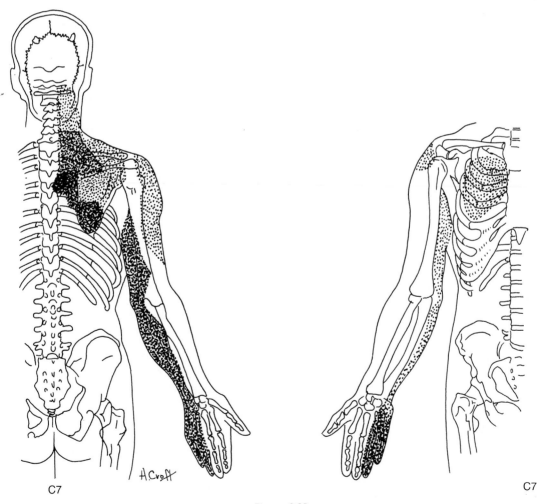

C7

C7

Figure 8.25.

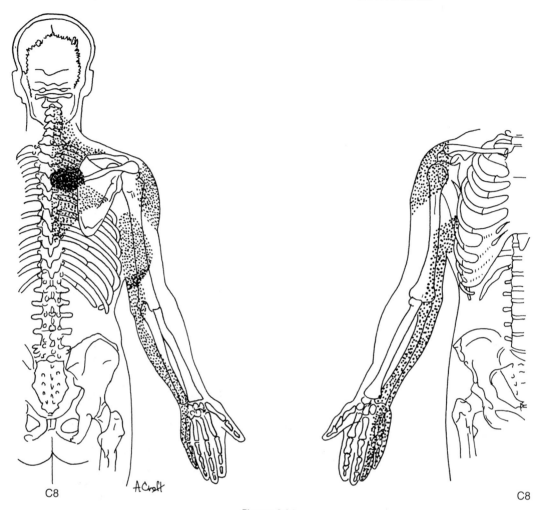

Figure 8.26.

patient. The patient should be positioned so that his or her neck is flexed slightly (Fig. 8.35). This form of traction is generally done with less weight (most water bags weigh 15–20 lb when full, although substituting sand or adding metal weights will increase this substantially). The advantage is one of convenience for the patient. Longer treatment times or multiple applications are possible with this method. The major disadvantage is that the halters provided with these units may adversely affect the temporomandibular joint and thus would be contraindicated in cases in which this disorder is a complicating feature.

The early concepts of cervical traction perhaps began with Sayre, an orthopaedic surgeon who hung his scoliosis patients by their necks temporarily while he applied plaster jackets to straighten thoracic scoliosis. His treatment, however, was not intended as cervical traction.

Many practitioners and therapists today still embrace and practice concepts of cervical traction that are overly simplistic. It is perhaps somewhat naive to suppose that the cervical spine is like a spring such that by pulling on one end, all interspaces can sequentially and uniformly be distracted. Therefore, it may be similarly unwise to use traction at forces that have been shown radiographically to distract intervertebral joints. These forces may serve to further injure joints that have already become hy-

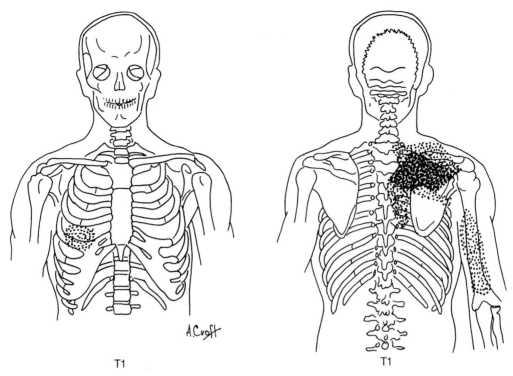

T1   T1

Figure 8.27.

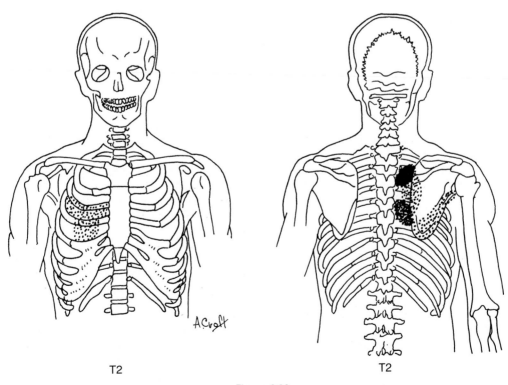

T2   T2

Figure 8.28.

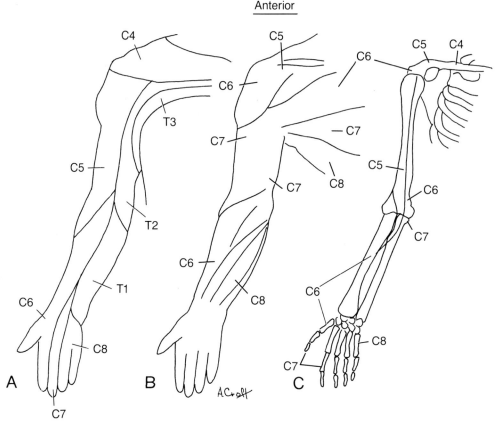

Figures 8.29 and 8.30. Anterior and posterior schematic drawings, respectively, of the segmental innervation first described by Inman and Saunders in 1944. **A.** Dermatomal pattern. **B.** Myotomal pattern. **C.** Sclerotomal pattern.

permobile due to either ligamentous instability from trauma or ligamentous laxity as a compensation for joint fixation at adjacent joints. Paradoxically, the tractional force sufficient to injure these hypermobile joints is often not adequate to successfully mobilize the hypomobile or fixated segments. This may explain some of the failures seen with conventional cervical traction.

Recently, Goodley (139) has devised a modification of the traditional cervical traction that allows careful placement of intersegmental traction along with any needed lateral flexion and rotational components, so that forces can be directed specifically at fixated segments. With this device, the patient, through foot pedal controls, can regulate the amount of force that is applied. This device can be used in a clinic or in the

patient's home. It can also be used in conjunction with conventional motorized traction. Goodley calls this new device the polyaxial cervical traction-mobilizer system; this form of traction appears promising. Clinical trials are currently in progress.

As with all physical medicine, the usual indications and contraindications should be carefully observed at all times. Accurate diagnosis and assessment of bony and soft tissue damage prior to the application of traction are essential. For example, marked disruption of the posterior elements is a definite contraindication for cervical traction, especially with forward flexion.

Many forms of medication are currently used to treat acute and chronic cervical spine injuries. The major categories of these drugs are analgesics, antiinflammatory drugs (both steroid and nonsteroid), tranquilizers, and muscle relaxants (some of which act on skeletal muscle directly, while others work on the CNS). Many physicians are also using antidepressants in low doses in combination with other drugs. This is claimed to be effective in cases of muscle contraction headaches.

Caution is the key word whenever the use of medication is considered. Narcotics and strong analgesics, because of the danger of habituation, should only be used in cases of moderate to severe pain. It must be remembered that these cases can last for several months and often for more than a year. And, as with visits to the physician, physical therapy sessions, and cervical collars, psychological dependency can also become a troublesome problem with this patient.

Muscle relaxants are effective when muscle spasm is present. That the phe-

nomena of both pain and muscle spasm serve a function in the aftermath of trauma and are not present simply to irritate the hapless victim of a hyperextension/hyperflexion injury should be kept in mind, however. These medications should be used in conjunction with the appropriate prescription for rest and bracing and not as a substitute. Otherwise, the well-intentioned physician may indirectly hamper the healing process by removing these important, albeit unpleasant, activity-inhibiting symptoms, thereby allowing the patient to move through ranges of motion that otherwise would have been limited by pain and spasm reflexes. And further microtrauma and delayed healing may result.

There are many muscle relaxants available today. I prefer to use a nonprescription preparation of *Passiflora* root, Valeriana root, and magnesium gluconate. It also

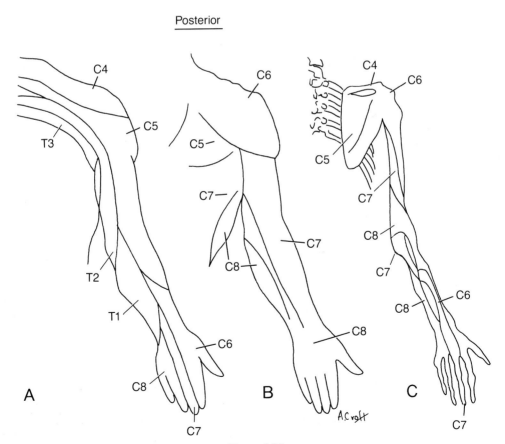

Figure 8.30.

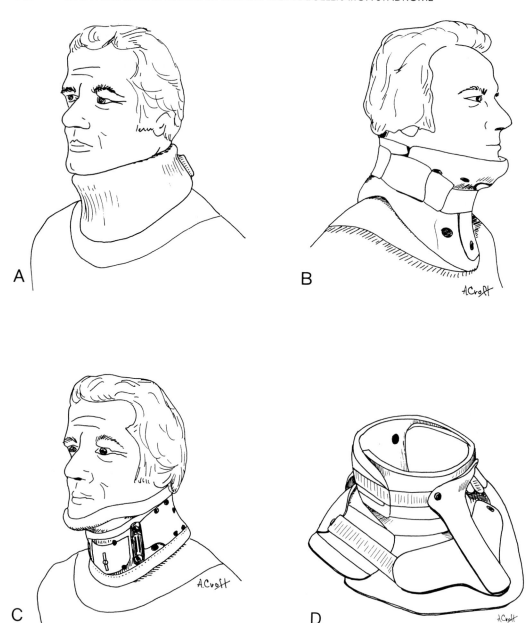

Figure 8.31. Cervical orthoses. **A.** Soft cervical collar with Velcro closure. **B.** Philadelphia collar. **C.** Rigid cervical collar. **D.** Modular, adjustable rigid cervical collar. **E.** Lerman Minerva spinal orthosis. **F.** Sternooccipital mandibular immobilizer. **G.** Thoracic cervical support. **H.** Anterior posterior rotational orthosis.

has a mild sedative effect and is surprisingly effective in about 80% of the cases of mild to moderate acceleration/deceleration trauma, especially when used in conjunction with salicylates or ibuprofen.

More popular in the realm of antiinflam-

matory drugs are the nonsteroidal antiinflammatory drugs. Ibuprofen is one of the most commonly used of these drugs.

Some authors (136, 140) have advocated the injection of steroids such as dexamethasone or cortisone in conjunction with local

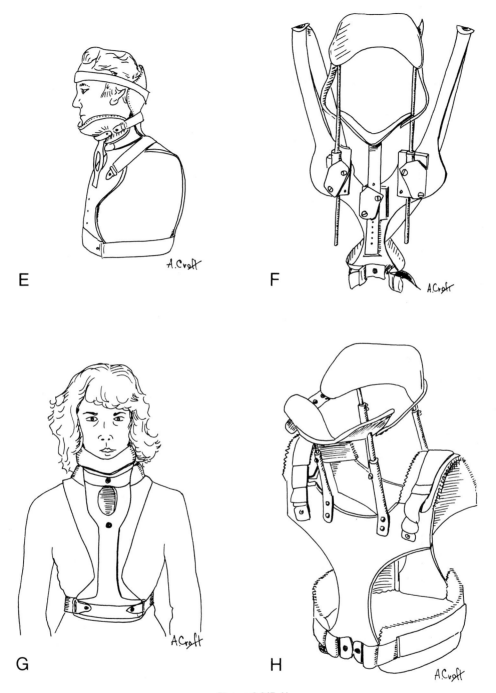

Figure 8.31E–H.

anesthetics such as lidocaine, procaine, or marcaine. It is suggested that infiltrating of painful trigger points in a muscle is often effective in breaking the painful cycle of pain and reflex muscle spasm. Although this is often effective, it is generally not a pleasant experience for the patient, and these trigger points can usually be relieved by noninvasive methods such as electro-acupuncture, ultrasound, transcutaneous

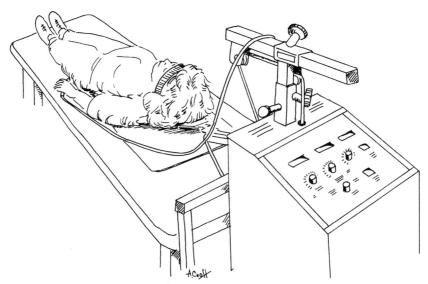

Figure 8.32. Cervical traction unit. Traction is applied from the base of the skull rather than from the jaw. The patient holds a "kill switch" and can shut off the machine if necessary.

electrical neural stimulation, and certain forms of deep massage. Some of these have been described by Travell and Simons (140).

As noted earlier, insomnia or restlessness at night is relatively common, especially in cases of postconcussion syndrome. This disorder is usually transient, although it may last for several months in some cases. The patient should be advised of this possibility and encouraged to retire to bed early, eat a small dinner, and reduce or eliminate his or her intake of caffeine and other stimulants during the day. Tryptophan (1000 mg) taken at bedtime may have a beneficial effect on sleep disorders (141, 142). It should be taken with a carbohydrate-rich and protein-poor meal. This increases insulin release which in turn, lowers the plasma levels of other neutral amino acids that compete for binding sites on carrier proteins. The protein-poor meal will further help to reduce the concentration of these amino acids, thereby selectively promoting transfer of tryptophan across the blood-brain barrier. Tryptophan is ultimately converted to serotonin. As one of the conversion steps is dependent upon pyridoxine (vitamin B6), this should be taken along with tryptophan.

Tryptophan is also important in the treatment of pain inasmuch as endogenous opioid-induced analgesia, which is produced by pain alone or by pain interacting with morphine, has been shown to depend on an increase in the uptake of tryptophan into the brain (143, 144). Clinical trials have shown it to be useful by itself in pain control. In one study (127), a regimen of 1000 mg of tryptophan 4 times a day along with high-carbohydrate and low-protein meals was used, and in another study (145), a regimen of 3000 mg of tryptophan given in 500-mg divided doses over a 24-hour period was used. Both proved effective. The use of hypnotics is not advisable because of the potential for habituation and dependence in cases that may last for weeks to months.

Other agents should also be considered in cases of soft tissue injury. Vitamin C is known to be important in wound healing inasmuch as it is needed for hydroxylation of proline and lycine. A considerable amount of the proline and lycine in collagen is hydroxylated (146). Vitamin C may also be required for incorporation of the hydroxylated amino acids into the polypeptides of the tropocollagen macromolecule (147). Another theory is that vitamin C plays a major role in the maintenance of the protein synthetic apparatus within the fibroblast (148). Jackson (149) has recom-

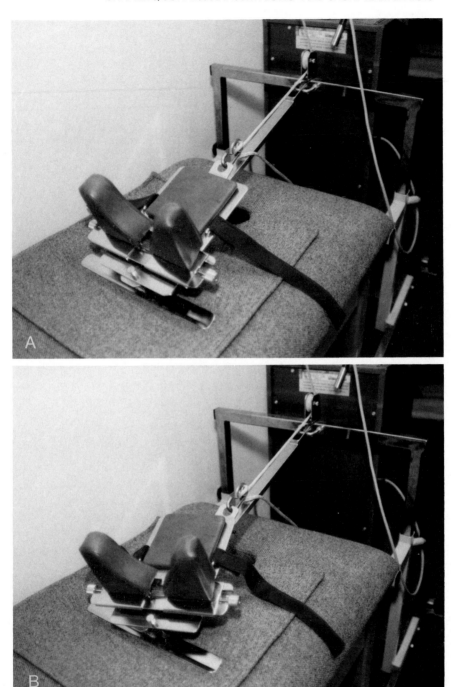

Figure 8.33. The traction plate rotates, thereby allowing the therapist to select one of several settings to facilitate selective asymmetric distraction.

mended time-release vitamin C in the early stages of the injury. Zinc is probably also important for wound healing (150).

Manipulation of the spine has been ad-vocated by Wickstrom and La Rocca (136), Maigne (151), Mennell (152), Jackson (153), Cyriax (154), Haldeman (155), Kirkaldy-Willis (156), and many others. In recent

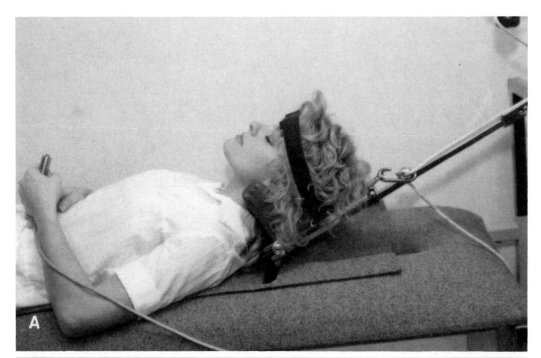

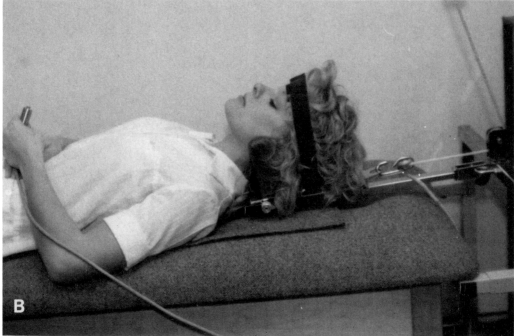

Figure 8.34.   A. The direction of pull has greater altitude, resulting in a greater concentration of distractive force at the lower cervical levels. **B.** A lower altitude traction pull directs forces at upper cervical levels.

studies, comparisons have been made between early mobilization by manipulation and the standard treatment—soft cervical collar, rest, and oral analgesics—in cases of whiplash trauma. In this single blind test, it was shown that early manipulation resulted in significantly less pain at both 4 weeks and 8 weeks (157). Manipulation is, of course, a large part of the practice of chiropractic and is practiced by many osteopaths as well.

The art and the science of spinal manipulation are not new. The earliest recorded evidence of manipulation dates back to the Aurignacian period (17,500 BC) in which prehistoric cave paintings clearly depict spinal manipulations being delivered (158). Manipulation is also known to have been practiced by the ancient Chinese, the ancient Greeks, the Polynesians, the Hindus, North, Central, and South American Indians, and the Egyptians.

Hippocrates himself wrote two entire books on the subject of manipulation, and another prolific writer, Galen, was given the title, "Prince of Physicians," when he reportedly corrected a paralysis in the hand of Eudemus, a prominent Roman scholar, by manipulating his cervical spine (159). Manipulation is one of the oldest forms of treatment still used today.

The indications, contraindications, and the various theories and applications of this form of therapy are beyond the scope of this book. Manipulation should only be used by those specifically trained in its use, however, because, although serious complications from cervical manipulation are not common (there have been less than 100 cases reported in the literature), they can be disastrous and can result in stroke, paralysis, and death. Many of the cases of complication reported in the literature were performed by practitioners who were untrained in this procedure. It is disturbing, therefore, that more and more workshops and seminars are being offered on the subject of spinal manipulation and are geared toward those with no formal training or background in this field. One can no more expect to master this practice in 1 or 2 weekends than a nonphysician could expect to master the art of surgery in the same time. As it was once put by a famous surgeon, "I could teach anyone to perform an appendectomy in about 1 hour, but it would take 4 years of medical school and 3 years of specialized training to teach him what to do when something goes wrong." A little bit of knowledge can be dangerous!

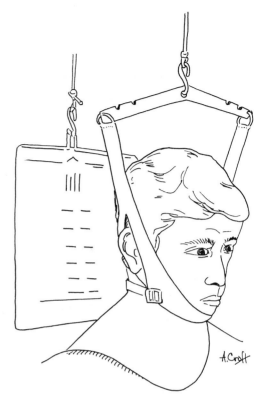

Figure 8.35. The home traction unit should be used with the head flexed slightly forward.

Activities of daily living is a subject that should always be addressed. Proper posture should be emphasized, and this should include posture during sleep. The subject of bedding should be explored, as bedding is often inadequate and, in some cases, may serve to aggravate the patient's condition rather than provide an environment for rest and recuperation.

The cervical spine should be maintained in alignment with the rest of the spine when the patient lies on his or her side. Some patients sleep with two or more pillows, or large, overstuffed pillows, or with pillows made of synthetic material with poor compressibility, while others sleep with very small pillows or without pillows. The implications to sleep posture are obvious. Jackson (159) has recommended the use of a cervical pillow to maintain proper sleep posture. This pillow is cylindrical and semisoft. Also available are pillows made of foam that are designed to maintain (*a*) the normal lordotic curve when used in the

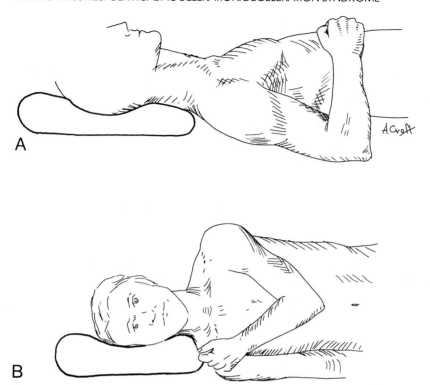

Figure 8.36.   Several manufacturers produce foam pillows designed to maintain the normal physiological lordotic curve of the cervical spine in the supine position (**A**). In the side-lying position (**B**), these pillows prevent unnatural lateral flexion.

supine position and (*b*) straight alignment in the coronal plane when used in the side-lying position (Fig. 8.36). I usually recommend a medium firmness down pillow, as it can accomplish the above objectives quite easily and is generally better tolerated by the patient. Sleeping in the prone position is to be discouraged, as it results in excessive rotational stresses, especially in the upper cervical spine.

Conclusion

About the time humans invented the automobile, physicians discovered a new disorder—the cervical acceleration/deceleration syndrome. Toward the end of the mid-century, researchers were busily probing the mysteries of this phenomenon. Although some isolated experimentation has been carried out on human volunteers, the majority of studies have been done on laboratory animals.

Scientists were initially surprised to find so much soft tissue injury in these animals, but the lesions produced experimentally have also been shown to occur in humans. These studies have, therefore, gone a long way toward explaining the constellation of perplexing and often bizarre symptomatology seen in the whiplash victim. Much remains speculative, however, and further testing and research are needed to understand the complexities of the lesion as well as to devise some standard of care in treating these individuals.

Our goal as health care practitioners should be: first, to properly diagnose the condition as specifically as possible; then second, to design a rational treatment program tailored to our patient's particular needs. One area that often seems to be neglected is that of communicating with the patient. This is especially true with regard to prognosis. From a statistical standpoint this injury can have far-reaching consequences, and the patient should be made to understand this as early as possible in the treatment. And although it may be argued that full disclosure may, at times, serve only to intensify a patient's anxiety or even worsen his or her condition through the power of suggestion, I believe that by duly warning the patient of any and all possible future residuals, the physician will secure the greatest amount of understanding, trust, and cooperation from the patient. In the long run, this will most benefit the patient who, with a full understanding of the importance of compliance in regard to treatment and rehabilitative exercise, is much more likely to follow through with the physician's recommendations. This assures the best possible prognosis.

In the studies that have been conducted to date, a large number of patients with chronic on-going symptomatology several years after a whiplash injury have been seen. When the large number of rear-end collisions with injuries that occur every year is taken into consideration, it is obvious there are a tremendous number of people suffering from these posttraumatic sequelae at any given time. For example, the National Safety Council estimated that in 1971 in the United States there were 3,800,000 rear-end collisions resulting in about 1,000,000 injuries. According to the National Highway Traffic Safety Administration, 73% of these injuries occurred in nontowaway crashes, and it was reported that the average insurance compensation for this injury (in 1981 dollars) was $2150.00 (160). Macnab (16) has conservatively estimated that 45% of those injured in hyperextension/hyperflexion trauma continue to be symptomatic 2 years after settlement of claims. That a significant number remain symptomatic 3 or perhaps even 5 years after settlement can also be assumed. Add to this the inestimable amount of long-term suffering from osteoarthritis and its plethora of symptomatology, which had its beginnings with biokinetic alterations secondary to acceleration/deceleration trauma and the resulting soft tissue disruption and ligamentous instability as described by Jackson (119), Turek (120) and Ehni (72), and as demonstrated in the research of Hohl (21), and it becomes clear that this problem

is of great magnitude. Assuming for the moment that the number of rear-end collisions with injuries has remained constant from 1971 to 1988 (it has undoubtedly increased) and using Macnab's statistics with interpolation, the following rough figures can be advanced:

1986—1,000,000 new whiplash injuries in the United States.
1987—1,000,000 new injuries + 750,000 residual injuries.
1988—1,000,000 new injuries + 750,000 residuals from 1987 + 450,000 (4.5 × 1,000,000) residuals from 1986 = 2,200,000.

Add to this

1. Increased number of probable accidents relative to an increase in total number of cars on the road in 1988 versus those on the road in 1971.
2. ? number of cases not reported.
3. ? number of residuals from 1985 and previous years, i.e., injuries lasting more than 2 years.
4. Permanent disability and/or osteoarthritis from all previous years.

In all probability, more than 1% of the population in the United States alone suffers from acute or chronic effects of the whiplash injury at any given time. The cost for this phenomenon is difficult to estimate but is staggering, especially when lost work days are considered. It probably well exceeds $2 billion/year.

These statistics point to a need for continued and aggressive research in the area of automotive traffic safety and crash protection. As discussed in Chapter 1, however, much has already been learned through this type of research, but automobile manufacturers have traditionally been slow to implement safety design changes, probably because of retooling and other manufacturing and marketing costs as well as perhaps out of fear of compromising the aesthetics of the finished product. Most safety design changes have, in fact, been the result of changes in Federal Motor Vehicle Safety Standards.

Summary

1. Early interest in the pathophysiology and biomechanics of the acceleration/deceleration injury led to experimentation with laboratory animals. Researchers were surprised at the number of soft tissue injuries resulting from this mechanism. Most of the injuries have also been seen clinically in humans.

2. Symptoms of acceleration/deceleration trauma are remarkably constant and have been associated with long-term disability. Studies have shown that these chronic injuries persist for years and are not related to "litigation neurosis," as has been suggested by some.

3. Possible explanations for some long-term disability include damage to the CNS, as demonstrated by laboratory experimentation as well as clinical evaluation by EEG. Scar tissue formation, an inevitable consequence of soft tissue injury, and altered biomechanics secondary to muscular and ligamentous instability are other probable mechanisms involved. Long-range changes include accelerated osteoarthritic changes.

4. The evaluation of pain requires an understanding of the normal anatomy, biomechanics, and neurology of the cervical spine. Other phenomena, which require an understanding of embryology, may also be operant. The concept of sclerotomal pain is useful in the understanding of many types of pain associated with soft tissue injury and helps to explain symptoms that occur distal to the site of injury that do not follow classical neurological patterns.

5. Early treatment with rest, immobilization, manipulation, physical therapy, and adjunctive nutritional supplementation will assure the best possible prognosis. Proper application of these principles by those treating this condition will result in a more favorable long-term outcome.

6. Recent studies have demonstrated the effectiveness of early manipulative mobilization on this type of cervical spine injury. This approach, however, should only be used by those with adequate training and experience in this area.

References

1. Farbman AA: Neck sprain. *JAMA* 223(9):1010–1015, 1973.
2. Macnab I: Acceleration injuries of the cervical spine. *J Bone Joint Surg* 46A:1797–1799, 1964.
3. Wickstrom J, Martinez J, Rodrigues R: Cervical sprain syndrome: experimental acceleration injuries of the head and neck. In: *Proceedings, Prevention of Highway Injury.* Ann Arbor, MI, Highway Safety Research Institute, University of Michigan, Ann Arbor, 1967, pp 182–187.
4. Wickstrom J: Effects of whiplash injury. *JAMA* 194:40, 1965.
5. Wickstrom J: Whiplash injury termed a problem. *Med Tribune* 8: June 15, 1967.
6. Unterharnscheidt F: Pathological and neuropathological findings in rhesus monkeys subjected to −Gx and +Gx indirect impact acceleration. In Sances A, Thomas DJ, Ewing CL, Larson SJ, Unterharnscheidt F (eds): *Mechanisms of Head and Spine Trauma.* Goshen, NY, Aloray, 1986.
7. Katayama K: Histopathological study of the whiplash injury. *J Jpn Orthop Assoc* 44:439–453, 1970.
8. Sances A, Myklebust J, Kostreva D, Cusick JF, Weber R, Houterman C, Larson SJ, Maiman D, Wassh P, Chilbert M, Unterharnscheidt F, Ewing C, Thomas D, Siegesmund K, Ho K, Saltzberg B: Pathophysiology of cervical injuries. In: *Proceedings, 26th Stapp Car Crash Conference.* New York, Society of Automobile Engineers, 1982, pp 41–70.
9. Sokoloff L: Relation between physiological function and energy metabolism in the central nervous system. *J Neurochem* 29:13–26, 1977.
10. Sokoloff L: Mapping of local cerebral functional activity by measurement of local cerebral glucose utilization with (^{14}C) deoxyglucose. *Brain* 102:653–668, 1979.
11. Sokoloff L: The deoxyglucose method; theory and practice. *Eur Neurol* 20:137–145, 1981.
12. Sokoloff L: Localization of functional activity in the central nervous system by measurement of glucose utilization with radioactive deoxyglucose. *J Cereb Blood Flow Metab* 1:7–36, 1981.
13. Sokoloff L, Reivich M, Kennedy C, Des-Rosiers MH, Patlak CS, Pettigrew KD, Sakurada O, Sohara M: The (^{14}C) deoxyglucose method for the measurement of local cerebral glucose utilization: theory, procedure, and normal values in the conscious and anesthetized albino rat. *J Neurochem* 28:897–916, 1977.
14. Lin YK, Wickstrom JK, Saltzberg B, Heath RG: Subcortical EEG changes in rhesus monkeys following experimental whiplash. *26th ACEMB,* 404, 1973.
15. Bocchi L, Orso CA: Whiplash injuries of the cervical spine. *South Ital J Orthop Traumatol Suppl* 171–181, November 9, 1983.
16. Macnab I: Acceleration extension injuries of the cervical spine. In Rothman RH, Simeone FA (eds): *The Spine,* ed 2. Philadelphia, WB Saunders, 1982, vol 2, p 653.
17. Macnab I: Acceleration extension injuries of the cervical spine. In Rothman RH, Simeone FA (eds): *The Spine,* ed 2. Philadelphia, WB Saunders, 1982, vol 2, p 648.
18. McKenzie JA, Williams JF: The dynamic behaviour of the head and cervical spine during whiplash. *J Biomech* 4:477–490, 1971.
19. Wickstrom J, La Rocca H: Trauma: head and neck injuries from acceleration-deceleration forces. In Ruge D, Wiltse LL (eds): *Spinal Disorders: Diagnosis and Treatment.* Philadelphia, Lea & Febiger, 1977, p 350.
20. Gotten N: Survey of one hundred cases of whiplash injury after settlement of litigation. *JAMA* 162(9):865–867, 1956.
21. Hohl M: Soft tissue injuries of the neck. *Clin Orthop Rel Res* 109:42–49, 1975.
22. Baily RW, Badgley CE: Stabilization of the cervical spine by anterior fusion. *J Bone Joint Surg* 42A:565, 1960.
23. Whitley JE, Forsyth HF: The classification of cervical spine injuries. *Am J Roentgenol* 83:633, 1960.

24. Wickstrom J, Martinez J, Rodriguez R: Quoted in Frankel VH: *Cervical Pain.* New York, Pergamon Press, 1972.
25. Webb JK, Broughton RBK, McSweeney T, Park WM: Hidden flexion injury of the cervical spine. *J Bone Joint Surg* 58B(3):322–327, 1976.
26. Green JD, Harle TS, Harris JH Jr: Anterior subluxation of the cervical spine: hyperflexion sprain. *AJNR* 2:243–250, 1981.
27. Evans DK: Anterior cervical subluxation. *J Bone Joint Surg* 58B(3):318–321, 1976.
28. Fielding JW, Cochran GVB, Lawsing JF III, Hohl M: Tears of the transverse ligament of the atlas. *J Bone Joint Surg* 56A(8):1683–1691, 1974.
29. Scher AT: Anterior cervical subluxation: an unstable position. *AJR* 133:275–280, 1979.
30. Holdsworth FW: Fractures, dislocations, and fracture-dislocations of the spine. *J Bone Joint Surg* 45B:6–20, 1963.
31. Backwinkel KD: Injuries from seatbelts. *JAMA* 205:305–307, 1968.
32. Carroll TB, Bruber FH: Seatbelt fractures. *Radiology* 91:517–518, 1968.
33. Fletcher BD, Brogdon BG: Seat-belt fractures of the spine and sternum. *JAMA* 200:167–168, 1967.
34. Garrett JW, Braunstein PW: Seat belt syndrome. *J Trauma* 2:220–237, 1962.
35. Haddad GH, Zickel RE: Intestinal perforation and fracture of lumbar vertebra caused by lap-type seat belt. *J Med* 67:930–932, 1967.
36. Howland WJ, Curry JL, Buffington CB: Fulcrum fractures of the lumbar spine. *JAMA* 193:240–241, 1965.
37. Steckler RM, Epstein JA, Epstein BS: Seat belt trauma to lumbar spine. *J Trauma* 9:508–513, 1969.
38. Chance GQ: Note on type of flexion fracture of spine. *Br J Radiol* 21:452–453, 1948.
39. Smith WS, Kaufer H: Patterns and mechanisms of lumbar injuries associated with lap seat belts. *J Bone Joint Surg* 51A:239–254, 1969.
40. Hurwitt ES, Silver CE: Seat-belt hernia. *JAMA* 194:829–831, 1965.
41. Sube J, Ziperman HH, Mclver WJ: Seat belt trauma to abdomen. *Am J Surg* 113:346–350, 1967.
42. Williams JS, Lies BA, Hale HW: Automotive safety belt: in saving life may produce intra-abdominal injuries. *J Trauma* 6:303–313, 1966.
43. Christian MS: Non-fatal injuries sustained by seat-belt wearers: a comparative study. *Br Med J* 2:1310–11, 1976.
44. Newman RJ: Chest wall injuries and the seat belt syndrome. *Injury* 16:110–113, 1984.
45. Hamilton JB: Seat-belt injuries. *Br Med J* 4:485–486, 1968.
46. MacLeod JH, Nicholson DM: Seat-belt trauma to abdomen. *Can J Surg* 12:202–206, 1969.
47. McRoberts JW: Seat belt injuries and legal aspects. *Ind Med* 34:866–869, 1965.
48. Bergquist D, Dahlgren S, Hedelin H: Rupture of the diaphragm in patients wearing seatbelts. *J Trauma* 18(11):781–783,1978.
49. Dawes REH, Smallwood JA, Taylor I: Seat belt injury to the female breast. *Br J Surg* 73:106–107, 1986.
50. Donegan WL, Spratt JS Jr (eds): *Cancer of the Breast,* ed 2. Philadelphia, WB Saunders, 1979, pp 35–36.
51. Wickstrom J, La Rocca H: Head and neck injuries from acceleration-deceleration forces. In Ruge D, Wiltse LL (eds): *Spinal Disorders: Diagnosis and Treatment.* Philadelphia, Lea & Febiger, 1977, p 349.
52. Gibbs FA: Objective evidence of brain disorder in cases of whiplash injury. *Clin Electroencephalogr* 2(2):107–110, 1971.
53. Hodge JR: The whiplash injury: a discussion of this phenomenon as a psychosomatic illness. *Ohio State Med J* 60:762–776, 1964.
54. Wickstrom J, La Rocca H: Trauma: Head and neck injuries from acceleration-deceleration forces. In Ruge D, Wiltse LL (eds): *Spinal Disorders: Diagnosis and Treatment.* Philadelphia, Lea & Febiger, 1977, p 351.
55. Macnab I: Acceleration extension injuries of the cervical

56. Macnab I: Acceleration extension injuries of the cervical spine. In Rothman RH, Simeone FA (eds): *The Spine,* ed 2. Philadelphia, WB Saunders, 1982, vol 2, p 652.
57. Robbins SL: Blood vessels. In Robbins SL (ed): *Pathologic Basis of Disease.* Philadelphia, WB Saunders, 1974, p 604.
58. Pollock RA, Apple DF, Purvis JM, Murray HH: Esophageal and hypopharyngeal injuries in patients with cervical spine trauma. *Ann Otol* 90:323–327, 1981.
59. Spenler CW, Benfield JR: Esophageal disruption from blunt and penetrating external trauma. *Arch Surg* 111:663–667, 1976.
60. Stringer WL, Kelly DL, Johnson FR, Holliday RA: Hyperextension injury of the cervical spine with oesophageal perforation. *J Neurosurg* 53:541–543, 1980.
61. Morrison A: Hyperextension injury of the cervical spine with rupture of the oesophagus. *J Bone Joint Surg* 42B:356–357, 1960.
62. Parkin GJS: The radiology of perforated oesophagus. *Clin Radiol* 24:324–332, 1973.
63. Love L, Berkon A: Trauma to the oesophagus. *Gastrointest Radiol* 2:305–321, 1978.
64. Wychulis AR, Fontana RS, Payne WS: Instrumental perforation of the oesophagus. *Chest* 55:184–189, 1969.
65. Berry BE, Ochner JL: Perforation of the oesophagus, a 30 year review. *J Thorac Cardiovasc Surg* 65:1–7, 1973.
66. Foster JL, Jolly PC, Sawyer JL, Daniel RA: Esophageal perforation: diagnosis and treatment. *Ann Surg* 161:701–709, 1965.
67. Schutt CH, Dohan FC: Neck injury to women in auto accidents. *JAMA* 206(12):2689–2692, 1968.
68. Braff MM, Rosner S: Symptomatology and treatment of injuries of the neck. *NY State J Med* 55:237–242, 1955.
69. Ebbs SR, Beckly DE, Hammonds JC, Teasdale C: Incidence and duration of neck pain among patients injured in car accidents. *Br Med J* 292:94–95, 1986.
70. Hohl M: Soft-tissue injuries of the neck in automobile accidents. *J Bone Joint Surg* 56A(8):1675–1682, 1974.
71. Norris SH, Watt I: The prognosis of neck injuries resulting from rear-end vehicle collisions. *J Bone Joint Surg* 65B(5):608–611, 1983.
72. Ehni G: Degenerative motion segment encroachments. In: *Cervical Arthrosis: Diseases of the Cervical Motion Segments.* Chicago, Year Book, 1984, p 54.
73. Cailliet R: Neck and upper arm pain. In: *Soft Tissue Pain and Disability.* Philadelphia, FA Davis, 1984, p 136.
74. Jacome DE, Risko M: EEG features in post-traumatic syndrome. *Clin Electroencephalogr* 15(4):214–221, 1984.
75. Haas DC, Pineda GS, Lourie H: Juvenile head trauma syndromes and their relationship to migraine. *Arch Neurol* 32:727–730, 1975.
76. Weil AA: EEG findings in a certain type of psychosomatic headache: dysrhythmic migraine. *Electroencephalogr Clin Neurophysiol* 4:181–186, 1952.
77. Bickerstaff ER: The basilar artery and the migraine-epilepsy syndrome. *Proc R Soc Med* 55:167–169, 1962.
78. Patten J: Headache. In: *Neurological Differential Diagnosis.* New York, Springer-Verlag, 1978, p 222.
79. Ford JS: Posttraumatic headache. *Med Recertification Associates* 4(1):3–11, 1985.
80. Patten J: Headache. In: *Neurological Differential Diagnosis.* New York, Springer-Verlag, 1978, p 244.
81. Rutherford WH, Merrett JD, McDonald JR: Sequelae of concussion caused by minor head injury. *Lancet* 1:1–4, 1977.
82. Ommaya AK, Faas F, Yarnell P: Whiplash injury and brain damage: an experimental study. *JAMA* 204:285–289, 1968.
83. Unterharnscheidt F, Higgins LS: Traumatic lesions of the brain and spinal cord due to non-deforming angular acceleration of the head. *Tex Rep Biol Med* 27(1): Spring 1969 (reprint).

84. Glaser MA, Shafer FP: Skull and brain trauma. *JAMA* 98:27, 1932.

85. Wechsler I: Trauma and the nervous system. *JAMA* 104:519, 1935.

86. Russell WR: Cerebral involvement in head injuries; a study of 200 cases. *Brain* 55:549, 1932.

87. Jackson H: A study of convulsions. *St Andrews Med Grad A Tr* 3:162, 1870.

88. Cloward RB: War injuries to the head. *JAMA* 118:267, 1947.

89. Torres F, Shapiro SK: Electroencephalograms in whiplash injury. *Arch Neurol* 5:28–35, 1961.

90. Shapiro SK, Torres F: Brain injury complicating whiplash injuries. *Minn Med* 43:473–476, 1960.

91. Denker PG, Perry GF: Postconcussion syndrome in compensation and litigation: analysis of 95 cases with electroencephalographic correlations. *Neurology* 4:912–918, 1954.

92. Denker PG: The postconcussion syndrome: prognosis and evaluation of the organic factors. *NY State J Med* 44:379, 1944.

93. Simons DJ, Wolff HG: Studies on headache: mechanisms of chronic posttraumatic headache. *Psychosom Med* 8:227–242, 1946.

94. Miller H: Accident neurosis. *Br Med J* 1:919–925, 1961.

95. Miller H, Cartilidge N: Simulation and malingering after injuries to the brain and spinal cord. *Lancet* 2:580–585, 1972.

96. Ellard J: Psychological reactions to compensable injury. *Med J Aust* 2:349–355, 1970.

97. Abbott HK: Neck sprain syndrome. *Med Arts Sci* 13:139–153, 1959.

98. Threadgill FD: Whiplash injury—end results in 88 cases. *Med Ann DC* 29:266–268, 1960.

99. Brenner C, Friedman A, Merritt HH, et al: Posttraumatic headache. *Neurosurgery* 1:379–391, 1944.

100. Coburn DF: Vertebral artery involvement in cervical trauma. *Clin Orthop* 24:61, 1962.

101. Dziob JS: Trauma and breast cancer, or the anatomy of an insurance claim. *R I Med J* 63:37–42, 1980.

102. Robbins SL: Inflammation and repair. In Robbins SL (ed): *Pathologic Basis of Disease.* Philadelphia, WB Saunders, 1974, p 68.

103. Robbins SL: Inflammation and repair. In Robbins SL (ed): *Pathologic Basis of Disease.* Philadelphia, WB Saunders, 1974, p 58.

104. Lewis GP: Plasma kinins and other vasoactive compounds in acute inflammation. *Ann NY Acad Sci* 116:846, 1964.

105. Spector WG, Willoughby DA: Vasoactive amines in acute inflammation. *Ann NY Acad Sci* 116:839,1964.

106. Robbins SL: Inflammation and repair. In Robbins SL (ed): *Pathologic Basis of Disease.* Philadelphia, WB Saunders, 1974, p 71.

107. Robbins SL: Inflammation and repair. In Robbins SL (ed): *Pathologic Basis of Disease.* Philadelphia, WB Saunders, 1974, p 90.

108. Reznick M: Origins of myoblasts during skeletal muscle regeneration. *Lab Invest* 20:353, 1969.

109. Hay ED: Skeletal muscle regeneration. *N Engl J Med* 284:1033, 1971.

110. Lehto M, Jarvinen M, Nelimarkka O: Scar formation after skeletal muscle injury. A histological and autoradiographical study in rats. *Arch Orthop Trauma Surg* 104(6):366–370, 1986.

111. Allbrook D, Baker WdeC, Kirkaldy-Willis WH: Muscle regeneration in experimental animals and in man. *J Bone Joint Surg* 48B(1):153–169, 1966.

112. Muir AR, Kanji AHM, Allbrook D: The structure of the satellite cells in skeletal muscle. *J Anat* 99:435, 1965.

113. Saunders JH, Sissons HA: The effect of denervation on the regeneration of skeletal muscle after injury. *J Bone Joint Surg* 35B:113, 1953.

114. Clark WE, Le Gras: An experimental study of the regeneration of mammalian striped muscle. *J Anat* 80:24, 1946.

115. Allbrook DB, Aitken JT: Reinnervation of striated muscle after acute ischaemia. *J Anat* 85:376, 1951.

116. Robbins SL: Inflammation and repair. In Robbins SL (ed): *Pathologic Basis of Disease.* Philadelphia, WB Saunders, 1974, p 92.

117. Jarvinen M: Healing of a crush injury in rat striated muscle. *Acta Pathol Microbiol Scand [A]* 83:269–282,1975.

118. Denny-Brown D: The influence of tension and innervation on the regeneration of skeletal muscle. *J Neuropathol Exp Neurol* 10:94–96, 1951.

119. Jackson R: Etiology. In Jackson R (ed): *The Cervical Syndrome,* ed 4. Springfield, IL, Charles C Thomas, 1977, p 121.

120. Turek SL: The cervical spine. In: *Orthopaedics: Principles and Their Application,* ed 3. Philadelphia, JB Lippincott, 1977, p 742.

121. Greenfield GB: The joints. In: *Radiology of Bone Diseases,* ed 3. Philadelphia, JB Lippincott, 1980, p 779.

122. Bland JH, Cooper SM: Osteoarthritis: a review of the cell biology involved and evidence for reversibility. Management rationally related to known genesis and pathophysiology. *Semin Arthritis Rheum* 2(14):106–133, 1984.

123. Radin EL: Mechanical aspects of osteoarthrosis. *Bull Rheum Dis* 26:862–865, 1976.

124. Videman T: Hypothesen zur Pathogenese der Osteoarthrose. *Med Sport* 20:367–368, 1980.

125. Hagberg M: Occupational musculoskeletal stress and disorders of the neck and shoulder: a review of possible pathophysiology. *Int Arch Occup Environ Health* 53:269–278, 1984.

126. Huskisson EC, Dieppe PA, Tucker AK, Cannel LB: Another look at osteoarthritis. *Ann Rheum Dis* 38:423–428, 1979.

127. Hedaya RJ: Pharmacokinetic factors in the clinical use of tryptophan. *J Clin Psychopharmacol* 4(6):347–348, 1984.

128. Radin EL, Paul IL: A consolidated concept of joint lubrication. *J Bone Joint Surg* 54A:607–616, 1972.

129. Kempson GE: The mechanical properties of articular cartilage. In Sokoloff L (ed): *The Joints and Synovial Fluid.* Orlando, FL, Academic Press, 1980, vol 2, pp 177–235.

130. Feinstein B, Langton JNK, Jameson RM, Schiller F: Experiments of pain referred from deep somatic tissues. *J Bone Joint Surg* 36A(5):981–997, 1954.

131. Inman Vt, Saunders JBdeCM: Referred pain from skeletal structures. *J Nerv Ment Dis* 99:660–667, 1944.

132. Feinstein B: Referred pain from paravertebral structures. In Buerger AA, Tobis JS (eds): *Approaches to the Validation of Manipulation Therapy.* Springfield, Charles C Thomas, 1977, pp 139–174.

133. Evans P: The healing process at cellular level: a review. *Physiotherapy* 66(8):256–259, 1980.

134. Dyson M, Suckling J: Stimulation of tissue repair by ultrasound—a survey of the mechanisms involved. *Physiotherapy* 64(4):105, 1978.

135. Jackson R: Treatment. In Jackson R (ed): *The Cervical Syndrome,* ed 4. Springfield, Charles C Thomas, 1977, p 284.

136. Wickstrom J, La Rocca H: Head and neck injuries from acceleration-deceleration forces. In Ruge D, Wiltse LL (eds): *Spinal Disorders: Diagnosis and Treatment.* Philadelphia, Lea & Febiger, 1977, p 352.

137. Jackson R: Treatment. In Jackson R (ed): *The Cervical Syndrome,* ed 4. Springfield, IL, Charles C Thomas, 1977, p 285.

138. Wickstrom J, La Rocca H: Head and neck injuries from acceleration-deceleration forces. In Ruge D, Wiltse LL (eds): *Spinal Disorders: Diagnosis and Treatment.* Philadelphia, Lea & Febiger, 1977, p 353.

139. Goodley PH: *A Clinical Manual on Cervical Traction and the Goodley Polyaxial Cervical Traction Mobilizer System.* Westbury, CT, E-2-EM Orthopedic Products, 1986.

140. Travell JG, Simons DG: *Myofascial Pain and Dysfunction: The Trigger Point Manual.* Baltimore, Williams & Wilkins, 1983.

141. Spring B: Recent research on the behavior effects of tryptophan and carbohydrate. *Nutr Health* 3(1–2):55–67, 1984.

142. Lindsley JG, Hartmann EL, Mitchell W: Selectivity in response to L-tryptophan among insomniac subjects: a preliminary report. *Sleep* 6(3):247–256, 1983.

143. Kelly SJ, Franklin KB: An increase in tryptophan in brain may be a general mechanism for the effect of stress on sensitivity to pain. *Neuropharmacology* 24(11):1019–1025, 1985.

144. Godefroy F, Weil-Fugazza J, Bineau-Thurotte M, Besson JM: The relationship between morphine analgesia and the activity of bulbo-spinal serotonergic system as studied by tolerance phenomenon. *Brain Res* 226(1–2):201–210, 1981.

145. Shpeen SE, Morse DR, Furst ML: The effect of tryptophan on postoperative endodontic pain. *Oral Surg Oral Med Oral Pathol* 58(4):446–469, 1984.

146. Ham AW: The cells of loose connective tissue and their functions. In Ham AW (ed): *Histology*, ed 7. Philadelphia, JB Lippincott, 1974, p 222.

147. Robbins SL: Inflammation and repair. In Robbins SL (ed): *Pathologic Basis of Disease*. Philadelphia, WB Saunders, 1974, p 100.

148. Ross R, Benditt Ed: Wound healing and collagen formation. IV. Distortion of ribosomal patterns of fibroblasts in scurvy. *J Cell Biol* 22:365, 1964.

149. Jackson R: Treatment. In Jackson R (ed): *The Cervical Syndrome*, ed 4. Springfield, IL, Charles C Thomas, 1977, p 333.

150. Pories WJ, Henzel JH, Rob CG, Strain WH: Acceleration of wound healing in man with zinc sulphate given by mouth. *Lancet* 1:121, 1967.

151. Maigne R: *Orthopaedic Medicine. A New Approach to Vertebral Manipulation*. Springfield, IL, Charles C Thomas, 1972.

152. Mennell JM: *Back Pain: Diagnosis and Treatment Using Manipulative Techniques*. Boston, Little, Brown, 1960.

153. Jackson R: Treatment. In Jackson R (ed): *The Cervical Syndrome*, ed 4. Springfield, IL, Charles C Thomas, 1977, p 280.

154. Cyriax J: *Textbook of Orthopaedic Medicine*, ed 11. London, Baillière-Tindall, 1984, vol 2.

155. Haldeman S: What is meant by manipulation? In Buerger AA, Tobis JS (eds): *Approaches to the Validation of Manipulation*. Springfield, IL, Charles C Thomas, 1977.

156. Kirkaldy-Willis WH: *Managing Low Back Pain*. Edinburgh, Churchill Livingstone, 1983.

157. Mealy K, Brennan H, Fenelon GCC: Early mobilization of acute whiplash injuries. *Br Med J* 292:656–657, 1986.

158. Schafer RC: The historic roots of chiropractic philosophy. In Schafer RC (ed): *Chiropractic Health Care*, ed 2. Des Moines, Foundation for Chiropractic Education and Research, 1977, p 9.

159. Schafer RC: The historic roots of chiropractic philosophy. In Schafer RC (ed): *Chiropractic Health Care*, ed 2. Des Moines, Foundation for Chiropractic Education and Research, 1977, pp 13–14.

160. *An Evaluation of Head Restraints*. Federal Motor Vehicle Safety Standard 202, NHTSA Technical Report, February 1982.

161. Jackson R: Treatment. In Jackson R (ed): *The Cervical Syndrome*, ed 4. Springfield, IL, Charles C Thomas, 1977, p 310.

162. Simeone FA, Rothman RH: Cervical disc disease. In Rothman RH, Simeone FA (eds): *The Spine*, ed 2. Philadelphia, WB Saunders, 1982, vol 1, p 454.

9

Nervous System Trauma

STEPHEN M. FOREMAN, DC, DABCO

Mechanisms of Trauma_____

DIRECT INJURY

The central nervous system, although encased within the protective skull and spinal column, is subjected to a variety of injuries. These neurological insults may be direct or indirect in nature, but both types adversely affect the function of the system. If the cranial vault is fractured, the patient usually suffers contusions or bruising of the brain. If the skull is fractured or penetrated, the patient may suffer a laceration of the brain or surrounding dura.

Contusions of the brain may be minimal, or large poolings of blood may form in the subdural space. Rupture of the middle meningeal artery or vein causes an extradural hematoma to form (Figs. 9.1 and 9.2). Both subdural and extradural hematomas may cause compression symptoms such as a loss of consciousness, nausea, or vertigo (1).

Compression injuries are particularly common in the spinal column because the spinal cord is often exposed to the excessive movements between two vertebrae (Fig. 9.3). This type of movement is more common in children (2). Their spines are typically more flexible, and the movement of the segments can injure the spinal cord, although, many times, abnormalities will not be seen on posttraumatic radiographic studies.

Other anatomical changes within the spinal canal may cause direct compression of the spinal cord. During a rapid deceleration, the cervical cord may strike the edge of a spondylophytic bar, vertebral fracture, or dislocated segment. The cord may also be subjected to aberrations in spinal canal size, such as ossification of the posterior longitudinal ligament, herniation of the nucleus pulposus, and infolding of the ligamentum flavum (3, 4).

Compression produced by hypertonic muscles or vascular malformations can also be a major cause of symptoms in the peripheral nervous system. Other causes

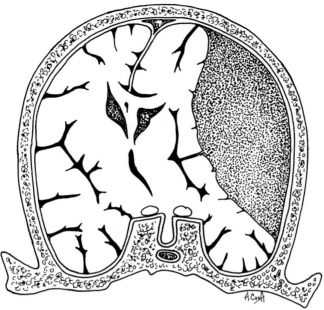

Figure 9.1.   Line drawing of a subdural hematoma. Note the shift in the neural contents. (Adapted from Chusid JG: *Correlative Neuroanatomy and Functional Neurology*, ed 17. Los Altos, CA, Lange Medical Publications, 1979.)

of peripheral entrapment include fibrous adhesion bands and accumulations of blood within fascial confines, termed compartment syndromes. This discussion centers on compression injuries arising from the bony confines of the intervertebral foramen.

There are two main methods of classifying injuries of the peripheral nervous system (5, 6). With each method, there has been an attempt to correlate the clinical picture with the degree of injury. In the classification put forth by Seddon (5), the injuries were grouped into the three categories defined below:

1. *Neuropraxia*—the mildest form of neuronal compression. Recovery from this lesion usually takes 3–6 weeks on account of the absence of wallerian degeneration.

2. *Axonotmesis*—a severe crushing injury of the peripheral nerve that causes wallerian degeneration. The transport and fibrous tubules, the epineurium, the perineurium, and the endoneurium are often damaged but remain intact. The long-term prognosis is favorable when these tubules are intact, but recovery may take up to 6 months. This delay is needed for the myelin sheath to regenerate (7).

3. *Neurotmesis*—a complete disruption of

both neural and fibrous elements. A return to proper function will depend on the ability of the previously mentioned neural tubules to reconnect. The long-term prognosis, even after surgical repair, is guarded.

The classification system proposed by Sunderland (6) is similar to that of Seddon's, except that he divides the stages of nerve injury into five categories. I prefer to use Sunderland's classification system on the effects of stretch injuries (discussed later in the chapter).

Another mechanism of trauma is excessive stretching of the spinal cord or brainstem. Rapid cervical hyperextension may pull and tear the pyramids at the junction of the medulla oblongata and the pons (8). The resultant hematoma at the base of the brain may cause a variety of symptoms, which are discussed later in the chapter.

INDIRECT INJURY

It must be remembered that the spinal cord is subject to a variety of indirect insults that may complicate the clinical picture in the acute stage or may affect the long-term prognosis. This occurs because most indirect injuries alter the vascular dynamics of the area.

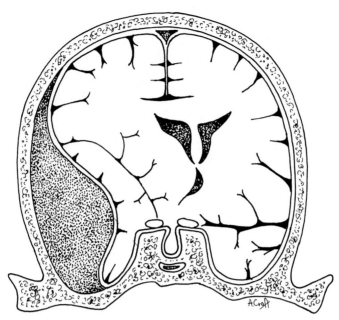

Figure 9.2.   Line drawing of an extradural hematoma. (Adapted from Chusid JG: *Correlative Neuroanatomy and Functional Neurology*, ed 17. Los Altos, CA, Lange Medical Publications, 1979.)

Ischemia or infarction of the spinal cord may be due to involvement of the intrinsic vessels, extrinsic vessels, or both (9–11). Involvement of the extrinsic vessels leading to the spinal cord may come from a variety of sources, the most common of which is probably thrombosis of the distal aorta (Table 9.1). This etiology obviously affects the lower portion of the spinal cord.

Intrinsic spinal cord artery involvement may come from syphilitic arteritis, diabetes mellitus or, rarely, polyarteritis nodosa and lupus erythematosus (12, 13). The use of certain drugs, such as the sulfonamides, and exposure to radiation therapy have also been cited as causes of intrinsic spinal cord vessel occlusion. The differentiation between spinal cord symptoms arising from ischemia and those caused by injury may be difficult.

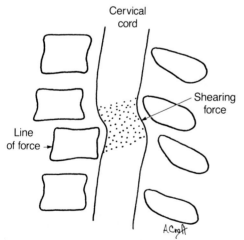

Figure 9.3.   Line drawing depicting the potential shift between the vertebral segments and the area of resultant cord damage. (Adapted from Raynor RB, Koplik B: Cervical cord trauma: the relationship between clinical syndromes and force of injury. *Spine* 10(3):193–197, 1985.)

Acute Central Nervous System Injury

The brain and the surrounding dura, as previously described, are subject to trauma within the cranial vault. Outward signs of trauma may not be present, and radiographic examination may be equivocal.

Most of the symptomatic picture after head trauma may be related to disruption of the cranial nerves. Anosmia, or loss of smell, occurs commonly and arises from

Table 9.1.
Extrinsic Vessel Involvement

Thrombosis of distal aorta

Erosion of atheromatous plaques in atherosclerotic aorta with repeated embolization

Dissecting aortic aneurysm affecting intercostal and lumbar arteries

Vertebral artery thrombosis and occlusion of the radicular arteries

the shearing forces that disrupt the nerve fibers from the olfactory bulb as they enter the cribriform plate (14). It is noteworthy that most of these patients complain of a "change of taste." The anosmia is almost always a permanent deficit.

Another sign of head injury is double vision. The increased cranial pressure seen in some cases of concussion may affect the sixth cranial nerve. This nerve is the most vulnerable to increased pressure because it has the longest intracranial course of all of the cranial nerves. When double vision is present, however, intracranial masses must be ruled out. A computed tomogram of the head is often required to rule out the presence of such a mass.

Subdural hemorrhage, as mentioned earlier, may follow relatively minor head injuries. The acute variety may be small and not require surgical intervention, whereas the chronic variety usually warrants treatment.

An extradural hemorrhage usually follows rupture of the middle meningeal artery or vein. A brief loss of consciousness is not uncommon. The bleeding may continue for a period of several days during which the patient continues to develop signs of increased intracranial pressure. Tests such as heel-to-toe walking and the finger-to-nose test are quite useful in the evaluation of this pressure change.

Brainstem Injury

Traumatic injury to the brainstem may be considered a rare clinical entity, since the majority of cases are fatal. Brainstem lesions typically affecting the rostral pyramids at the level of the medulla oblongata

and the pons are usually produced by dislocations of either the occiput or C1 or may arise from severe hyperextension of the neck. Those patients who survive such an injury are subject to a variety of symptoms.

Klingele et al. (15) described several cases of pontine gaze paresis occurring after hyperextension injuries. They noted that several patients were unable to move their eyes in a lateral plane after a hyperextension accident. This clinical presentation is most commonly associated with tumors affecting the brainstem.

Another observer (8) found that the damage sustained by the pyramids, combined with secondary hematoma formation, may result in tetraplegia without a loss of consciousness. A similar clinical entity is seen in the shaken infant syndrome in which a young child is subjected to violent flexion-extension. The muscles of the cervical region in the young child are not able either to protect the cervical spine or to maintain the head in a neutral position. Common postmortem findings in children with this injury are subdural hematomas, brainstem tears, and intraocular bleeding. Those children who survive will often suffer mental retardation and permanent impairment of both vision and hearing (16).

The most commonly encountered brainstem lesion is infarction secondary to occlusion of the vertebral artery. The clinical picture of vertigo, nausea, vomiting, unsteady gait, Horner's syndrome, horizontal nystagmus, ipsilateral loss of pain and temperature sensation on the face, and contralateral loss of pain and temperature in the body is indicative of a lateral medullary syndrome. This condition, also known as Wallenberg's syndrome, is produced by either occlusion or rupture of the vertebral artery as it runs up the foramen transversarium or the posterior inferior cerebellar artery. It is usually encountered after any excessive flexion and rotation. This same syndrome has been observed in isolated cases following cervical manipulation.

Cord Injury

The spinal cord is subject to injury via compression, stretch, and torque mechanisms as described earlier. Its position within the spinal column gives adequate protection during normal ranges of motion, but damage often occurs when the spinal cord is subjected to severe forces, as is described in Chapter 1.

Many studies and observations have been made regarding the effects of trauma on the cervical spine. Most of these efforts have described various symptomatic patterns, and these clinical pictures have been divided into four separate syndromes.

The first of these is the *root syndrome*. In this syndrome, all of the symptomatic changes are related to one or more nerve roots. The typical clinical picture is characterized by the presence of either motor or sensory deficits. The motor deficit can vary from slight weakness to total paralysis of a muscle group, depending on the severity of injury and the levels involved. Sensory deficits are typified by the loss of pain perception within a specific dermatome. Early suppression of the deep tendon reflexes in the upper extremities is also a typical finding.

The second clinical entity is the *central cord syndrome*. This syndrome is typically associated with the more severe automobile accidents. Vertebral body fracture would not be an uncommon radiographic finding. The neurological pattern of this syndrome is associated with the function of the central portion of the cord, particularly pain, temperature sensation, and voluntary motion of the upper extremities. The patient usually experiences symptoms in the upper extremities, as described previously, and neurological dysfunction of the bladder and bowel.

The third and even more clinically significant lesion is termed the *anterior spinal artery syndrome*. The syndrome is so named because the original investigators believed that the resultant clinical picture was caused by ischemia secondary to occlusion of the anterior spinal artery. These patients suffer major neurological changes including an immediate and complete paralysis distal to the lesion. Patients with this syndrome present with hypesthesia and hypalgesia in the affected areas, but there is preservation of other cord function such as light touch, joint position, and some vibration sense (17). These neurological functions are

relatively spared, as they are primarily seated within the posterior columns.

The last and fourth syndrome is *complete transection of the cord*. There is no neurological function distal to the injury level, and recovery does not occur. The clinical picture is characterized by flaccid paralysis and painless retention of urine resulting from reflex closure of the sphincter. After 4–6 weeks, the patient experiences an increase in muscle tone and will eventually develop spastic paralysis, hyperreflexia, and clonus. The spastic paralysis, if left untreated, will progress, causing the patient to assume the fetal position. Extensive physical and occupational therapy in the early stages can often prevent these deforming contractures (18).

At first glance, these four syndromes seem quite separate and unrelated. The first three seem to involve separate areas of the cord. It was originally assumed, therefore, that their etiologies were different. The earliest clinical studies promoted spinal cord compression as the source of neurological symptoms. It was assumed that direct pressure resulted from either vertebral fracture fragments or a herniated nucleus pulposus, and although this was often found to be the case upon surgical inspection, sometimes no source of pressure was found.

The lack of direct spinal cord compression in some cases caused investigators to explore the possibility of vascular damage or compromise as the source of the patient's symptomatology. Some animal studies supported the theory that spinal cord ischemia arising from occlusion of either the spinal cord arteries or the arteries leading to the cord could result in this neurological picture.

Other studies seemed to validate the concept of vascular compromise. Autopsy studies by Hashizume et al. (19) revealed extensive damage to the gray matter, compared with damage to the white matter, and although the white matter did demonstrate demyelination and axon loss with status spongiosus, the gray matter underwent tissue necrosis and cavity formation. Secondary circulation damage due to compression of the anterior spinal artery may also be significant in the pathogenesis of spinal cord damage (20).

These concepts, i.e., various spinal cord compression and vascular ischemia, as pointed out by Raynor and Koplik (21), have several "disturbing problems." Both the motor pathways and the lateral and ventral spinothalamic tracts are part of the same vascular network supplied by the anterior spinal artery. If vascular occlusion was truly responsible for the clinical picture, these investigators contend, the patient would also exhibit a loss of the pain and light touch functions provided by the lateral and ventral spinothalamic tracts (1, 22). These two functions, pain and light touch, are mediated by different types of fibers. The pain fibers are predominantly of the small unmyelinated C variety, while those supplying light touch are of the large myelinated A type (11). It is this difference, these investigators claim, that helps to disprove the theories about ischemia and spinal artery occlusion. Studies have shown that pain fibers such as those already described are more susceptible to trauma and anoxia, yet the function of these fibers is usually maintained (23).

The last objection that Raynor and Koplik have to the vascular occlusion model is the marked sparing of neurological function in the posterior columns. The common blood supply of these structures, from both the anterior and posterior spinal arteries, would not make them immune to functional loss (21). It is possible, of course, that the anterior columns are also spared. The preservation of light touch, believed to be mediated through the ventral spinothalamic tract (1), is usually intact in anterior spinal artery syndromes. This assertion, namely, that the anterior columns are spared, is difficult to confirm, however, as there are no accurate clinical tests to evaluate the vestibulospinal and tectospinal tracts.

It has recently been theorized that these four separate syndromes are really only one entity, with variations in the force and the direction of the impact being the differentiating factor (21). Raynor contends that the force applied to the spinal cord tends to be concentrated somewhere in the region of the middle third of each half of the spinal cord (Fig. 9.4).

Injuries of lower amplitude and force generally only affect the anterior and posterior horn areas. The crossing pain and

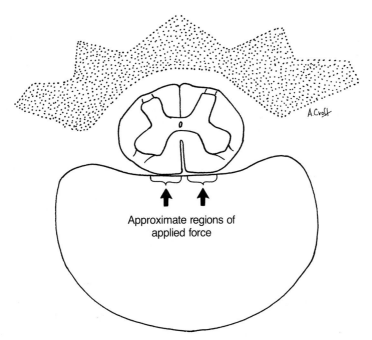

Figure 9.4.   Line drawing demonstrating how the shearing force, applied in an anterior-posterior direction, affects the middle third of each half of the cord. (Adapted from Raynor RB, Koplik B: Cervical cord trauma: the relationship between clinical syndromes and force of injury. *Spine* 10(3):193–197, 1985.)

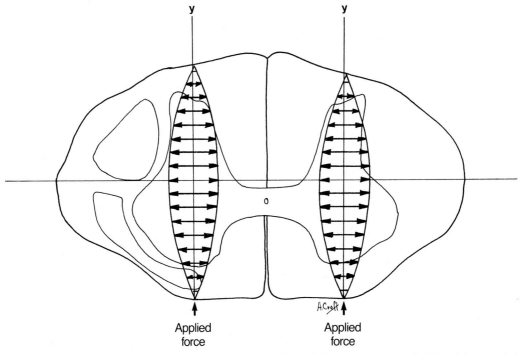

Figure 9.5. Line drawing depicting a root syndrome. The *elliptical area* on each side of the y axis is affected by the applied force and causes the clinical picture. (Adapted from Raynor RB, Koplik B: Cervical cord trauma: the relationship between clinical syndromes and force of injury. *Spine* 10(3):193–197, 1985.)

temperature tracts may be affected. This concentration of forces on the anterior and posterior horns is believed to be responsible for root syndromes (Fig. 9.5). The production of a nerve root syndrome, as previously described, may be unilateral or bilateral, depending on the angle or direction of force applied to the area and the position of the head during impact.

The central cord syndrome has the same etiology and mechanism of trauma described for the root syndrome. If the applied force is increased, the area of internal cord damage or "shock" increases (Fig. 9.6). This enlarged "shock area" now includes the anterior horn cell for the upper extremities along with the corticospinal tracts. The *shaded area* in Figure 9.6 also includes the anteromedial gray matter that controls bladder function. This would make the proposed areas of injury consistent with the clinical picture seen in central cord syndromes.

It becomes apparent that as the applied force increases, the anterior cord syndrome involves a greater portion of the cord (Fig.

9.7). Note that in Figure 9.7, the area of the posterior white matter is still relatively preserved. As pointed out previously, the function of the anterior white matter should also be intact. The gray matter seems to take the majority of the impact in all of the cases, especially in the last case presented. This finding is consistent with the observations by Cawthon et al. (24) who noted that the "gray matter seems to undergo a sharp contusion with rapid, long-lasting effects, while white matter acts as if it sustained a blunt contusion with delayed and variable effects on blood flow."

In Raynor and Koplik's (21) study, several cases in which the force of the injury came from the oblique position were documented. In these select cases, a Brown-Séquard syndrome consisting of either an actual or a physiological hemisection of the spinal cord was observed. The clinical picture is typified by an ipsilateral impairment of proprioception, vibration, two-point discrimination, and joint sensation along with a contralateral loss of pain and temperature as well as by a local ipsilateral lower motor

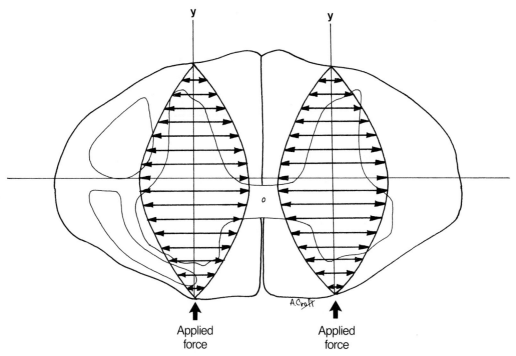

Figure 9.6. Line drawing depicting a central cord syndrome. The *elliptical area* on each side of the y axis is larger in this syndrome than in the root syndrome depicted in Figure 9.5. (Adapted from Raynor RB, Koplik B: Cervical cord trauma: the relationship between clinical syndromes and force of injury. *Spine* 10(3):193–197, 1985.)

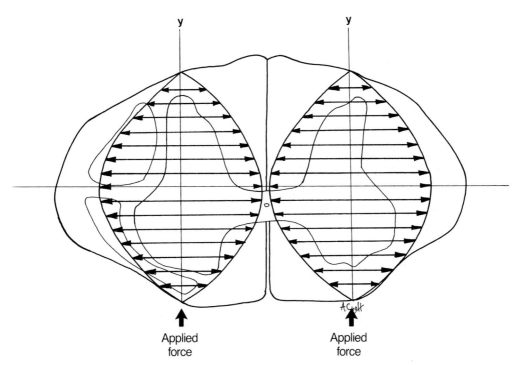

Figure 9.7. Line drawing depicting an anterior cord or spinal artery syndrome. The affected area (*elliptical area*) is now at its largest (compared with the area shown in the root and the cord syndrome) and yet still spares the anterior and posterior white matter. (Adapted from Raynor RB, Koplik B: Cervical cord trauma: the relationship between clinical syndromes, and force of injury. *Spine* 10(3):193–197, 1985.)

neuron lesion at the level of injury and an ipsilateral upper motor neuron motor paralysis below the lesion. These losses are distal to the injured spinal cord. One of these cases also presented with unilateral facet dislocation. The oblique line of force (Fig. 9.8) causes all of the stress to be applied to one side of the spinal cord. This effectively includes the lateral corticospinal and lateral spinothalamic tracts responsible for the clinical changes.

Peripheral Nervous System Trauma

Damage to the peripheral nerves is one of the unfortunate aspects of cervical injuries. These nerves are subject not only to compression at the intervertebral foramen but also to severe stretch injuries and peripheral entrapment by other anatomical structures.

The peripheral nerve is a complex composite structure composed of nerve fibers, their Schwann cells, and the endoneurium, perineurium, and epineurium tubes.

Peripheral nerve compression, like that exerted on the spinal cord, produces narrowing of the axons, anoxic block of both ionic and axonal transport, and intraneural edema (7). These neuronal changes are also seen in cases of nerve root traction.

The combination of compression and traction adversely affects the vascular function of the nerve root and may cause either a partial or a complete ischemia (3). The pressure on a nerve needed to cause stasis of the intraneural blood flow is slight. Rydevik et al. (25) demonstrated stasis in the rabbit tibial nerve with pressures as low as 20–30 mm Hg. Increasing the pressure to 60–80 mm Hg caused total ischemia in the nerve.

Controlled elongation in the absence of compression produces a similar effect. Lundborg and Rydevik (26) demonstrated venous stasis when the nerve was stretched 8% longer than its original length. Complete ischemia occurred when the nerve was stretched to 15% more than its original length.

It is of clinical importance to realize that

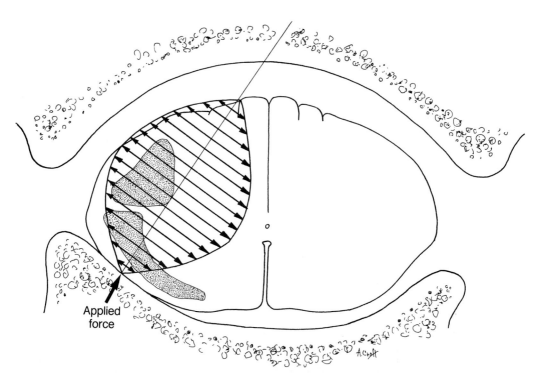

Figure 9.8.   Line drawing depicting an oblique line of applied force. The resulting damage is limited to one half of the spinal cord and causes a Brown–Séquard syndrome. (Adapted from Raynor RB, Koplik B: Cervical cord trauma: the relationship between syndromes and force of injury. *Spine* 10(3):193–197, 1985.)

acute compression of a normal nerve root causes localized ischemia and may produce numbness of a dermatome, or an entire limb, but usually does not cause pain (3). It appears that posttraumatic irritation of the affected nerve root is the prerequisite for the development of radicular pain that arises from nerve compression (27, 28).

This important concept was demonstrated by Howe et al. (29) when they surgically compressed normal nerve roots that induced short duration impulses, which is typical of normal function, without pain. In other studies, Howe et al. irritated nerve roots with chromic gut ligatures; 2–4 weeks later, the same compression was reapplied, which induced a long nerve firing pattern typically seen in a damaged nerve, with pain. The authors concluded that the long firing pattern was consistent with and represented pain from compression.

Tractional or stretch injuries may also affect the nerve roots or cords. The damage is typically produced when the head and neck are laterally flexed and the shoulder depressed beyond the normal limit. The damage and stages of injury described by Sunderland (30) (Fig. 9.9) are listed below:

Stage 1. The initial stretch tears the axon only. All other neural structures are left intact.

Stage 2. This is a continuation of stage 1, in that the distal axon degenerates.

Stage 3. The axon and its complex sheath and endoneurium are disrupted.

Stage 4. An increase in force causes all of the previously described damage and a separation of the perineurium. The function of the nerve is not normal.

Stage 5. Complete disruption of the nerve and a cessation of function have occurred.

Pathology within the intervertebral foramen and spinal canal may cause compression, traction, or both. Some of the causes for nerve compression include neurofibromas, destructive lesions of the vertebral body, hypertrophic changes in the ligaments, osteophytic encroachment, and apophyseal capsule swelling (30). The most common cause of intervertebral stenosis is the bony encroachment secondary to degeneration of the intervertebral disc. The loss of height causes hypertrophic changes in both the uncovertebral and facet joints.

A herniated anulus fibrosus or nucleus pulposus of a cervical disc may cause extreme pain, and its occurrence after a whiplash accident is becoming more frequently recognized. Nevertheless, although it may have the same traumatic etiology as a central cord syndrome, it should not be mistaken for such. Clinically, the patient with an acute cervical disc herniation presents with nerve root symptoms including motor and sensory deficits. The pain is often severe and persistent; the neck is usually spastic in an attempt to limit cervical motion. The central cord syndrome is indicated by the hypalgesia/hyperpathia due to a damaged spinothalamic tract (31).

The tractional or stretch injuries previously outlined may affect only one or multiple levels in the spinal cord. The area of injury is then localized to the plexus, rather than to the root, that is damaged. Electrodiagnostic tests are more difficult to perform on a patient with an injured plexus than on a patient with an injury in any other area of the peripheral nervous system (32). This lack of diagnostic specifity is the reason it is common to see general terms such as "plexopathy or plexitis" used in reference to either disease or injury to this area.

The plexus may also be damaged by compression or vascular disorders. One of the best known is the thoracic outlet syndrome. Despite the extensive attention received by this condition in the literature, it is still difficult to locate an anatomic cause. This situation is further complicated by the lack of a specific electrodiagnostic test (33). This is why I believe that the diagnosis will often be one of exclusion. Several sources of local compression, such as a cervical rib, elongated cervical transverse process, and abnormally positioned scalene muscles, have been identified in the literature. Bonney (34) has implicated the presence of a hypertrophic suprapleural membrane (Sibson's fascia) as the cause of compression, particularly if a deep part of the anterior scalene runs behind the subclavian artery and in front of the lower trunk from the seventh cervical transverse process to the first rib.

Despite the lack of a specific electrodi-

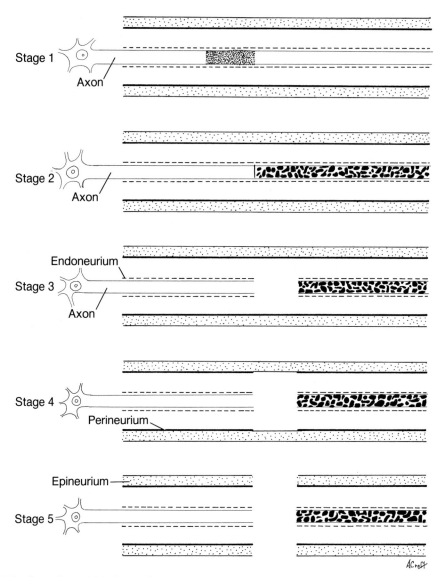

Figure 9.9. Depiction of Sunderland's classification of nerve injury based on the effects of stretching. (Adapted from Sunderland S: The anatomy of the intervertebral foramen and the mechanisms of compression and stretch of nerve roots. In Haldeman S (ed): *Modern Developments in the Principles and Practice of Chiropractic.* New York, Appleton-Century-Crofts, 1980, p 56.)

agnostic test for thoracic outlet syndrome, the clinician still has a variety of procedures available to aid in the establishment of a correct diagnosis. The majority of these, such as Adson's test and Wright's test, provide for the reproduction of vascular occlusion and help confirm the physician's clinical impression.

The clinical picture of thoracic outlet syndrome typically consists of vascular symptoms such as achy pain and paresthesias or coldness in the extremity. According to Kline et al. (33), the differential diagnosis should include "cervical disc and spondylotic disease; . . . tumor (such as a Pancoast's tumor) originating from or compressing the plexus or more peripheral nerves; . . . ulnar or median nerve entrapment; and . . . brachial plexitis."

Individual nerves arising from the brachial plexus may also suffer peripheral entrapment. In the following sections, each nerve and its primary entrapment syndromes are briefly discussed and then the onset of these syndromes is related to the occurrence of a cervical acceleration/deceleration syndrome injury.

MEDIAN NERVE

Anomalous muscles, pressure from tortuous or aberrant vascular formations, and fascia in the area of the clavicle can affect the median nerve. Clinical symptoms often occur after hyperabduction of the arm, which may stretch the median nerve around the previously described anatomical structures. This syndrome, termed *intraclavicular median nerve entrapment* (35), may also be caused by compression of the pectoralis minor muscle against the coracoid process. This is especially true in patients who are hypermobile and able to markedly hyperabduct their shoulders.

All of the muscular and fascial structures in the pronator arch have been implicated in median nerve compression. The *pronator syndrome*, as it is called, produces a graded weakness in the extrinsic and intrinsic muscles of the hand, which are innervated by the median nerve. There is also a diminished sensory function associated with this particular syndrome (36).

The *anterior interosseous syndrome*, also known as the *Kiloh-Nevin syndrome* (37), consists of peripheral entrapment of the anterior interosseous nerve that arises from the posterior aspect of the median nerve as it exits the cubital fossa. The clinical picture is one of motor involvement only. The patient is unable to flex the distal joints of the index finger and thumb. This is known as the pinch sign. There is also a weakness in pronation when the elbow is flexed. Surgery for the anterior interosseous and the pronator syndrome is reserved for those patients who do not improve or who worsen over a period of 3–6 months (38, 39).

The most widely known median nerve lesion is *carpal tunnel syndrome*. First recognized by Sir James Paget in 1865 (40), it is the most common example of peripheral nerve entrapment. Clinical symptoms include numbness and tingling of the index, long, and ring fingers; it occurs most often in middle-aged women. The symptoms are vague at first, and it is not unusual to have the patient relate a history of being awakened at night by burning pain in the hands or wrist, which the patient relieves by either rubbing or shaking the wrists.

The etiology of carpal tunnel syndrome is complex. It may be caused by trauma, inflammatory diseases, endocrine changes, tumors, and extremes of wrist position. These are only the "categories" of etiology, and many conditions may fit into each category.

Diagnosis of carpal tunnel syndrome is accomplished, to a large degree, by the history related by the patient. Although electrodiagnostic tests such as those described in Chapter 3 may be used, I advocate that the diagnosis be one of exclusion. Neurological tests such as Phalen's and Tinel's may reproduce the symptoms and help confirm the problem. Another useful test is a modified Phalen's which reproduces the symptoms with a forceful flexion of the thumb, index, and long fingers while the wrist is flexed (35).

Sensory testing should include pinprick, light touch, two-point discrimination, and vibratory testing. In a recent study, Dellon (41) showed that application of a 256-cycle/sec tuning fork to the digital pulp of the finger could help indicate early compressive lesions. He further noted that 72% of his test group reported a significant difference in their vibratory sensibility in the affected extremity. His results suggest that this loss of vibratory sensation is a more reliable indication of carpal tunnel syndrome than are both Phalen's and Tinel's test. The patient's sensitivity to vibration returned to normal within several weeks after surgical decompression of the carpal tunnel. Each extremity should be tested when these evaluations are made.

More than 30% of patients with a true carpal tunnel syndrome respond to conservative care consisting of rest, cock-up splints, and anti-inflammatory medications (35). Patients with evidence of motor weakness or thenar atrophy have a poorer prognosis and often require surgical decompression of the tunnel (42).

ULNAR NERVE

The ulnar nerve classically originates from the C8 and T1 nerve roots that form the lower trunk and medial cord of the brachial plexus (Fig. 9.10). Active compression produces motor weakness of the intrinsic or interosseous muscles of the hand. Sensory deficits in ulnar nerve lesions produce numbness of the dorsal and volar aspects of the little and ring fingers. When the muscle is being tested, the patient may, when attempting to pinch, try to substitute the flexor pollicis longus and flexor profundus of the index finger for the paralyzed ulnar intrinsic muscles. This substitution is known as Froment's sign and is considered pathognomonic of an ulnar lesion (35).

The most common point of entrapment of the ulnar nerve is the cubital tunnel; thus this condition is termed the *cubital tunnel syndrome* (43, 44). The nerve travels through a tunnel composed of the medial epicondyle and an aponeurotic band that serves to bridge the dual origin of the flexor carpi ulnaris. Its superficial location causes it to be subjected to external compression or tethering when the elbow is flexed.

The cubital tunnel syndrome is usually found in those patients who have either suffered previous trauma to the elbow or have an increased susceptibility to nerve damage because of concurrent conditions such as diabetes, alcoholism, leprosy, or hereditary neuropathy (35). The chief clinical symptom is numbness in the small and

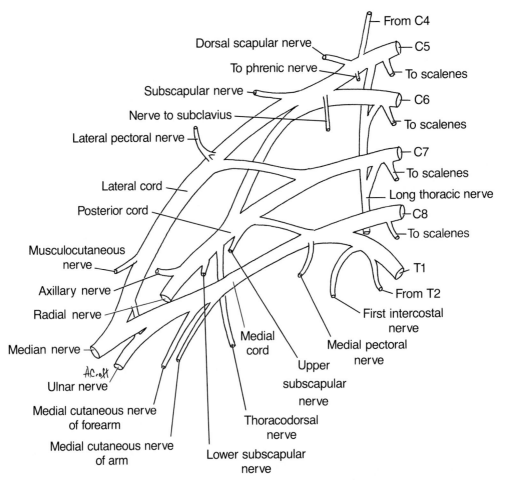

Figure 9.10. Anatomy of the brachial plexus. (Adapted from Warwick R, Williams PL: *Gray's Anatomy*, Br ed 35. Philadelphia, WB Saunders, 1975, p 1038.)

ulnar side of the ring fingers. Higher levels of pressure may cause weakness of the interosseous muscles.

Symptomatic lesions of the ulnar nerve, on occasion, develop a number of years after an injury to the elbow. This delayed clinical manifestation is termed a "tardy ulnar palsy." The delayed onset is the result of direct pressure on the ulnar nerve by the posttraumatic degenerative changes around the elbow.

The ulnar nerve may also become entrapped in the wrist by the pisiform, hook of the hamate, or Guyon's canal. This is five times less common than the cubital tunnel syndrome, however, and should be considered a rare clinical condition.

RADIAL NERVE

The radial nerve may be compressed, and the symptoms are usually divided into either the *Saturday night palsy*, the *posterior interosseous syndrome*, or the *superficial radial nerve entrapment syndrome*. Saturday night palsy is caused by pressure on the proximal-medial portion of the arm. Patients with this syndrome often drape their arm over the edge of a table or chair back for several hours without interruption. The prolonged compression results in a neuropraxia that will usually respond to conservative care.

The posterior interosseous nerve syndrome may be considered the reverse of the anterior interosseous syndrome of the median nerve. Caused by compression of the radial nerve just distal to the elbow, it limits a patient's ability to extend both the thumb and the metacarpophalangeal joints. There is no sensory involvement. Most cases are caused by prior episodes of elbow trauma or fibrous bands that entrap the nerve.

Unlike the other radial nerve syndromes, superficial radial nerve entrapment comes from an external rather than an internal compression. Pain and paresthesias of the web of the thumb are the clinical findings, and a tight cast or watchband is the most likely cause (45).

GANGLIONEUROPATHIES

Ganglioneuropathies, more commonly termed the *double crush syndrome*, were originally described by Upton and McComas (46) in their 1973 study. According to the double crush theory, "multiple or serial impingements upon a peripheral nerve can act in a cumulative manner and cause a symptomatic distal entrapment neuropathy."

Each nerve possesses a certain margin of safety designed to accommodate some chronic compression without causing symptoms. When this mildly compromised nerve is subjected to compression at another level, the safety margin is exceeded and symptoms are manifested. Hurst et al. (47) noted that "cervical arthritis causing mild proximal impingement in combination with mild carpal tunnel syndrome may cause symptoms which would not be present if either one of these mild impingements were acting alone [Fig. 9.11A–E]."

With this concept of the double crush syndrome kept in mind, the various peripheral entrapments of the ulnar, radial, and median nerves can now be associated with whiplash injury. With this injury, the compressed or damaged nerve root, which may have been a minor symptomatic area in the normal patient, has now become a major source of extremity pain in the patient with a subclinical peripheral entrapment. This concept may help to explain situations in which (a) the pain in the upper extremity is out of proportion to the cervical injury, (b) the pain in the elbow or wrist after a cervical injury does not conform to a specific dermatome pattern, and (c) there is prolonged elbow or wrist pain after the cervical spine becomes asymptomatic.

Autonomic Nervous System Trauma

The autonomic nervous system is composed of efferent nerves through which all of the visceral organs, glands, intrinsic muscles of the eyes, and hair follicles are innervated. This system is divided into the functional components of the sympathetic and the parasympathetic nervous system. Both of these, especially the sympathetic nervous system, are related in some manner to the cervical area.

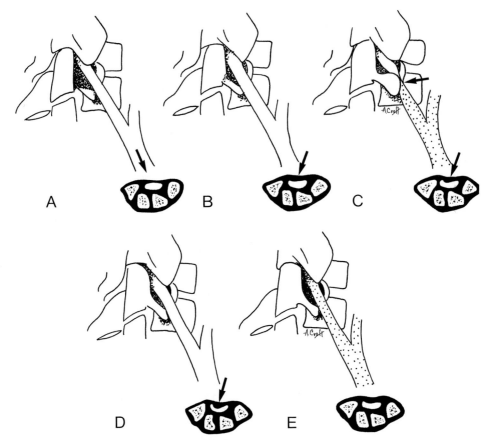

Figure 9.11. **A.** Line drawing depicting a normal cervical intervertebral foramen (IVF) and carpal tunnel. The *arrow* indicates the direction of the axoplasmic flow and the normal nerve root and ovoid shape of the median nerve. **B.** The axoplasmic flow has not been altered despite the mild pressure being exerted on the median nerve (*arrow*). This patient would still be asymptomatic. **C.** The axoplasmic flow has been altered (represented by the *dots* within the nerve) because of pressure on the exiting nerve root (*upper arrow*) and mild compression on the median nerve (*lower arrow*). The combination of proximal and distal impingement has caused the symptomatic threshold to be surpassed. Denervation now exists. **D.** The axoplasmic flow is normal in the nerve, but a carpal tunnel syndrome exists because of the denervation distal to the flexor retinaculum. Note a normal IVF and nerve root but severe pressure and deformity of the median nerve (*arrow*). **E.** The axoplasmic flow has been altered by the combination of mild distal pressure and peripheral neuropathy. The most common cause of this type of neuropathy is diabetes. (Adapted from Hurst LC, Weissberg D, Carrol RE: The relationship of the double crush to carpal tunnel syndrome: an analysis of 1,000 cases of carpal tunnel syndrome. *J Hand Surg* 10B(2):202-204, 1985.)

The sympathetic nervous system extends from the cranium to the coccyx, and generally each ganglion in this sympathetic chain is segmentally related to the spinal cord, except in the cervical spine. In the cervical spine, the ganglia are located between the transverse processes and the carotid arteries. These ganglia include the inferior, the intermediate, the middle, and the superior cervical. The inferior cervical ganglion is often fused with the first tho-racic ganglion to form the cervicothoracic or stellate ganglion. Each of the ganglia supplies innervation to the cervical nerves via the gray rami.

The parasympathetic nervous system in the cervical spine area is limited to the vagus nerve as it travels from the medulla to the viscera. Specific syndromes associated with injury to the vagus nerve from an acceleration/deceleration accident have not been documented in the literature. This may be because injury to the cervical spine could overshadow the vagal dysfunction.

SYMPATHETIC NERVOUS SYSTEM

The stellate ganglion is connected to C7 and C8 nerve roots by the gray rami. The inferior cervical sympathetic cardiac nerve extends from the stellate ganglion to the cardiac plexus. This ganglion also supplies innervation to the common carotid, vertebral, and subclavian arteries.

The fifth and sixth cervical nerves supply innervation to the middle cervical sympathetic ganglion. This middle cervical ganglion innervates the cardiac plexus and inferior thyroid artery.

The superior cervical sympathetic ganglion is the largest of the cervical ganglia. It receives preganglionic fibers through the sympathetic chain from the T1–T4 nerve roots. Sympathetic fibers also arise from the body of the ganglion and supply the C1–C4 nerve roots. Fibers from this superior ganglion also make up the major portion of the internal carotid plexus.

The cervical sympathetic ganglia within the cervical spine also supply various structures within the head. Included among these structures are the salivary glands, the intrinsic muscles of the eye, and the mucous membranes of the nose and pharynx. Of equal importance is the vascular supply that extends into the head and is also innervated by the sympathetic nervous system. The vestibular and cochlear portions of the ear, for example, are supplied by the labyrinthine artery and the stylomastoid branch of the posterior auricular artery. The former is fed by the anterior inferior cerebellar artery that arises from the basilar artery. The latter is supplied by the external carotid artery.

The various vascular supplies and neurological innervations explain the wide variety of symptoms seen in some cervical injuries. For example, the symptoms associated with the *posterior cervical syndrome*, also knows as the *Barré-Lieou syndrome* (48), include vertigo, blurred vision, tinnitus, transitory deafness, and shoulder pain. The sympathetic nervous system damaged during the accident can alter the vascular flow rate into the head or affect the innervation, especially to the eyes, and produce the symptoms listed in Table 9.2.

Another more commonly encountered disorder of the sympathetic nervous system is the *shoulder-hand syndrome* or *reflex sympathetic dystrophy* (49). DeTakats and Miller (50) were the first to use the term reflex sympathetic dystrophy to describe painful nutritional changes in the upper extremity that were induced by circulatory and neural disturbances in their series of 33 trauma patients. The characteristic clinical progression of this sign may be divided into three stages (51):

Stage 1. Stage 1 is characterized by an insidious onset of shoulder and arm pain. The fingers are swollen, and the normal range of motion is decreased in all of the affected joints. Stage 1 lasts 3–6 months.

Stage 2. Stage 2, showing progression of this disorder over the subsequent 3–6 months, is characterized by stiffness and flexion deformities in the fingers as the swelling subsides.

Stage 3. Stage 3 is marked by trophic changes in the hand. There is a continuation of tendinous contraction, especially on the ulnar side.

The shoulder-hand syndrome may be seen in conditions other than cervical trauma. Myocardial infarction and cervical spondylosis with narrowing of the intervertebral foramen are the most common etiologies (52). Because of these other, nontraumatic etiologies, the condition is found bilaterally in about 30% of cases.

Table 9.2.
Signs and Symptoms of Posttraumatic Headache Syndrome

Head pain
Neck pain
Insomnia
Irritability
Mood changes
Anxiety
Memory loss
Changes in sleep patterns
Difficulty concentrating
Intolerance to alcohol

Chronic Conditions: Posttraumatic Syndrome___

A common complication of closed head injury is the persistence of headache and other cranial symptoms. This situation has been the source of controversy in medical circles over the years and has been complicated by our increasingly litigious society. The point of contention in these cases concerns the degree of difference frequently observed between the symptomatology and the degree of injury. Some authors have even implied an inverse relationship between the two factors. The symptomatic picture has some degree of variability, but the salient features are headache, dizziness, irritability, and difficulty with sleep and concentration (14). For a more detailed discussion, see Chapter 8.

This syndrome is a chronic source of pain for many patients. Brenner et al. (53) found that 40–60% of the patients hospitalized for closed head injury experienced headaches for longer than 2 months. Denker's (54) study found that one third had pain for more than 1 year and 15% had pain for more than 3 years. Many of these patients were labeled "neurotic" because of the apparent lack of an anatomical lesion responsible for symptoms. This situation, however, is slowly changing. The courts and juries are now, more than ever, recognizing the presence of soft tissue injuries and their ability to produce long-term pain.

In 1961, Strich (55) described degeneration in the cerebral white matter, noted at autopsy, in patients who had died weeks or months following severe head injury. This process was attributed to the shearing of axons and is now termed diffuse axonal injury (56). It is believed that the axon death is a primary manifestation of trauma and is not secondary to hypoxia or edema.

It was later postulated that the same type of axonal degeneration occurred in minor episodes of head trauma (56). It is, however, quite difficult to prove this contention without autopsy studies. There are some animal studies that lend credibility to this theory, however. Gennarelli et al. (57)

demonstrated that head acceleration in primates, without impact, can produce a coma that has the same pathological appearance as a true concussion.

Povlishock et al. (58), using electron microscopy, later demonstrated early evidence of damage. In their study, cats were subjected to very minor head trauma and were later shown to manifest an evolution of changes beginning with early axonal damage and ending with the more classical picture of diffuse axonal injury.

Viewed together, all of these studies indicate that minor head injury, possibly insufficient to cause a loss of consciousness, may result in subtle brain damage. This would explain the uniformity in symptoms of automobile accident victims over the decades.

The clinical picture is usually quite uniform in nature (Table 9.2). Three separate types of posttraumatic headaches were originally described by Simons and Wolff (59), and their classification remains accurate today (59). These types—generalized, focal, and unilateral—may be readily applied to most patients.

Generalized posttraumatic headaches, the most common form, produce a constant discomfort that waxes and wanes (60). Focal headaches, by definition, are limited to a specific area and are thought to arise from localized scar formation or periostitis.

Unilateral headaches mimic vascular headaches but represent only a small percentage of the actual cases encountered. Like migraine, the pain is characterized by throbbing, is episodic, and is unilateral.

Seizures have long been associated with closed head injuries, such as those encountered in some automobile accidents. These seizures do not seem to favor any particular age group or sex. There is, however, a definite increase in the frequency of seizures in the posttraumatic population compared with the normal population. Annegers et al. (61) followed the progress of 2747 patients who suffered head trauma and found that they experienced 3.6 times more seizures than the control groups. These seizures may respond to medication and can be expected to continue for years.

Summary

1. The nervous system may be injured by either direct or indirect trauma. Direct trauma may cause either neuropraxia, axonotmesis, or neurotmesis. Indirect trauma is usually due to injury or disease of the vascular supply to the spinal cord or peripheral nerve.

2. Direct trauma to the spinal cord may cause the various cord syndromes that were previously believed to be caused by vascular occlusion. The variable in these syndromes is the degree of cord compression occurring during the injury.

3. Damage to peripheral nerves, classified as stages 1–5, may cause either motor or sensory deficits. Subclinical peripheral nerve damage may become symptomatic when it is combined with distal nerve entrapment.

4. Automobile accidents may cause a postconcussion syndrome hallmarked by headaches, dizziness, irritability, and difficulty with sleep and concentration.

References

1. Chusid JG: *Correlative Neuroanatomy and Functional Neurology*, ed 17. Los Altos, CA, Lange Medical Publications, 1979, pp 335–336.
2. Babcock JL: Spinal Injuries in children. *Pediatr Clin North Am* 22(2):487–500, 1975.
3. Foreman SM: Nerve root ischemia and pain secondary to spinal stenosis syndrome: technical and clinical consideration. *J Manipulative Physiol Ther* 8(6):81–86, 1985.
4. Raynor RB, Koplik B: Cervical cord trauma: the relationship between clinical syndromes and force of injury. *Spine* 10(3):193–197, 1985.
5. Seddon H: Three types of nerve injury. *Brain* 66:237, 1943.
6. Sunderland S: *Nerves and Nerve Injuries*. Baltimore, Williams & Wilkins, 1968.
7. Bora WF, Osterman AL: Compression neuropathy. *Clin Orthop* 163:20–31, 1982.
8. Lindenberg R, Freytag E: Brainstem lesions characteristic of traumatic hyperextension of the head. *Arch Pathol* 90:509–515, 1970.
9. Fieschi C, Gottlieb A, De Carolis V: Ischemic lacunae in the spinal cord of arteriosclerotic subjects. *J Neurol Neurosurg Psychiatry* 33:138–146, 1970.
10. Garland H, Greenberg J, Harriman DGF: Infarction of the spinal cord. *Brain* 89:645–662, 1966.
11. Herrick MK, Mills PE: Infarction of the spinal cord. Two cases of selective gray matter involvement secondary to asymptomatic aortic disease. *Arch Neurol* 24:228–241, 1971.
12. Penn AS, Rowan AJ: Myelopathy in systemic lupus erythematosus. *Arch Neurol* 18:337–349, 1968.
13. Schrire V, Asherson RA: Arteritis of the aorta and its major branches *Q J Med* 33:439–463, 1964.
14. Ford JS: Post-traumatic headache: keeping current in the treatment of headache. *NY Med Recertification Assoc* 4(1): 3–11, 1985.
15. Klingele TG, Schultz R, Murphy MG: Pontine gaze paresis due to traumatic cervicocranial hyperextension. *Neurosurgery* 53:249–251, 1980.
16. Caffey J: The whiplash shaken infant syndrome: manual shaking by the extremities with whiplash induced intracranial and intraocular bleedings, linked with residual permanent brain damage and mental retardation. *Pediatrics* 54(4):396–403, 1974.
17. Schneider RC: The syndrome of acute anterior spinal cord injury. *J Neurosurg* 12:95–122, 1955.
18. Gilroy J, Meyer JS: *Medical Neurology*, ed 3. New York, Macmillan, 1979.
19. Hashizume Y, Iijima S, Kishimoto H, Yanagi T: Pathology of spinal cord lesions caused by ossification of the posterior longitudinal ligament. *Acta Neuropathol* 63(2):123–130, 1984.
20. Foreman SM: Ossification of the posterior longitudinal ligaments: a cause of spinal stenosis syndrome. *J Manipulative Physiol Ther* 8(4):251–255, 1985.
21. Raynor RB, Koplik B: Cervical cord trauma: the relationship between clinical syndromes and force of injury. *Spine* 10(3):193–197, 1985.
22. Crosby EC, Humphrey T, Lauer EW: The spine. In: *Correlative Anatomy of the Nervous System*. New York, Macmillan, 1962.
23. Raynor RB: Severe injuries of the cervical spine treated by early anterior fusion and ambulations. *J Neurosurg* 28:311–316, 1968.
24. Cawthon DF, Senter HJ, Stewart WB: Comparison of hydrogen clearance in C-antipyrine autoradiography in the measurement of spinal cord blood flow after severe impact injury. *J Neurosurg* 52:801–807, 1980.
25. Rydevik B, Lundborg G, Bagge V: Effects of graded compression on intraneural blood flow: an in-vivo study on rabbit tibial nerve. *J Hand Surg* 6:3–12, 1981.
26. Lundborg G, Rydevik B: Effects of stretching the tibial nerve of the rabbit: a preliminary study on the intraneural microcirculation and the barrier function of the perineurium. *J Bone Joint Surg* 55B:390–401, 1973.
27. Macnab I: The mechanism of spondylogenic pain. In Hirsch C, Zotterman Y (eds): *Cervical Pain*. New York, Pergamon Press, 1972, pp 89–95.
28. Smyth MJ, Wright V: Sciatica and the intervertebral disc: an experimental study. *J Bone Joint Surg* 40A:1401–1418, 1958.
29. Howe JF, Loeser JD, Calvin WH: Mechanosensitivity of dorsal root ganglia and chronically injured axons: a physiological basis for the radicular pain of nerve root compression. *Pain* 3:25–41, 1977.
30. Sunderland S: The anatomy of the intervertebral foramen and the mechanisms of compression and stretch of nerve roots. In Haldeman S (ed): *Modern Developments in the Principles and Practice of Chiropractic*. New York, Appleton-Century-Crofts, 1980, chap 3, pp 45–65.
31. Scoppetta C, Vaccario ML: Hypertension injuries of the cervical spine. *Lancet* 1:1054, 1978 (letter).
32. Daube JR: *An Electromyographer's Review of Plexopathy: Syl-*

labus on Neuromuscular Disease as Seen by the Electromyog-rapher. Rochester, MN, American Association of Electro-myography and Electrodiagnosis, 1979.

33. Kline DG, Hackett ER, Happel LH: Surgery for lesions of the brachial plexus. *Arch Neurol* 43:170–181, 1986.
34. Bonney G: Some lesions of the brachial plexus. *Ann R Coll Surg Engl* 59:298–306, 1977.
35. Bora WF, Osterman AL: Compression neuropathy. *Clin Orthop* 163:20–32, 1982.
36. Muckart RD: Compression of the common peroneal nerve by ganglions. *J Bone Joint Surg* 58B:241, 1976.
37. Kiloh LG, Nevin S: Isolated neuritis of the anterior inter-osseous nerve. *Br Med J* 1:850, 1952.
38. Nakano KK, Lundergan C: Anterior interosseous nerve segments: diagnostic methods and alternative treat-ments. *Arch Neurol* 34:477, 1977.
39. Spinner M: Management of peripheral nerve problems. In Spinner M (ed): *Injuries to the Major Branches of the Peripheral Nerves of the Forearm,* Philadelphia, WB Saun-ders, 1980, p 582.
40. Phalen GS: The carpal tunnel syndrome: 17 years experi-ence in diagnosis and treatment. *J Bone Joint Surg* 48A:211, 1966.
41. Dellon AL: Clinical use of vibratory stimuli to evaluate peripheral nerve injury and compression neuropathy. *Plast Reconstr Surg* 65:466, 1980.
42. Gelberman RH, Aronson D, Weisman MH: CTS: a pro-spective trial of steroid injection and splinting. *J Bone Joint Surg* 62A:1181, 1980.
43. Feindel W, Stratford J: Cubital tunnel compression. *Can Med Assoc J* 78:351, 1958.
44. Wadsworth TG: The external compressor syndrome of the ulnar nerve in the cubital tunnel. *Clin Orthop* 124:189, 1977.
45. Braidwood AS: Superficial radial nerve neuropathy. *J Bone Joint Surg* 57B:380, 1975.
46. Upton ARM, McComas AJ: The double crush in nerve entrapment syndromes. *Lancet* 2:359–361, 1973.
47. Hurst LC, Weissberg D, Carrol RE: The relationship of the double crush to carpal tunnel syndrome: an analysis of 1,000 cases of carpal tunnel syndrome. *J Hand Surg* 10B(2):202–204, 1985.
48. Barré JA: Sur un syndrome sympathique cervical poster-ieur et sa cause frequente, l, artrite cervicale. *Rev Neurol (Paris)* 1:1246–1248, 1926.
49. Wainapel SF: Reflex sympathetic dystrophy following traumatic myelopathy. *Pain* 18:345–349, 1984.
50. DeTakats G, Miller D: Post-traumatic dystrophy of the extremities. *Arch Surg* 46:467, 1943.
51. Steinbrocker O: Shoulder-hand-syndrome. *Am J Med* 3:402, 1947.
52. Oppenheimer A: Swollen atrophic hand. *Surg Gynecol Obstet* 67:446, 1938.
53. Brenner C, Friedman A, Meritt HH, et al: Post-traumatic headache. *Neurosurgery* 1:379–391, 1944.
54. Deuker PG: The postconcussive syndrome: prognosis and evaluation of the organic factors. *NY State J Med* 44:379–384, 1944.
55. Strich S: Shearing of nerve fibers as a cause of brain dam-age due to head injury. *Lancet* 2:443–448, 1961.
56. Thomlinson BE: Brainstem lesions after head injury. *J Clin Pathol* 23:154–165, 1970.
57. Gennarelli TA, Thibault LE, Adams JH, Graham DI, Thompson CJ, Marcincin RP: Diffuse axonal injury and traumatic coma in the primate. *Ann Neurol* 12:564–574, 1982.
58. Povlishock JT, Becker DP, Cheng CLY, Vaughn GW: Ax-onal change in minor head injury. *J Neuropathol Exp Neurol* 42:225–242, 1983.
59. Simons DJ, Wolff HG: Studies on headache: mechanisms of chronic post-traumatic headache. *Psychosom Med* 8:227–242, 1946.
60. Raskin N: Posttraumatic headache. In: Raskin N, Appen-zeller A (eds): *Headache.* Philadelphia, WB Saunders, 1980.
61. Annegers JF, Grabbow JD, Groover RV, Laws ER Jr, Elve-back LR, Kurland LT: Seizures after head trauma: a pop-ulation study. *Neurology* 30:683–689, 1980.

10

Temporomandibular Joint Injuries

LAWRENCE A. WEINBERG, DDS, MS, FACD, FICD

In order to understand the pathome-chanics of whiplash injury on the tempo-romandibular joint (TMJ) and its effect on diagnosis and treatment, a review of TMJ anatomy and biomechanics of movement is necessary. It is also extremely important to understand how previously existing subclinical TMJ dysfunction and/or disc derangement can influence the tissue re-sponse to whiplash injury and therefore the diagnosis and treatment of the joint itself as well as of the cervical spine.

Normal Anatomy and Biomechanics of TMJ

The TMJ is a sliding hinge joint, but its function is so intimately related to its op-posing side and the teeth that it should not be thought of as a single functioning unit. The head of the lower jaw (condyle) is po-sitioned within the fossae by the balance in muscle tonus of all the muscles of mastica-tion (bilaterally) when the mandible is in the resting position and there is a small space between the teeth. When the teeth are occluded, however, they dominate condylar position in the fossae. When a malocclusion is present, it *disarticulates* the joints three dimensionally despite the disc being interposed between the articulating surfaces (1–15). The temporomandibular ligament is directed downward and back-ward (Fig. 10.1) and cannot resist this con-dylar displacement. Research has shown that the factors that influence condylar po-sition in the fossae (when the teeth are apart) are primarily muscular (6–11) rather than ligamentous in nature, as was origi-nally thought (12). As is subsequently dis-cussed, the condylar position in the fossae *before* the injury takes place has a profound

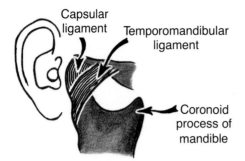

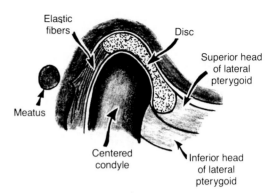

Figure 10.1. The temporomandibular ligament is directed downward and backward.

Figure 10.2. When the condyle is centered, the superior portion of the fossae contains the posterior portion of the disc, with the narrowed central portion against the posterior portion of the eminentia. The anatomical relationships are shown.

influence on the tissue response, treatment, and prognosis.

DISC

The articular disc is biconcave with thickened borders around its circumference. It is made of fibrocartilage with no nerve fibers or blood vessels within its body, which indicates its stress-bearing function. When the condyle is positioned in the middle of the fossae, the superior portion of the fossae contains the posterior portion of the disc, with the narrowed central portion against the posterior portion of the eminentia (Fig. 10.2). The disc is attached to the condyle on the medial and lateral poles only. The anterior portion of the disc is attached to the upper head of the lateral pterygoid muscle, which serves to pull the disc forward, while the elastic

fibers that form the posterior attachment of the disc function to pull the disc posteriorly when they are stretched (Fig. 10.3). During physiological opening, both condyles move forward with the discs closely attached to the condyles and interposed between the bony surfaces (Fig. 10.3). Within the normal range of opening (about 35–40 mm), the condyles move anteriorly to, but not beyond, the crest of the articular eminence (Fig. 10.3). During the closing movement of the mandible, the elastic fibers pull on the disc posteriorly while, as recent research has revealed, the upper head of the lateral pterygoid tenses to provide coordi-

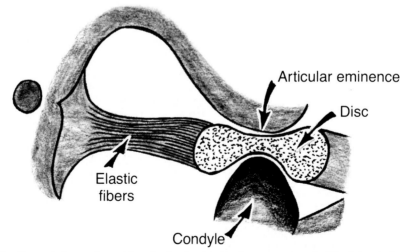

Figure 10.3. The anterior portion of the disc is attached to the upper head of the lateral pterygoid muscle which serves to pull the disc forward, while the elastic fibers when stretched function to pull the disc posteriorly.

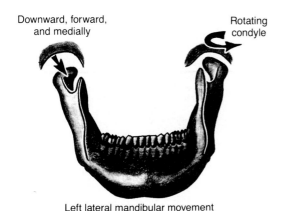

Downward, forward, and medially

Rotating condyle

Left lateral mandibular movement

Figure 10.4. Lateral mandibular movement is accomplished by having one condyle rotate and move slightly laterally while the opposite side moves downward, forward, and medially.

nated posterior movement (13) rather than relaxation, as was previously thought.

LATERAL MANDIBULAR MOVEMENT

Lateral mandibular movement is accomplished by having one condyle rotate and move slightly laterally while the opposite side moves downward, forward, and medially (Fig. 10.4). The medial wall of the fossa is slightly more inclined than the anterior wall of the fossa formed by the eminentia. The significance of this anatomic fact is discussed in relation to disc derangements.

JOINT NOISES

In the past, joint noises were shrugged off as insignificant because almost 40% of the population demonstrated one form of them or another (14), they were painless, not much was known about the cause and effect, and there was no definitive treatment. With the advent of soft tissue imaging and increased awareness of disc pathology, it has generally been accepted that any joint noise, i.e., popping, clicking, and gritting, is a sign of disc derangement and of possible pathological bony changes. If a new joint noise were to develop after whiplash injury, its timing and character may help establish that a disc derangement occurred as a result of the trauma.

SWALLOWING

During normal swallowing, the teeth are braced together to form a mandibular platform from which some of the extrinsic muscles of the tongue and hyoid bone receive positional support. The tip of the tongue is placed behind the upper anterior teeth, and a wave of muscular contraction moves upward and backward against the palate, propelling the bolus or liquid into the pharynx.

Abnormal Anatomy and Biomechanics of TMJ

The field of TMJ dysfunction pain (or craniomandibular pain) is somewhat controversial because of the multicausality of the syndrome, stress factors, and the difficulty of isolating single etiological factors for study in the human being. Most variation of opinion can be found in methods of treatment by dentists. These methods are described and, in general terms, are related to the whiplash injuries observed primarily by chiropractors, medical practitioners, and physiotherapists.

DISC DERANGEMENT

The anatomic weakness of the condyle-disc assembly is the relatively weak ligamentous attachment of the disc to the condyle only at the medial and lateral poles. This attachment can be easily stretched or torn by trauma or long-term posterior condylar displacement which results in disc derangement. The clinical sign of disc derangement is joint noise characterized by popping or clicking during movement. Almost one third of the "normal" population (without pain symptoms) have posterior condylar displacement (15, 16). This is extremely important in relation to joint injuries because a joint with a previously painless disc derangement does not respond as well to injury (or treatment) as does a normal joint. Indeed, this type of joint should be treated differently, which would call for a differential diagnosis established by the dentist. A protective splint should be constructed if a neck collar or traction is indicated.

A normal lateral transcranial TMJ radio-

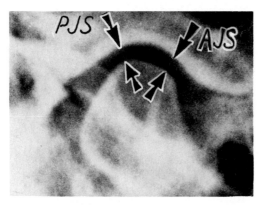

Figure 10.5. A normal lateral transcranial TMJ radiograph is shown which was taken with teeth together. The joint spaces (posterior (*PJS*) and anterior (*AJS*) are relatively equal, so that the condyle is said to be centered within the superior portion of the fossae.

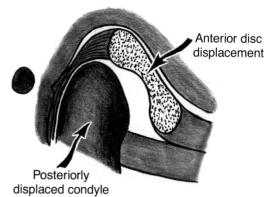

Figure 10.7. The condyle is displaced posteriorly by the teeth. The disc is displaced anteriorly from its normal relationship to the condyle.

graph is shown in Figure 10.5. This radiograph was taken with the teeth together. The joint spaces are relatively equal, so that the condyle is said to be centered within the superior portion of the fossae. On the lateral transcranial TMJ radiograph seen in Figure 10.6, on the other hand, a posterior displaced condyle is illustrated, since the posterior joint space is much smaller than the anterior joint space. When the condyle is displaced posteriorly by the teeth, there is no space in the fossae for the disc to follow in its normal relationship to the condyle (Fig. 10.7). As a result, the ligaments stretch or are torn, producing an anteriorly displaced disc relative to the condyle. This

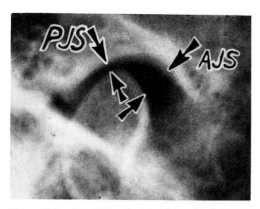

Figure 10.6. A posterior displaced condyle is shown; the posterior joint space *(PJS)* is much smaller than the anterior joint space *(AJS).*

is usually characterized by an immediate click on opening and closing the teeth together. This is caused by the condyle moving posteriorly past the posterior thickness of the disc on closure (Fig.10.7). Conversely, on opening, the slight anterior movement of the condyle over the same posterior thickness of the disc produces the second click. This has been called reciprocal clicking (17); it is almost always present when radiographs of the TMJ show posterior condylar displacement. *Thus, the combination of reciprocal clicking and posterior condylar displacement as seen in the radiographs is sufficient evidence* (without soft tissue imaging) *to warrant protective splints* if traction or a neck brace is indicated. (All radiographs are taken with the teeth in maximum occlusion.)

The reciprocal clicking is clinical evidence that the condyle is *self-reducing*; it is not necessarily associated with limitation of motion or pain. As a result of trauma or long-standing anterior disc displacement, however, the disc can fold on itself and become *dislocated* anterior to the condyle (Fig. 10.8), which will usually result in limitation of movement of the condyle on that side and *no* joint noise. The derangement cannot be reduced without manipulation and/or surgery. Only 5% of TMJ cases require surgery (17), but surgery is indicated only after conservative treatment has proven to be unsuccessful (18). Soft tissue imaging with modalities such as arthrography (19), computed tomography (CT), or

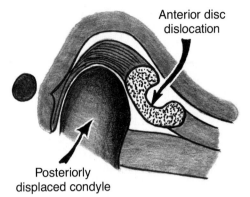

Anterior disc
dislocation

Posteriorly
displaced condyle

Figure 10.8.   When the disc folds on itself, it becomes *dislocated* anterior to the condyle. (Adapted from Weinberg LA: An evaluation of occlusal factors in TMJ dysfunction pain syndrome. *J Prosthet Dent* 41:198, 1979.)

magnetic resonance imaging (MRI) can confirm this condition.

CREPITUS

Crepitus usually is produced by a hole in the disc which most often is located on the lateral portion (14). Nature attempts to adapt to the pathology by a growth of soft tissue from the head of the condyle, which corresponds to the location of the damaged disc; this growth is later followed by bony breakdown on the adjacent surface of the fossae (20). These localized arthritic bony changes are thought to be responsible for the gritting and grinding noises (crepitus) that are usually painless and require no specific treatment other than the maintenance or rehabilitation of proper occlusal support. The existence of crepitus, per se, has no particular significance for the treatment of whiplash injury other than the aforementioned maintenance of occlusion.

WIDE OPENING CLICK (OR POP)

Some patients have exaggerated opening (of about 55 mm) present from youth, which represents a "chronic hyperextension anteriorly." The condyle moves beyond the crest of the articular eminence (Fig. 10.9), loosening the ligamentous attachment of the condyle-disc assembly. The condyle passes over the thickened anterior portion of the disc, producing a loud click or pop. The subluxation is self-reducing, producing another closing click as the head of the condyle passes posteriorly over the thickened anterior portion of the disc, returning to the thinner middle portion. If the condition worsens, and the condyle moves superiorly (due to the upward pull of the elevator muscles), the condyle can become dislocated anterior to the eminentia and is not considered self-reducing. In this case, the mandible has to be reduced

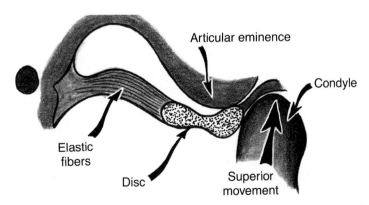

Articular eminence

Condyle

Elastic
fibers

Disc

Superior
movement

Figure 10.9.   When the condyle moves beyond the crest of the articular eminence, the condyle passes over the thickened anterior portion of the disc, producing a loud click or pop. If the condyle moves superiorly, it can become dislocated anterior to the eminentia and is not self-reducing. (Adapted from Weinberg LA: An evaluation of occlusal factors in TMJ dysfunction pain syndrome. *J Prosthet Dent* 41:198, 1979.)

by manipulation downward and backward to recapture the disc. The condition can be controlled by patient awareness and reduced opening as well as by simultaneous bilateral chewing that limits condyle translation. No surgical or dental treatment is usually recommended, other than patient-controlled limitation of motion. The origin of exaggerated motion can be contributed to by a shallow fossae, exaggerated opening habits, impact trauma, professional singing, and congenital looseness of other body joints.

Exaggerated opening disc derangement can exist with or without the reciprocal derangement previously described, which can be looked upon as "hyperextension posteriorly" on closure. Of course, this can be observed as posterior condyle displacement on TMJ radiographs or as clinical clicking on immediate opening and closing, which would be significant in the treatment of whiplash, although joint noise on wide opening would not be significant.

SIGNIFICANCE OF SUDDEN CHANGE IN OCCLUSION

After whiplash injury, particularly in a patient with a previously existing subclinical disc derangement, a sudden change in occlusion usually indicates that the disc has been dislocated traumatically. The mandible can be manipulated downward and forward in an attempt to recapture the disc. The incidence of disc dislocation in a normal joint, as a result of whiplash injury, is minimal. As is subsequently discussed, however, the patient should always be questioned after any injury to the jaw, be it whiplash or direct trauma, to establish if the teeth do not fit together normally.

ABNORMAL SWALLOWING

Clinical experience of over 30 years (unpublished observations) has indicated that posterior condylar displacement is associated with "pathological swallowing"; i.e., while swallowing, the patient prevents the mandible from coming into occlusal contact in an unconscious physiological attempt to prevent the condyles from being displaced posteriorly. The joint capsule is

richly innervated with sensory proprioceptive fibers (21) that are apparently overstimulated when the posterior condylar displacement causes disc derangement and violates the normal joint position sense as well. One of the diagnostic factors then would be to check the patient's swallowing to determine whether the teeth occlude during deglutition whenever reciprocal clicking (on immediate opening and closing) occurs. Under these circumstances, TMJ radiographs are indicated to verify posterior condylar displacement.

Pathomechanics of Whiplash Injury

During whiplash injury, the head is thrust backward so suddenly that inertia causes the mandible to remain where it was in space, causing *anterior mandibular displacement* as the mouth opens (Fig. 10.10). Contradictory as it may seem, initially during whiplash the posterior thrust of the head causes *Anterior* rather than posterior joint injury. Internal joint injury may consist of tearing of the lateral and medial ligamentous attachment of the disc to the condyle, disc derangement, disc displacement, and bleeding and inflammation within the joint.

Most often there is also a sudden stopping of the vehicle after the first impact, causing the head to be thrust forward while inertia causes the mandible to be suddenly thrust *posteriorly*, traumatically closing the mouth (Fig. 10.11). This sudden mandibular closure can cause injury to the teeth themselves, such as a cusp fracture or chipping of the anterior teeth without actual direct impact trauma to the jaw itself. The teeth usually prevent overclosure and posterior injury to the joint itself. In rare cases of patients who are missing a complete lower denture, however, overclosure is possible with subsequent injury of the posterior portion of the joint as well. Although this is rare, denture patients should be questioned to ascertain whether both dentures were worn during the accident and whether one or both dentures popped out of the mouth on first impact.

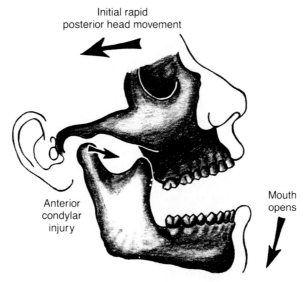

Figure 10.10. During whiplash injury, the head is thrust backward so suddenly that inertia causes the mandible to remain where it was in space, causing *anterior mandibular displacement* as the mouth opens.

TISSUE RESPONSE TO INJURY

Intracapsular inflammation stimulates the sensory innervation of the capsule, belonging to the same nerve as the motor innervation to the muscles that move the joint. These muscles go into reflex spasm, effectively splinting the joint (22). This produces pain and trismus (limitation of motion) which is one of the cardinal signs of

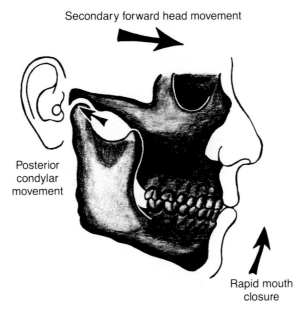

Figure 10.11. After the first impact in an automobile rear-end collision, the head is then tossed forward while inertia causes the mandible to be suddenly thrust *posterior*, traumatically closing the mouth.

acute TMJ dysfunction pain. Usually, the intraincisal opening is less than 24 mm, and the patient has pain on movement, pain on chewing and, the most significant sign of all, pain on opening which is pathognomonic. Intrajoint inflammation will cause pain on complete closure, and on a cursory history the examiner may falsely record that the patient has said something (the occlusion) feels different. This can be due to the *pain itself* rather than the dislocated disc. This distinction can be made when, if no disc is dislocated, the teeth can be occluded even in the presence of pain. In a true disc dislocation, however, the teeth cannot be occluded normally, regardless of the pain. The diagnostic and treatment procedures are different in both cases; therefore, it is important to elicit the history carefully.

General Signs and Symptoms

The general signs and symptoms of TMJ injuries are indicated in Figure 10.12.

PAIN ON OPENING

Pain on opening is pathognomonic of TMJ dysfunction. It results from muscle spasm due to overstimulation of the neuromuscular system, which can be caused by malocclusion, stress clenching, or muscle splinting due to intracapsular inflammation caused by injury.

```
GENERAL SIGNS & SYMPTOMS CHART

   1) Pain on opening
   2) Trismus
   3) Joint noises
   4) Pain on chewing
   5) Tenderness in TMJ
   6) Change in occlusion
   7) Headache
   8) Muscle palpation
```

Figure 10.12. General "signs and symptoms" chart.

TRISMUS

Limitation of motion (trismus) can be caused by all of the factors indicated under "Pain on Opening." The converse is not true, however, namely, that trismus must be present with acute TMJ dysfunction pain. Patients with chronic TMJ pain usually have a *history* of trismus but not necessarily at the time of examination. Patients with TMJ pain as a result of whiplash injury, however, might be expected to have a higher incidence of trismus because of the nature of the injury which may precipitate intracapsular inflammation. On the other hand, patients with chronic TMJ pain may have trismus associated with muscle spasm without intracapsular inflammation. It is necessary for the dentist to make this distinction because it will affect the choice of treatment appliances, occlusal adjustment, choice of drugs, palliative treatment, definitive treatment, and prognosis.

JOINT NOISES

Joint noises, per se, are *not* pathognomonic of acute TMJ dysfunction pain, even after whiplash injury, although the incidence is very common in all acute cases. It cannot be used as a criterion for diagnostic purposes. The main diagnostic function of joint noise must, therefore, be used in conjunction with other symptoms to delineate the nature of injury to determine whether the disc derangement is significant and how it affects treatment. In summary, joint noise only demonstrates a disc derangement, while the other symptoms, such as trismus, pain on opening, pain on chewing, joint pain, changes in occlusion, and face pain, determine whether TMJ dysfunction has been produced as a complication to cervical injury.

PAIN ON CHEWING

Pain on chewing, in the muscles of mastication, is a strong indication of acute TMJ involvement. The patient usually gives a history of pain on chewing hard food or perhaps on any functional movements. Pain that remains *after* chewing, without movement, is a common complaint. Many times, the patient will reveal that he or she feels pain after talking a great deal. All these symptoms indicate TMJ involvement.

TENDERNESS OF TMJ

Over 60% of all patients with acute TMJ involvement reveal that they feel tenderness and pain in this area (23). This symptom is, therefore, reliable as a diagnostic factor in determining whether the joint is involved in whiplash injuries. Neuralgic pain can be eliminated if the patient does not reveal a history of tenderness to light touch which triggers a painful response.

CHANGE IN OCCLUSION

As discussed previously, a sudden change in occlusion after whiplash injury can indicate disc dislocation. This change must be distinguished from changes in occlusion that are merely caused by discomfort. If the patient cannot occlude the teeth normally, regardless of discomfort, disc dislocation must be regarded as a likely cause, in which case soft tissue imaging may be required to establish a differential diagnosis.

HEADACHE

Headache can be caused by many systemic conditions. If this symptom is newly established after a whiplash injury, however, it is likely that the cause is referred pain from the cervical area and/or TMJ dysfunction pain syndrome. In this case, differential diagnosis of TMJ involvement is important.

EAR SYMPTOMS

Occasionally, tinnitus is a complaint. Its etiology and relationship to TMJ dysfunction are unknown, however. More frequently, the patient will reveal pain "in the ear," which is usually referred, and stuffiness and loss of equilibrium associated with posterior condylar displacement.

General Examination Procedure: Patient Pain History

It is helpful to have a visual chart of the location of the patient's subjective pain (24) (Fig. 10.13). Some patients only complain of pain in the TMJ area and perhaps also the temporal region. These data should be recorded for comparison with the location of the pain on palpation. Often, what seems like a simple unilateral problem confined to the one joint area reveals itself as not only bilateral but also extended to many of the

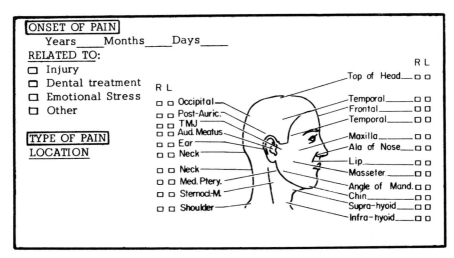

Figure 10.13. Patient pain history and location of the patient's subjective pain. (Adapted from Weinberg LA: The etiology, diagnosis, and treatment of TMJ dysfunction-pain syndrome, Parts I–IV. *J Prosthet Dent* 42:654, 1979; 43:58, 1980; 43:186, 1980.)

muscles of mastication. Conversely, on rare occasions no pain is elicited on palpation. This is very unusual in patients with acute TMJ dysfunction, and the possibility of referred pain from the cervical area, trigger points, neuralgia, neoplasm, atypical TMJ pain, idiopathic pain, or malingering must be considered.

In patients with long-standing TMJ dysfunction, the pain elicited on palpation is usually bilateral. This is most often because what may have started out as muscle spasm on one side may have altered the mandibular position and the occlusion that contributes to muscle pathology on both sides. In patients with acute TMJ dysfunction brought about by whiplash injury, however, the pain may be unilateral, particularly on the side where there was a dysfunctional joint mechanism subclinically before injury, which increased susceptibility on that side.

Factors Useful in Establishing TMJ Dysfunction

Factors useful in establishing the diagnosis of TMJ dysfunction are listed in Figure 10.14. It is essential to deemphasize a chron-

ological history of events and emphasize the translation of the patient's symptoms into medical language that will help to differentiate a TMJ disorder from a neurological or other medical problem. The specific characteristics of the pain symptoms will easily isolate patients with TMJ dysfunction from those with other medical problems.

Although many patients with TMJ dysfunction may experience symptoms (pain chiefly) on only one side, symptoms may be elicited bilaterally on palpation of muscle (23). In the dental literature, unilateral TMJ pain dysfunction has been termed (myofascial pain dysfunction) (MPD) (25) in order to deemphasize the role of occlusion and the joints themselves and to emphasize muscle spasm as the main etiological agent. Once the condition becomes bilateral or one TMJ is sensitive to palpation or is painful, however, the patient is classified as having the more complicated TMJ dysfunction pain. I believe that this distinction between MPD and TMJ dysfunction pain is somewhat artificial and confuses rather than clarifies the diagnosis and treatment of this condition, since the results of one study revealed that the majority (58%) of 128 patients had bilateral pain and/or joint involvement and, therefore, were

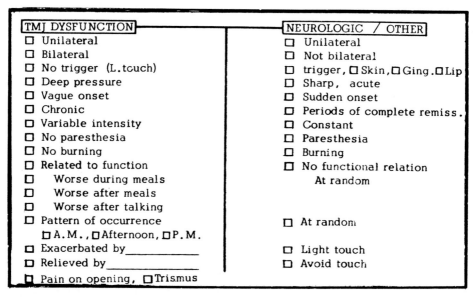

TMJ DYSFUNCTION	NEUROLOGIC / OTHER
□ Unilateral	□ Unilateral
□ Bilateral	□ Not bilateral
□ No trigger (L.touch)	□ trigger, □ Skin, □ Ging. □ Lip
□ Deep pressure	□ Sharp, acute
□ Vague onset	□ Sudden onset
□ Chronic	□ Periods of complete remiss.
□ Variable intensity	□ Constant
□ No paresthesia	□ Paresthesia
□ No burning	□ Burning
□ Related to function	□ No functional relation
□ Worse during meals	At random
□ Worse after meals	
□ Worse after talking	
□ Pattern of occurrence	□ At random
□ A.M., □ Afternoon, □ P.M.	
□ Exacerbated by_____	□ Light touch
□ Relieved by_____	□ Avoid touch
□ Pain on opening, □ Trismus	

Figure 10.14.   List of factors useful in establishing the diagnosis of TMJ dysfunction. (Adapted from Weinberg LA: The etiology, diagnosis, and treatment of TMJ dysfunction-pain syndrome. Parts I–IV. *J Prosthet Dent* 42:654, 1979; 43:58, 1980; 43:186, 1980.)

classified as having TMJ dysfunction (23). Furthermore, I believe that just because MPD is merely an early manifestation of TMJ dysfunction pain does not justify the use of separate terminology, etiology, and treatment basis. The only usefulness of this distinction is that patients identified as having early (1–2 weeks) TMJ dysfunction, in contradistinction to those identified as having chronic TMJ dysfunction (several months or years), might be treated palliatively without appliances or occlusal adjustments.

UNILATERAL VERSUS BILATERAL PAIN

Although the patient with TMJ dysfunction pain can have unilateral as well as bilateral symptoms, usually neurological or other medical etiology is limited to one side. There are exceptions, of course, such as "tension" headaches or headaches caused by hypoglycemia, which will be devoid of functional associated pain. In other words, a total pain history is necessary in order to come to definitive conclusions.

TRIGGER POINTS

The patient should be asked to "show the doctor" where it hurts. If the patient keeps his or her fingers a discrete $\frac{1}{2}$ inch from the skin, the patient may have a neuralgic trigger point involvement, with or without TMJ pathology. The patient should be asked if the skin or scalp is tender to the touch so that combing the hair, shaving, or washing the face causes discomfort.

QUALITY OF PAIN

TMJ pain is usually characterized by a sensation of deep pressure pain associated with muscles and joints, rather than a sharp surface pain which is typical of neuralgic symptoms.

ONSET OF PAIN

For the most part, TMJ pain is not of sudden onset, as, for example, is the pain experienced with neuralgia. The symptoms begin more vaguely, not suddenly as when a trigger point is stimulated. When a patient with suspected TMJ dysfunction reveals a sudden onset of pain, it is appropriate to ask whether a "functional movement" such as opening or chewing had immediately preceded the pain. Often, these patients will reveal that some functional movement produces a noise (disc derangement) which is immediately followed by pain. This type of information is very convincing evidence of TMJ dysfunction.

CHRONICITY OF PAIN

TMJ pain is chronic, characterized by variation in intensity, and, depending on the pain threshold of the patient, sometimes expressed as "tightness." Often there is low-grade background discomfort in the later stages that is exacerbated on functional movement. Neuralgia, on the other hand, is characterized by sudden onset, either by stimulation of a trigger area or spontaneously with no relation to function, time, or behavior. Often there are long periods of complete remission, in contradistinction to the TMJ patient whose pain is daily or is at least severe several times per week.

CONSTANCY OF PAIN

Some patients will reveal that pain is absolutely constant, like a dial tone on a phone, without change in intensity or remission (other than with the use of drugs) and with no relation to function of any kind. This is not usually characteristic of TMJ disorders.

PARESTHESIA AND BURNING

Paresthesia can be a symptom of a neoplasm pressing on a nerve; it is medicolegally important to eliminate this symptom, which could possibly indicate a life-threatening tumor, before treating symptoms of pain. TMJ patients will, however, often complain of a "fullness" or "tingling" in their musculature. This can be caused by changes in circulation within the musculature. To my knowledge, burning sensation is idiopathic, although vitamin supplements may have some effect. The possibility of hypochondriasis should be checked in these instances, as sometimes the tongue becomes a focus of conscious activity just as in other patients hyperocclusal awareness can drive the patient and dentist to distraction.

SYMPTOMS ASSOCIATED WITH FUNCTION

Neurological or medically caused pain is not usually associated with function. In TMJ patients, however, the examiner should ask whether the patient avoids eating when he or she has the pain. Does the patient limit chewing to soft foods? Does chewing make the pain worse, or bring it on? Often the patient will say the pain is also worse after chewing and motion stop. Quite often the patient will reveal that the pain is worse after talking a lot, or if he or she coughs during a bad cold. Sometimes, patients with high thresholds of pain will say it only hurts when chewing hard food. The examiner should not associate the severity of subjective symptoms necessarily with the expected degree of pathology because of the differences in perception of pain and the emotional response of the individual to pain.

PATTERN OF OCCURRENCE

The pain of neurological or medical etiology does not usually have a recognizable pattern of occurrence, whereas the pain from TMJ dysfunction will most often have a recognizable pattern; namely, the patient usually experiences pain upon arising in the morning (which indicates clenching or bruxism while sleeping) and pain late in the afternoon (which is associated with occupational stress-related clenching). The examiner must be careful in taking the history because some patients will not eat solid food, which exacerbates the pain, until the evening.

EXACERBATION OF PAIN

It is always good to summarize those factors that make the pain worse because sometimes another factor will come up and it provides a clear picture of the factors that produce pain. Neuralgia and medical pain most often occur at random and are not associated with function in the TMJ area.

PAIN RELIEF

That the patient complains of pain on function and obtains relief with heat and muscle relaxants helps to further identify the pathology, namely, that the pain is coming from the muscles.

PAIN ON OPENING

Pain on opening is pathognomonic of TMJ dysfunction. Trismus, however, usually follows injury of the joint. The latter does not have to be present to indicate that the patient has a TMJ problem.

Ear Symptoms

It is common for TMJ patients to have ear symptoms directly associated with joint dysfunction (Fig. 10.15). Stuffiness can be associated with posterior condylar displacement, as can dizziness which, upon questioning, is really a transient loss of equilibrium that is usually chronic. Pain can be referred to the ear from muscle trigger points. Ringing of the ears, however, is more elusive and quite perplexing to the clinician. It has been my experience that changes in vertical dimension between the two dental arches can vary the intensity and pitch of the noise but can only rarely eliminate the symptoms completely. In other patients, there is no dental manipulation that has any effect on symptoms. These patients will usually reveal that when they are distracted, they do not notice the intensity of the sound, but that when they are not preoccupied, it becomes loud. It is convenient for the clinician to ascribe to all unknown phenomena the label "psychosomatic." I prefer the more accurate description "idiopathic response," since many of these patients are as well adjusted to their environment as the clinician is to his or hers. We simply don't know.

Joint Noise

Joint noise (clicking, popping, gritting) (Fig. 10.15)) is not pathognomonic for acute TMJ dysfunction pain, although it is present in the majority of these patients. The presence of joint noise, since it occurs in 40% of asymptomatic patients (14), cannot be used as a clinical criterion for acute TMJ dysfunction when it occurs in whiplash injuries. In other words, joint noises, per se, quite definitely indicate disc derangement, which may or may not be significant as a factor in determining whether a specific patient has TMJ complications to whiplash injury.

```
┌─────────────────────────────────────────────────────────────────────┐
│  ┌EAR SYMPTOMS┐              ┌JOINT NOISE┐ (Pat. Aware)               │
│  □ Ringing      □R  □L        □ Clicking  □R,   □L                    │
│  □ Stuffiness   □R  □L        □ Popping   □R,   □L                    │
│  □ Dizziness    □R  □L        □ Gritting  □R,   □L                    │
│  □ Pain         □R  □L                                                │
│  ┌TRISMUS┐ (Pat. Aware)      ┌ASSOCIATED PAIN AREAS┐                  │
│  □         Onset date____     □ Head                                  │
│  □ Trigger mechanism          □ Neck                                  │
│  □         Injury             □ Shoulders                             │
│  □         Dentistry          □ Back                                  │
│  □         Stress             □ Other_____                       │
│  □ Pain,       □No pain                                               │
└─────────────────────────────────────────────────────────────────────┘
```

Figure 10.15. Ear symptoms, joint noise, trismus, and other associated pain areas are part of the pain history. (Adapted from Weinberg LA: The etiology, diagnosis, and treatment of TMJ dysfunction-pain syndrome, Parts I–IV. *J Prosthet Dent* 42:654, 1979; 43:58, 1980; 43:186, 1980.)

Trismus

Trismus (limitation of opening) (Fig. 10.15) is a definite sign of acute TMJ dysfunction; many patients with this TMJ dysfunction will not, however, demonstrate the symptoms at the time of examination. Usually trismus occurs immediately after injury, with pain on opening. Limitation of opening, however, can be transitory with or without pain. Most often the limitation of opening is due to the effect of pain rather than a restriction of actual movement. Evaluation in this situation is difficult, but the distinction should be made (limitation of opening due to pain), if possible, in order to delineate muscle spasm pain as a cause of trismus, rather than disc dislocation which mechanically prevents full range of condylar motion.

Associated Pain Areas

Occasionally, a patient will exhibit all the symptoms of acute TMJ dysfunction pain syndrome, but upon further examination it will be revealed that he or she has pain symptoms in *many areas of the body* (Fig. 10.15). In this case, the TMJ symptoms are a minor part of the broader clinical picture which is usually designated as a "chronic pain." Most physicians believe that the pain from any injury that does not heal in 6–8 weeks should be considered chronic. All too often this is a euphemism for psychosomatic pain. Most dentists, who work in unphysiological body positions all day long, go home with back pain associated with work-related dysfunction. The symptoms do not disappear as long as the bone-joint-muscle relationship is unphysiological. Many acute TMJ pain patients have unphysiological relationships between the TMJ and musculature, due to the occlusion, which will produce painful symptoms (precipitated by whiplash injury or not) for many years without *any psychosomatic etiology whatsoever*. The anatomical relationship between joints, muscles, and the occlusion can perpetuate painful symptoms for years without the patient introducing any psychosomatic factors whatsoever.

Life-Style Habits

It is important to explore life-style habits as an etiological factor in TMJ dysfunction pain (Fig. 10.16). It has been established that clenching contributes to TMJ dysfunction pain symptoms (26). It is, therefore, appropriate to question the patient about life-style habits that may be a significant factor contributing to symptoms in association with injury.

OCCLUSAL HABITS

Many patients express stress release orally. This would include biting objects (such as eyeglasses, pencils, nails), clenching, or bruxism (grinding) during waking or sleeping hours (Fig. 10.16). When occlusal disharmony triggers this response, the prognosis for correction is favorable. If,

LIFE-STYLE HABITS	DENTAL HISTORY
☐ Biting (objects)	☐ Orthodontics
☐ Clenching	☐ Length of treatment___yrs.
☐ Bruxism	☐ Surgery
☐ Head position	☐ Restoration
☐ Hand pressure	☐ Dentures ☐ FU, ☐ FL
☐ Sleeping	☐ Partial Dentures ☐ U, ☐ L
☐ Occupation	☐ Other_____
☐ Singing	TMJ TREATMENT (previously)
☐ Musical Instrument	☐ Treated, ☐ Not treated
☐ Stress	☐ Drugs___ ☐ Occl. adj.
☐ Other_____	☐ Appliances_____
	☐ Results_____
MEDICAL HISTORY	PSYCHOLOGICAL SCREENING
☐ Previous illnesses_____	☐ Previous history_____
☐ Operations_____	☐ Current treatment_____
☐ Drugs_____	☐ Consultation recommended
	☐ Attitude: ☐ good, ☐ poor

Figure 10.16.   A detailed history of the patient's life-style habits, dental history, medical history, and psychological screening completes the patient's verbal interview. (Adapted from Weinberg LA: The etiology, diagnosis, and treatment of TMJ dysfunction-pain syndrome, Parts I–IV. *J Prosthet Dent* 42:654, 1979; 43:58, 1980; 43:186, 1980.)

however, owing to early childhood conditioning the oral habit is deeply ingrained as the main avenue of stress release, occlusal disharmonies play a subordinate role and the prognosis is unfavorable. From a clinical point of view, this is almost impossible to predict, in that long-standing pain can cause behavioral changes associated with neurosis which is a dangerous assumption.

What we are dealing with is a human variable, which is almost impossible to define accurately. Years of experience in dealing with TMJ dysfunction patients make this distinction intuitive rather than scientific. For the general dentist or nondental specialist, the stress evaluation factor would be almost impossible to judge. Occasionally in the specialty practice concerned with TMJ dysfunction pain, a clinical trial with an intraoral appliance can help make this distinction easier, in conjunction with palliative treatment such as moist heat, soft diet, and muscle relaxant drugs. When there is no change whatever in symptoms, the diagnosis of acute TMJ dysfunction pain is in question. In this event, medical, referred pain, psychosomatic causes, or medical-legal factors must be strongly considered.

HEAD POSITION FACTORS

Occupational factors that alter normal head position, such as all-day phone usage with the head tilted to hold the phone against the ear, can produce head and neck pain (Fig. 10.16). Sometimes, patients have habits such as reading while leaning on one hand against the mandible. This can cause many hours of positioning the teeth together rather than the rest position which separates the teeth. In those patients with posterior condylar displacement, joint discomfort can be produced, by the same mechanism as clenching the teeth together or wearing a neck brace for whiplash injury.

Many patients sleep on two pillows, which can cause abnormal head and neck positioning. Patients who have occupations that require long hours of tilted head positions, such as artists, architects, etc., may develop occupationally induced head and neck pain. It is quite common for professional singers who vocalize several hours a day to develop TMJ symptoms from the excessive muscular activity required to open the airway. This usually takes place if there is excessive opening in combination with predisposing factors such as condylar displacement and/or disc derangement or with injury.

It is quite common for violinists to have many special neuromuscular symptoms associated with the head and neck as well as the arm and shoulders. Some musicians use special braces to take the strain off the arm while practicing; the position of the jaw against the instrument, however, can cause serious mandibular deviation and subsequent TMJ dysfunction pain. Similarly, wind instrument players are required to assume special mandibular positions that can cause dysfunction and occupational pain disorders. It is extremely important to elicit this type of information during the history taking, since it may have a direct bearing on symptoms that may be incorrectly attributed to TMJ dysfunction or whiplash injury when, in fact, they may be occupation or life-style habits.

Stress itself or a life crisis can induce muscular pain or behavioral mannerisms (such as clenching) that, in turn, can produce muscle spasm pain. Some dentists (a minority) believe that TMJ dysfunction pain is stress induced without occlusal factors (25). These dentists usually have little experience in the field of restorative dentistry in which it is common to observe that the slightest alteration of the bite can trigger TMJ dysfunction pain. Their limited experience in reconstructing occlusions, in combination with the observation of a minority of patients where stress clenching is the major casual agent, can lead to narrowed opinion on etiology. TMJ dysfunction is usually of multicausal etiology, with stress aggravating the condition and playing a varied role, depending on the individual patient. In summary, stress can vary in its etiological role from none, to contributory, to a singular cause in TMJ dysfunction pain. In the vast majority of patients, stress plays a contributory role.

Dental History_____

It is very appropriate to question a whiplash injury patient who manifests possible TMJ pain to determine whether he or she has had recent dental treatment (Fig. 10.16). The TMJ symptoms could be related to orthodontics, surgery, prosthetics, or other dental treatment that happens to be coincidental to the injury but may play a major underlying role. And, quite obviously, the possibility of a preexisting TMJ condition that may or may not have been treated by a dentist, as well as the nature and results of such treatment, need to be explored further.

Medical History_____

Occasionally, a patient will reveal a medical history of previous illnesses which will suggest hyprochondriacal background, stress-related diseases or dysfunction, neurological symptoms, symptoms of hypoglycemia, and generalized undiagnosed muscle, joint, or chronic pain, all of which may suggest that more than the original trauma (Fig. 10.16) and its effects are happening in this patient. The medications and/or "recreational" drugs the patient uses can also indicate a great deal about the patient physiologically or psychologically that bears directly on diagnosis and prognosis.

Psychological Screening_____

When a patient has long-standing chronic pain from a legitimate dysfunction, such as TMJ pain, the pain itself can cause a superimposed neuralgia (or vice versa), emotional response, and behavioral changes as a *response to the pain* rather than its cause. After several years it is difficult to separate cause and effect, and the patient's emotional response to chronic pain becomes part of the disease itself. Only if one experiences long-standing pain that is considerably higher than the pain threshold can one really understand the *emotional exhaustion* that results. The emotional effect resembles neurosis. The patient's defenses are down, and he or she becomes increasingly defensive as a response to frustration at the patronizing attitude of doctors to, for instance, the typical female patient who bursts into tears when describing her symptoms. Many patients with TMJ dysfunction pain have been told it is due to stress and they have to learn to live with it. Perhaps in some instances a stress is indeed the single cause, or the patient seems to be emotionally disturbed. It is inappropriate, however, to jump to these conclusions without considerable study, before the patient is advised to learn to live with this problem.

These comments may seem editorial in nature, but in the field of TMJ dysfunction pain (craniomandibular pain), controversy is a reality because of multiple causality, medical systemic influences and, most of all, patient variability in resistance and susceptibility to diseases and dysfunction. A given malocclusion, for instance, may produce pain in one patient, while in another it does not. This fact goes against most of the training of those in the dental community for whom cause and effect are prerequisite to diagnosis and treatment. With medical problems, perhaps the opposite is true, since a good portion of the time many factors are operating simultaneously, with some unknown, which is a given in the diagnosis and treatment of the whole patient. It is important for the nondental specialist to be aware of the cross-section of opinion in the dental community in order to evaluate the responses of dental referrals. The controversy within the dental profession is due to lack of knowledge or interest in TMJ problems and the difficulty in handling these patients. There is little organized undergraduate or postgraduate training in this area, which is the underlying root cause, and change is slow. It is, therefore, important for chiropractic and medical specialists to refer patients to qualified specialists* in TMJ dysfunction rather than untrained (albeit otherwise knowledgeable) dentists.

Brief psychological screening questions (Fig. 10.16) will provide the examiner with a quick psychological background of the patient, which might not come to light un-

less the patient is asked this specific information. This type of questioning is very valuable to coincide with the onset of TMJ symptoms or perhaps to indicate why the patient is not responding in the expected way to treatment as a result of whiplash injury. Often, stress can decrease the level of cure or improvement, and if the patient and doctor are aware of this before treatment, a better relationship will be produced. Malpractice litigation often has its roots in the patient's lack of knowledge and *acceptance* of his or her own emotional or physical contribution to the disorder and its cure. The patient's unrealistic expectations and the consequent hostility resulting from failure are transferred to the patient's attempt to *get even* because of these dashed hopes. Volumes can and have been written about the psychological background of this type of patient, but in the main, most patients honestly want to be helped and are reasonable. However, it is the nature of TMJ problems, which fall somewhere between chiropractic, medicine, and dentistry, and the controversial nature of its etiology and treatment that make this particular specialty prone to misunderstanding. Much progress is being made in the scientific investigation of craniomandibular pain, and in a relatively short period of time these pitfalls will be eliminated.

Clinical Examination

The pain history will usually reveal, with great accuracy, that the patient has TMJ involvement or that the pain is not due to the specific characteristics of this clinical entity. The clinical examination will confirm this conclusion and will indicate to the dentist the appropriate methods of treatment. (The greatest variation in this field is in the method of treatment rather than in the diagnosis).

MUSCLE PALPATION

One of the strongest indications for acute TMJ dysfunction is pain on muscle palpation. The results of one study revealed over 50% of patients with acute TMJ dysfunc-

---

*A source of referrals is the American Academy of Craniomandibular Disorders, Secretary, Donald F. Fournier, DDS, 199 East Monterey Way, Phoenix, AZ 85012.

tion had muscle palpation tenderness of the TMJ area itself, the buccinator, the insertion of the temporal muscle on the coronoid process of the mandible, and the lateral pterygoid muscle and approximately 30% had involvement of the remaining muscles of mastication (23). It is, therefore, important to be familiar with the location of these muscles and to chart the location of their tenderness to palpation (Fig. 10.17).

The areas that are tender to palpation should be charted in color for quick visual reference, rather than by the written word which requires volumes to describe and is painstaking and time-consuming to review (24) (Fig. 10.17). The joint area anterior to the ear and the temporal muscle are familiar areas of palpation. So too is the sternocleidomastoid muscle; the internal pterygoid at the angle of the mandible, however, also is a frequent area of complaint. These areas, as well as the masseter, are familiar to most professionals treating whiplash injuries; when palpation is extended intraorally, however, these muscles are not examined as frequently as they should be.

The insertion of the temporal muscles is on the coronoid process of the mandible

(Fig. 10.18) which is best palpated intraorally superior and lateral to the teeth in the retromolar area. The lateral pterygoid can be palpated intraorally as far posterior and superior as possible lateral to the location of the upper wisdom tooth. Most often the patient must move the mandible laterally to provide access to this region. As previously mentioned, these two intraoral areas (insertion of the lateral pterygoid and temporal muscles) as well as the masseter have an incidence of over 50% involvement in acute TMJ dysfunction cases (23). Therefore, it is advisable for the clinician to be familiar with intraoral examination procedures.

It is significant that when the patient complains of temporal pain, for instance, no discomfort is elicited on palpation. Pain referral and a long list of medical causes could be responsible, complicating the diagnosis. How simple it is when the patient complains of muscle pain in a specific area, and upon palpation this area is found to be tender! This information, when correlated with the pain history, can confirm whether there is TMJ dysfunction or no TMJ involvement at all. The diagnosis and the

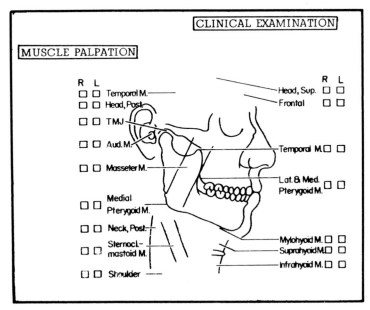

Figure 10.17.   Clinical examination of muscle palpation pain areas will support the pain history and indicate the appropriate methods of treatment. (Adapted from Weinberg LA: The etiology, diagnosis, and treatment of TMJ dysfunction-pain syndrome. Parts I–IV. *J Prosthet Dent* 42:654, 1979; 43:58, 1980; 43:186, 1980.)

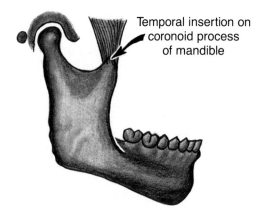

Temporal insertion on coronoid process of mandible

Figure 10.18. Insertion of the temporal muscles is on the coronoid process of the mandible.

JOINT NOISES

It is important to record objective joint noise in order to delineate the type of sound (clicking, popping, crepitus) and its timing (Fig. 10.19*A*). This information will indicate what type of disc derangement is present, how it is associated with condylar po-

treatment of atypical TMJ dysfunction patients are discussed subsequently.

sition, and if dental prosthesis is necessary if traction or a neck brace is contemplated. As discussed previously, a click or a pop is caused by the condyle moving over the posterior or anterior thickening of the disc. This obviously implies that the ligamentous attachment of the disc to the condyle has been stretched or torn. If the joint noise preceded the whiplash injury, in all probability a chronic subclinical TMJ dysfunction was present, and its significance would not be as alarming as if there were no joint noise *before* the trauma. In either case, however, joint noise of any kind would suggest a dental referral and TMJ radiographs to determine whether there is posterior condyle displacement (protective appliance therapy is required if traction or a neck brace is utilized). If joint noise was *not* present before the trauma or if trismus is present, it must be determined whether the lack of opening has been caused by muscle splinting or disc dislocation which would *not* have joint noise on the affected side. In the latter case, no joint noise would occur *and a sudden change in occlusion would present*. In this case, soft tissue imaging (arthrography, CT, or MRI) would be required to confirm the diagnosis.

The timing of the joint noise is signifi-

A. JOINT NOISE ☐ none	B. INTEROCCLUSAL DISTANCE
☐ click, ☐pop, ☐grit; ☐R, ☐L	☐ Freeway space (___ mm.)
☐ preceded pain onset	☐ wide opening (___ mm.)
☐ simultaneous with pain	☐ lat. deviation ☐R, ☐L
☐ after pain onset , ☐unknown	draw_____
OCCURRENCE	
☐ on immediate opening	C. MANDIBULAR POSTURE
☐ on immediate closure	☐ speaking space (mm.)
☐ R, ☐ L, Lateral opening	☐ clenched position
☐ on wide opening	☐ other_____
D. MASTICATION & DEGLUTITION	E. OCCLUSION
☐ mastication, bilateral ☐	☐ C.R.&C.O. identical
☐R, ☐L, Anterior ☐	☐ C.R. deflective slide
☐ deviate swallower	☐ forward(mm.)
☐ anterior open occlusion	☐ V.D.change (mm.)
	☐ Lat.dev.(mm.) ☐R, ☐L
	☐ bal. defl., ☐R, ☐L

Figure 10.19. The clinical examination is completed by recording the joint noise, interocclusal distance, mandibular posture, mastication factors, and occlusal relationships. (Adapted from Weinberg LA: The etiology, diagnosis, and treatment of TMJ dysfunction-pain syndrome. Parts I–IV. *J Prosthet Dent* 42:654, 1979; 43:58, 1980: 43:186, 1980.)

cant. If the clicking is immediate on opening or closing the teeth together, it is almost always associated with posterior condylar displacement. Joint noise on lateral or wide opening can be caused by condylar hypermobility which produces a *wide opening click*. Crepitus (gritting sounds) is associated with a hole in the disc and, unless posterior condylar displacement is present, would not require a protective occlusal splint if traction is necessary.

INTEROCCLUSAL DISTANCE

Normally, the resting position of the mandible with the patient in a upright position would create a small space of about 1–3 mm between the upper and lower teeth. This space is called the freeway space or speaking space (Fig. 10.19*B*). The maximum opening at the time of examination, as measured between the edges of the front teeth, should be between about 35 mm and 40 mm. Either side of this number is significant, in that the lower range of opening represents the possibility of muscle splinting (trismus) or disc dislocation as a result of the trauma. Lateral deviation indicates that the joint on the side of the deviation is involved and that the contralateral joint is not or is involved to a lesser extent.

MANDIBULAR POSTURE

The position of the mandible is a significant factor in acute TMJ dysfunction pain. A normal 2–3 mm of freeway (or speaking space) should be present between upper and lower teeth (Fig. 10.19*C*). In some patients, stress causes the patient to have the teeth constantly in contact in a clenched position. This can be a primary cause of acute TMJ pain, and if present *after* whiplash injury, even if no prior TMJ condition was present, the prognosis for cure is unfavorable. This would be particularly true if condylar displacement (in any direction) was present. One of the problems in joint injury is the intracapsular inflammation that requires protection from pressure on the joint. This is responsible for the fact that some patients avoid placing the teeth together after injury. They usually want to protrude the mandible to create more intra-joint space. This move is counterproductive, however, because it requires continual contraction of the lateral pterygoid muscles to produce the anterior condylar adaptation. Hyperactivity of this muscle, which is usually injured in trauma, can quickly produce spasm pain, making the patient considerably worse. An occlusal onlay prosthesis covering all of the lower teeth is the recommended dental appliance therapy, which protects the joint from pressure and widens the joint space (without requiring lateral pterygoid contraction) by opening the vertical dimension between the two jaws. This is discussed later under "Treatment Procedures."

OCCLUSION

Although the section of the clinical examination concerned with occlusion is intended primarily for the dentist, it is useful to understand what the dentist is looking for in his or her examination of the patient's occlusion and how it might be useful in understanding the dental aspects of whiplash injury. I therefore describe this part of the clinical examination in general (nondental) terms (Fig. 10.19).

Normal Hinge Mandibular Closure

When the normal mandibular hinge closure produces a harmonious intercuspation, the teeth occlude normally without clashing during closure of the mandible. The muscles are usually in their most relaxed balanced state. If there is no condylar displacement or disc derangement, this type of closure would represent the most optimal functional joint relationship between the condyle-disc assembly, the musculature, and the teeth. This optimum four-part system (condyle, disc, musculature, and teeth) is rarely in balance or in the optimum relationship to each other. If this is true, why isn't there more pathology and TMJ complaints without injury? The answer and its implications are vital for this discussion. The TMJ is the most complicated joint in the body because it is a sliding hinge. In addition, the two joints and all the complicated musculature must work together. Nature builds into the system a great deal of tolerance, so that the patient can have pain-free function even though the parts of the system have a derangement in relation to each other and the opposite side.

For example, 40% of the population have some type of joint noise (14), indicating the existence of disc derangement or, to a lesser extent, disc perforation, but only 24% have some form of head and/or face pain, with 12% having pain on opening (14). Pain on opening is pathognomonic of acute TMJ dysfunction, which means that the incidence of acute TMJ dysfunction is somewhere between 12 and 24%. That is an enormous portion of the population to have such a controversial condition that is not effectively taught in undergraduate or postgraduate courses in dental schools. More important statistically, there is a 12–24% chance that a typical whiplash injury patient had an acute TMJ dysfunction *before* the trauma. Second, there is a 40% chance that this patient also had a disc derangement before the trauma. The conclusion can be drawn that the physiological tolerance built into the TMJ and its associated structures masks previously existing subclinical conditions that are superimposed on whiplash injuries. Since a third of the asymptomatic (nonpain) patients have posterior condylar displacement and the concurrent disc derangement (15), it would be appropriate to have a TMJ specialist referral in most whiplash injuries to establish two essential factors. First, is an acute TMJ dysfunction present? Second, is there a chronic posterior condylar displacement that requires a preventive occlusal onlay appliance whenever traction or a neck brace is contemplated? Medicolegally, it would also make sense to rule out TMJ dysfunction before extensive (nondental) cervical treatment is initiated and also to lessen the length of treatment if a TMJ disorder is present.

Deflective Hinge Closure

Most often there is a clashing of the teeth as the jaws close in a muscular balanced hinge-like closure. The jaw slides to accommodate, which is called the habitual occlusion or acquired occlusion. These descriptive terms are significant in describing what is happening. The jaw accommodates itself to the clashing teeth by a proprioceptive feedback mechanism in the periodontal membranes of the teeth that provide a sensory reflex arc to the spinal cord. This establishes a muscle programming that becomes reinforced every time the patient swallows (700 times/day) and the teeth come together in a noninjurious acquired or habitual position. The majority of asymptomatic patients have this discrepancy between the relaxed hinge closure and the maximum occlusion of all the teeth (2). Disc derangement is not necessarily involved, as the mandibular displacement is usually anterior and in the normal direction of movement. Therefore, in normal situations the disc moves along with the condyle without a derangement. It is when the condyle is displaced *posteriorly* that disc derangements occur and the mechanism for pathology is completely different.

In summary, patients tolerate the clashing of teeth that are not in harmony with the joints by a reflex muscular adaptation into a bite that is called the habitual or acquired occlusion. This muscle programming activity can be so overstimulated in stress or joint injury that the neuromuscular system is overwhelmed, causing the patient's resistance to TMJ dysfunction pain to be reduced. The treatment is obvious, to bring about harmony between the three struggling systems—namely, the joints, muscles, and teeth—which would decrease the noxious neuromuscular overstimulation and reduce muscle spasm pain. Psychotherapy and/or muscle relaxants usually do not effectively stop the pain-spasm-pain cycle once it has been established. Palliative as well as causative correction is usually required.

Magnitude of the Occlusal Discrepancy

The dentist records the magnitude of the occlusal discrepancy and its direction three dimensionally. Both factors are of help in evaluating the displacement of the condyles observed in the TMJ radiographs.

Lateral Transcranial TMJ Radiographs

Although for TMJ evaluation the use of lateral transcranial radiography versus other forms of hard structure imaging, such as tomography, is controversial, I prefer lateral transcranial radiography because it is an *in-office technique* that can be easily accomplished with existing dental x-ray equipment and a head positioner (27) and that has been proven to be statistically accurate to within ±0.2 mm (28). (Several types of head positioners are available from different manufacturers.) The dentist is the optimum clinician to ensure the proper occlusal position of the teeth when the radiographs are being taken. Many times during tomography the patient forgets to keep the teeth in the required intercuspal position, which can delay or even mislead the diagnostician. For TMJ evaluation, the condylar position in the fossae while the teeth are in maximum occlusion, not just bone pathology, is essential. With a referral radiographic technique, there is little assurance as to the position of the teeth when the radiographs are taken.

TOMOGRAMS VERSUS LATERAL TRANSCRANIAL RADIOGRAPHS

As long as the teeth are guaranteed to be in the maximum occlusal position, tomograms are of similar value in determining condylar position in the fossae. The lateral transcranial radiograph is a cross-section of the lateral third of the condyle and fossa (27), and most often only the lateral third (the same cross-section) of the tomograms is clear (29). The more medial sections are usually not clear, so that any study of duplicability would not be possible because of the poor resolution. There has been discussion that the condylar position may not be the same through various sagittal sections of the joint. Mongini (30), however, has shown that there is a general agreement between the results of the two techniques. To be fair to the opposing point of view, Mongini points out that when there is superimposition of the condyle on the lateral transcranial radiograph, indicating a rotated condyle, tomograms are indicated. I am in perfect agreement with this conclusion. Some maintain that only corrected tomograms are of value (submental-vertex x-rays are used to determine the exact angle of the condyle to the sagittal plane) in order to ensure that the central x-ray is perpendicular to the axis of the condyle itself (31).

I believe that sometimes the profession can become so involved with parochial opinions (which are usually unproven) on the superiority of one technique over the other that the main issue of what needs to be determined and what modality will satisfy that need, is lost in the heated dialog. I reiterate that I prefer an in-office TMJ radiographic technique (lateral transcranial) because of its high resolution, assured condylar position, and excellence in evaluating bony pathology. Tomograms and/or corrected tomograms are suitable to obtain this information. It is a matter of clinician preference most of the time. If there is a chance of neoplastic change within the joint, tomographic study is indicated.

TMJ Radiographic Findings

The condylar positions and pathological findings should be charted for quick reference (Fig. 10.20). The condyles are concentrically located in the fossae if the anterior and posterior joint spaces are equal (Fig. 10.21). When the anterior joint space is smaller than the posterior joint space, the condyle is displaced anteriorly (Fig. 10.22). Posterior condylar displacement is shown in Figure 10.23 in which the posterior joint space compared with the anterior joint space is reduced. There is no "normal" ideal joint space; therefore, in order to evaluate an individual situation both sides have to be compared. A reduced joint space is illustrated when the joint space in Figure 10.24 is compared with that of the opposite left side (Fig. 10.25). Often a widened joint space can be produced by pathological bone change (Fig. 10.26). Flattening of the condylar head is indicative of the pathological remodeling (Fig. 10.27) usually associated with displacement. Long-standing degenerative osteoarthritis is characterized by a thinning of the joint space, flattening of the condylar head so that bony lipping or a "beak-like" projection is observed anteriorly (Fig. 10.28). Many times, a flattening eminentia can be produced in several pathological situations, such as degenerative osteoarthritis (Fig. 10.28), long-standing anterior condylar displacement, which usually also causes a flattening condylar

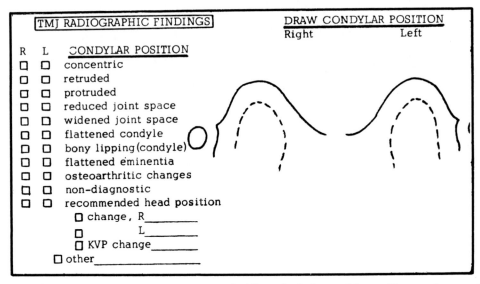

Figure 10.20. TMJ radiographic findings are recorded. These include condylar position, any bone pathology, and possible changes that may be required to improve the diagnostic value of new radiographs. (Adapted from Weinberg LA: The etiology, diagnosis, and treatment of TMJ dysfunction-pain syndrome. Parts I–IV. *J Prosthet Dent* 42:654, 1979; 43:58, 1980; 43:186, 1980.)

head (Fig. 10.29), and acute osteoarthritis (Fig. 10.26). The head of the condyle should have a fine mosaic of bone (Fig. 10.21). Any radiopaque areas are representations of osteoarthritic activity. Different stages of osteoarthritic activity are illustrated in Figures 10.30 and 10.31.

NONDIAGNOSTIC RADIOGRAPH

Most head positioners are created for the average person. In about 10–15% of the time, the cranial bone is superimposed into the image of the TMJ, rendering the radiograph *nondiagnostic*. The central x-ray passes through a "window of bone" created by the petrous portion of the temporal bone, which looks like a radiopaque structure passing at an angle inferior to the image of the condyle and fossa (Fig. 10.32). The anterior superimposition of cranial bone is the posterior clinoid process (Fig. 10.32) of the sphenoid bone which houses the pituitary. It is not appropriate to discuss radiographic correction techniques here, except to say that corrective head positioning can move these common cranial superimpositions away from the image of the joint, thus converting what would be a nondiagnostic radiograph (Fig. 10.32) into a use-

ful one (Fig. 10.33) which can be repeated subsequently if more radiographs are necessary (27). These corrective head position changes, as well as alterations in kilovolt peaks for improved density, are noted on Figure 10.20.

Etiology

Craniomandibular pain can be caused by numerous dental, cervical, stress, and medical factors that can operate in combination. For simplicity, this discussion of the etiology of craniomandibular pain is limited to pertinent dental factors, in order to provide background and the current thinking concerning this area and allow for informed discussion of dental treatment to correct TMJ dysfunction pain.

HISTORICAL BACKGROUND

Costen (32), in 1934, first described what has become known as the TMJ dysfunction pain syndrome. He said the pain was due to posterior condylar displacement caused by a loss of posterior teeth with subsequent impingement on the auriculotemporal nerve. The recommended treatment was to increase the vertical dimension to relieve

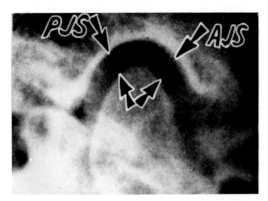

Figure 10.21. The condyles are concentrically located in the fossae if the anterior *(AJS)* and posterior *(PJS)* joint spaces are equal. (Adapted from Weinberg LA: The etiology, diagnosis, and treatment of TMJ dysfunction-pain syndrome. Parts I–IV. *J Prosthet Dent* 42:654, 1979; 43:58, 1980: 43:186, 1980.)

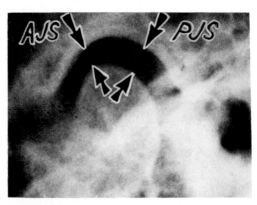

Figure 10.22. When the anterior joint space *(AJS)* is smaller than the posterior joint space *(PJS)*, the condyle is displaced anteriorly. (Adapted from Weinberg LA: The etiology, diagnosis, and treatment of TMJ dysfunction-pain syndrome. Parts I–IV. *J Prosthet Dent* 42:654, 1979; 43:58, 1980: 43:186, 1980.)

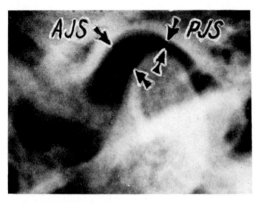

Figure 10.23. Posterior condylar displacement is shown where the posterior joint space *(PJS)* compared with the anterior joint space *(AJS)* is reduced. (Adapted from Weinberg LA: The etiology, diagnosis, and treatment of TMJ dysfunction-pain syndrome. Parts I–IV. *J Prosthet Dent* 42:654, 1979; 43:58, 1980: 43:186, 1980.)

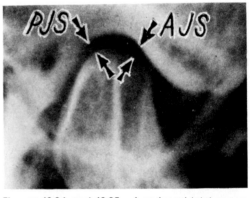

Figures 10.24 and 10.25. A reduced joint space must be compared with that on the opposite side. (Adapted from Weinberg LA: The etiology, diagnosis, and treatment of TMJ dysfunction-pain syndrome. Parts I–IV. *J Prosthet Dent* 42:654, 1979; 43:58, 1980: 43:186, 1980.)

this impingement (33). It should be noted that the empirical use of plastic appliances onlayed over the upper or lower teeth is, by far, the most common form of treatment to this day. The etiology and diagnostic implication was to look for a loss of vertical dimension in the occlusion. Subsequently, Sicher (34), who was an anatomist, pointed out that direct impingement of the auriculotemporal nerve was not anatomically plausible but left open the possibility of soft tissue pressure upon the nerve. The main

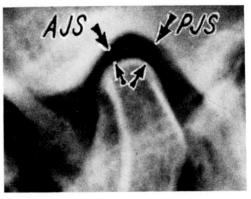

Figure 10.25.

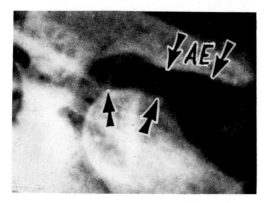

Figure 10.26. A widened joint space can be produced by pathological remodeling due to an acute osteoarthritis which has healed after a year of pathological bone change. (Adapted from Weinberg LA: The etiology, diagnosis, and treatment of TMJ dysfunction-pain syndrome. Parts I–IV. *J Prosthet Dent* 42:654, 1979; 43:58, 1980: 43:186, 1980.)

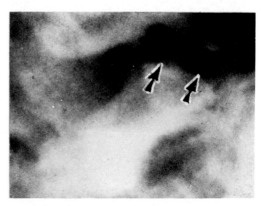

Figure 10.27. Flattening of the condylar head is indicative of pathological remodeling usually associated with displacement. (Adapted from Weinberg LA: The etiology, diagnosis and treatment of TMJ dysfunction-pain syndrome. Parts I–IV. *J Prosthet Dent* 42:654, 1979; 43:58, 1980; 43:186, 1980.)

dental diagnostic and treatment approach, however, has centered on lost vertical dimension and its effect on the *TMJ itself.*

In 1955, Schwartz and Cobin (35) presented the results of their landmark work, which attributed TMJ pain to muscle spasm and not directly to the joint itself. This spawned the concept that emotional stress, rather than occlusion, which mainly affected women, was the actual cause of the

syndrome. The diagnostic procedures were, therefore, directed to finding personality emotional traits common to the majority of patients, who were thought to be women between 20 and 30 years of age. Since TMJ dysfunction pain is multicausal, it is easily subject to well-meaning controversial debate. And on first examination it would seem logical to wonder how, since most TMJ patients were women, could the occlu-

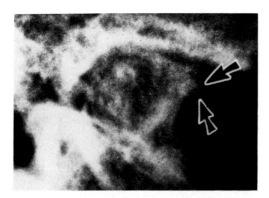

Figure 10.28. Long-standing degenerative osteoarthritis is characterized by a thinning of the joint space and flattening of the condylar head so that bony lipping or a "beak-like" projection is observed anteriorly. (Adapted from Weinberg LA: The etiology, diagnosis, and treatment of TMJ dysfunction-pain syndrome. Parts I–IV. *J Prosthet Dent* 42:654, 1979; 43:58, 1980: 43:186, 1980.)

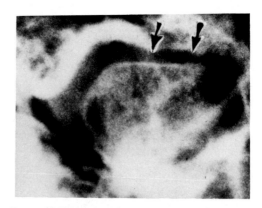

Figure 10.29. A flattened eminentia can be produced by long-standing anterior condylar displacement which usually also causes a flattened condylar head. (Adapted from Weinberg LA: The etiology, diagnosis, and treatment of TMJ dysfunction-pain syndrome. Parts I–IV. *J Prosthet Dent* 42:654, 1979; 43:58, 1980; 43:186, 1980.)

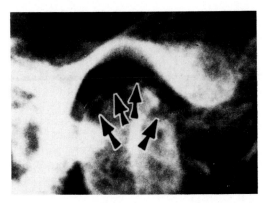

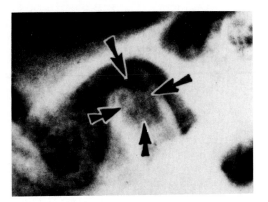

Figures 10.30 and 10.31.   The head of the condyle should have a fine mosaic of bone. Any radiopaque areas represent osteoarthritic activity. (Adapted from Weinberg LA: The etiology, diagnosis, and treatment of TMJ dysfunction-pain syndrome. Parts I–IV. *J Prosthet Dent* 42:654, 1979; 43:58, 1980; 43:186, 1980.)

Figure 10.31.

sion be the cause? First, it has been shown that females are more prone to seek clinical intervention for their symptoms than are males (36). Females are more prevalent in *any* dental practice. Second, evidence that TMJ symptoms are not overwhelmingly found exclusively in the female population has been presented (37),

Finally, Laskin (25) introduced the term myofascial pain dysfunction (MPD), which was an attempt to eliminate "joint" from the name of the disorder. In his article, he described MPD as unilateral in nature and specifically not involving the joint itself. If either of these factors were present, the condition was not to be considered MPD because the joint was only secondarily involved. As discussed previously, over 58% of the 139 patients in one study had pain that was bilateral in nature and the joint itself was involved (23). I consider MPD to be a very early manifestation of TMJ dysfunction which may be treatable by only palliative means. When the symptoms persist beyond 4–6 weeks, particularly without response to pure palliative treatment, the more complicated TMJ dysfunction pain syndrome is involved, and treatment usually requires therapeutic changes in the occlusion.

I have reported that in over 320 patients with acute TMJ dysfunction pain, condylar

displacement had an incidence of 90%, while in the controls it had an incidence of less than 50% (15, 23, 38). Similar findings have been subsequently reported (39, 40), establishing condylar displacement as a factor associated with TMJ symptoms. The Rieder report (40) was a 10-year study on almost 1000 patients that established a direct relationship between condylar displacement and the seriousness of symptoms. Those that oppose condylar displacement as a factor in TMJ symptoms claim that the evidence was gained by the use of lateral transcranial radiographs which they believe are not accurate despite statistically valid data that the radiographs are duplicable to ±0.2 mm (28). Similar clinical research on condylar position with

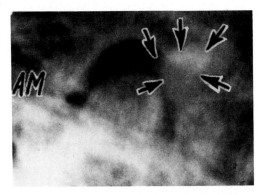

Figure 10.32.   The anterior superimposition of cranial bone on the TMJ radiograph is the posterior clinoid process of the sphenoid bone. (Adapted from Weinberg LA: Technique for temporomandibular joint radiographs. *J Prosthet Dent* 28:284, 1972.)

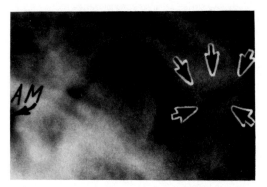

Figure 10.33. Corrective head positioning can move this common cranial superimposition away from the image of the joint, thus converting a non-diagnostic radiograph into a useful one. (Adapted from Weinberg LA: Technique for temporomandibular joint radiographs. *J Prosthet Dent* 28:284, 1972.)

other radiological methods has not been done to justify this position.

At the same time, Farrar (17) has introduced the concept of anterior disc displacement and/or dislocation as an important factor in etiology. (Soft tissue imaging is necessary to confirm the position of the disc (19).) Among those who accept this concept, however, there is debate over the cause of the disc displacement. It is generally agreed that direct trauma can cause disc displacement; in most patients, however, this condition takes place chronically, and there is considerable controversy over whether the anteriorly displaced disc causes posterior condylar displacement or whether posterior condylar displacement produces anterior disc displacement. It has been found that the condyle is displaceable superiorly when nonsupported occlusal force is applied (1, 2), which indicates that the disc does not resist condylar displacement. Anterior disc displacement is *rarely found* without posterior condylar displacement. Therefore, the evidence points to the posterior condylar displacement as a cause of the stretching of the ligamentous attachment to the disc on the medial and lateral pole of the condyle, since there is no space posterior to the central portion of the fossae to accommodate both the condyle and the disc. Therefore, the mechanical force generated by the occlusal disharmony displaces the condyle posteriorly, *causing* anterior disc displacement. Although this

concept may be only theory, its application seriously affects treatment and is, therefore, significant.

In summary, acute TMJ dysfunction pain was originally described as caused by a loss in vertical dimension produced by missing posterior teeth. In the middle 1950's, the concept of muscle spasm pain caused by emotional factors became popular. Additional information produced by improved transcranial radiographic technique and data relating condylar position to symptoms suggested that condylar displacement in *any direction* is an etiological factor. Recently, the focus has been on disc derangement as an important factor in etiology. Diagnosis and treatment would, therefore, depend on the conceptual understanding of the syndrome by the clinician.

WHAT IS A JOINT PATHOLOGY?

Pathological bone changes are observable on most good radiographic images of the TMJ, regardless of the particular technique (Figs. 10.21–10.31). There is relatively little that can be done dentally, however, other than establishing a sound occlusion for such situations. Dental treatment shows promise of being most effective in the area of dysfunction and its associated muscle and joint pain. To establish sound occlusion, the four parts of the functional TMJ system must be brought into harmony: condylar position in the fossae, muscle function, the occlusal-joint relationship, and a healthy condyle-disc assembly.

SIGNIFICANCE OF RESISTANCE AND SUSCEPTIBILITY

In dentistry, the concept of resistance and susceptibility has been overlooked, which has polarized etiological concepts unnecessarily and has led to confusion within and outside of the profession. That TMJ dysfunction pain is multicausal adds to the controversy. It is very easy to blame stress or emotional factors when a given degree of condylar displacement and malocclusion produces acute symptoms in one patient but no subjective symptoms in another. In medicine, resistance and susceptibility are givens in most diseases and disorders. In the human body, stress can cause symptoms in a characteristic target organ that is the weak link in one individual patient, which in another individual will be different. For instance, one patient may develop colitis, while another patient under the same stress may have skin lesions, headaches, blood pressure increases, ulcers, and/or behavioral changes.

Thus, when there is no one cause and effect relationship, such as a bacterium that causes a specific disease, or when the mechanism is unknown, empirical data must be collected over a long period of time (and will remain controversial) until the statistics in favor of one diagnosis over another are overwhelming. For instance, there is little doubt that smoking is an etiological agent in lung cancer, even though there are many patients who smoke who do not have lung cancer, as well as nonsmokers who have lung carcinoma. These cases do not invalidate the data associating the high incidence of lung cancer with smoking, nor do they establish that resistance and susceptibility play a significant role in the outcome of pathology. The incidence of condylar displacement associated with TMJ symptoms is twice as great as condylar displacement without symptoms; therefore, diagnosis and treatment are described on this basis. Stress is included as a secondary (contributing) factor within that context.

Diagnostic Procedures

EVALUATION OF OCCLUSION

Occlusion can cause dysfunction pain in several ways, which are described in "nondental" terms. When the patient closes in a relaxed "center" bite, the teeth may not mesh properly, requiring the patient to reflexly move the jaw forward to an acquired or habitual occlusion. This is not usually harmful within the joints because the forward movement of the condyle in the fossae is within the normal range of movement. In fact, most patients have this arrangement within reasonable limits of 1–2 mm. With a susceptible patient perhaps undergoing stress-caused clenching, the muscles are overactive in order to arrive at this acquired jaw position 700 times/day

during swallowing and during parafunctional clenching and grinding. In these patients, the noxious overstimulation of the neuromuscular system produces muscle spasm pain. Administration of tranquilizers and muscle relaxants usually does not eliminate the once-tolerated malocclusion, and reduction of symptoms requires occlusal adjustment to bring about harmony between the musculature, joints, and articulation of the teeth (3).

Another simple cause of occlusal trauma is the *tripping* of the contacting surfaces as they rub against each other in forward or sideward movements. The roughened or tripping surfaces are very traumatic to the neuromuscular system and trigger reflex rubbing of the traumatic surfaces, one against the other, without the patient's becoming aware of it. Nocturnal clenching or bruxism (rubbing) brought on by stress and/or irritating biting surfaces is a universally accepted cause of TMJ dysfunction pain.

The most damaging malocclusion is one in which the condyle is displaced posteriorly when the teeth mesh in maximum occlusion as is shown in Figure 10.23. This should be considered as a posterior hyperextension of the joint which is not intended physiologically. It causes stretching or tearing of the ligamentous attachment of the disc to the lateral and medial poles of the condyle. When the teeth occlude, the condyle moves posterior to the thickened posterior border of the disc, producing a clicking that occurs on immediate closure and opening.

In summary, the intraoral type of malocclusion is observed and noted on the patient's diagnostic form to be later correlated with the condylar position in the fossae on the TMJ radiographs. This correlation will determine the required definitive occlusal treatment. The three basic types of occlusal disharmony are: (*a*) deflective contacts that occur during relaxed closure, which causes the mandible to be deflected anteriorly, producing anterior condylar displacement; (*b*) roughed or tripping occlusal surfaces that are noxious to the neuromuscular mechanism and that instigate clenching and bruxism; and (*c*) maximum occlusal contact of the teeth, which produces posterior condylar displacement and disc derangement. (Superior condylar displacement can be found in less than 5% of patients with TMJ dysfunction.

ATYPICAL TMJ DYSFUNCTION

Occasionally, a patient with an atypical TMJ involvement may present with symptoms that (*a*) are conflicting and that may indicate that more than one disorder is operating simultaneously or (*b*) are mimicking TMJ dysfunction. In this case, nerve blocks can be used to differentiate referred pain, muscle relaxant drugs can be prescribed, and/or an intraoral appliance that usually decreases TMJ dysfunction pain can be provided. The use of such noninvasive palliative techniques to evaluate their effect can aid in establishing the diagnosis. More than 2 weeks of treatment usually removes the placebo effect, and if not one of the usually effective means produces diminution of symptoms, the presence of TMJ dysfunction pain is in serious doubt. An extensive pain history usually will delineate this type of patient. As a general rule, if the patient has no pain on function, no pattern of occurrence, and no pain from muscle spasm on palpation, a therapeutic noninvasive trial of palliative treatment is indicated. This procedure is thoroughly explained to the patient and should be noted in writing in the patient's records. It should be emphasized that stress alone can produce legitimate pain symptoms, but typical clinical dysfunction signs are present in this instance. Stress patients should not be confused with those who have pain symptoms that are *not* characteristic of TMJ disorders or medical pathology.

Treatment Procedures___

PALLIATIVE SYMPTOMS TREATMENT

The treatment for acute TMJ pain consists of the clinical management of cause and effect. The effects are pain and dysfunction (pain on chewing or movement, pain on opening, limitation of motion). Palliative treatment consists of procedures that are aimed at symptom relief only and should not be considered definitive treat-

ment in themselves. If the symptoms go away and the causes have not been removed, they can return at any time, and the uncorrected causes can make effective treatment at a later date more difficult and the results less effective. The only exception would be if the symptoms are only a few weeks in duration and caused by stress or by a sudden opening exclusive of trauma.

MUSCLE PAIN

If the pain is muscular in origin, several clinical procedures are indicated. Soft diet is suggested to limit functional stress and range of motion. Moist heat is used to increase circulation. Muscle relaxants, such as Valium, are used in very low doses (2 mg) 4 times a day or at the hour of sleep if the patient resists drug therapy. This is particularly indicated if the history reveals a pattern of pain in the morning. The appliances used in this therapy are generally of two types. One covers all the teeth in one arch and is designed to increase the vertical dimension (Fig. 10.34). The other is called a bite plate which fits over the upper anterior teeth only and is designed to *disocclude* the posterior teeth (Fig. 10.35). Research (41) and my own clinical experience of over 30 years has led me to favor the anterior bite plate in patients with TMJ pain of *nontraumatic* etiology. It has been shown that the disocclusion of the poste-

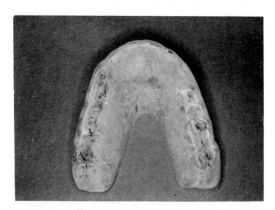

Figure 10.34. An occlusal onlay appliance covers all the teeth in one arch and is designed to increase the vertical dimension. (Adapted from Weinberg LA: Treatment prostheses in TMJ dysfunction-pain syndrome. *J Prosthet Dent* 39: 654, 1978.)

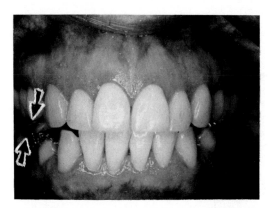

Figure 10.35. A bite plate fits over the upper anterior teeth only and is designed to *disocclude* the posterior teeth. (Adapted from Weinberg LA: Treatment prostheses in TMJ dysfunction-pain syndrome. *J Prosthet Dent* 39: 654, 1978.)

rior teeth decreases the myographic activity of the masseter and temporal muscles (41). This appliance can be constructed with the least amount of vertical dimension increase between the teeth that can be added within the patient's normal "speaking space" so that it will not be in contact when the patient's jaw is in the relaxed position.

TRISMUS (LIMITATION OF OPENING)

Trismus often accompanies traumatic as well as nontraumatic TMJ dysfunction pain. Usually, patients with long-term chronic TMJ dysfunction will give a history of trismus at some time during the course of the disorder but not necessarily at the time of examination. With injury of the direct trauma type, such as whiplash, trismus is a common finding. It is possible to have the disc dislocated anteriorly, which would limit motion on the effected side. Most often, however, the trismus is due to muscle splinting of the injured joint. To break the spasm-pain cycle, a soft diet, moist heat, salicylates, and muscle relaxants are immediately recommended. A bite plate (posterior disoccluding appliance), as previously described (Fig. 10.35), is prescribed for use 24 hours/day, except when the patient is eating. This type of appliance is most effective at trismus reduction and is utilized for 2–3 weeks. In patients with nontraumatic TMJ dysfunction pain, the appliance is worn during sleeping hours

only after the trismus has been reduced. In patients with traumatic TMJ dysfunction pain, the bite plate is preferred in order to break the trismus pattern and should then be followed by long-term use of the occlusal onlay appliance (10.34)

SIGNIFICANCE OF INCREASES IN VERTICAL DIMENSION

The occlusal onlay appliance has been overused as a treatment modality. Paradoxically, increases in vertical dimension between the teeth beyond the normal resting position of the mandible have decreased the myographic activity of the temporal and masseter muscles (42, 43). As a result, the short-term benefit of the appliance is effective. These same researchers, however, caution the long-term use of increases in vertical dimension as a treatment procedure (42, 43). In fact, the same author who originally described the decrease in myographic activity with increases in vertical dimension beyond the resting position of the jaw did long-term experiments on monkeys that showed that in 36 months the original space between the teeth was reestablished by intruding the teeth into the sockets (44). Clinically, this is frequently observed in humans. The patient seen in Figure 10.36 has an appliance in position that increases the vertical space

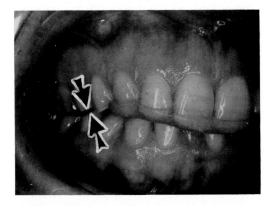

Figure 10.36. A patient is shown with an appliance in position that increases the vertical space between the jaws beyond the normal space. (Adapted from Weinberg LA: Treatment prostheses in TMJ dysfunction-pain syndrome. *J Prosthet Dent* 39:654, 1978.)

between the jaws beyond their normal space. With the appliance out of the mouth (Fig. 10.37), the remaining anterior teeth maintain contact, illustrating the degree of intrusion of the posterior teeth into the sockets.

CONCLUSION ON VERTICAL DIMENSION INCREASES

An increase in vertical dimension decreases symptoms but is dangerous in the long term. It should not be used in nontraumatic cases as a general rule. The reverse is true in patients who have suffered trauma. In these latter patients, *intracapsular edema* resulting from joint injury is treated by salicylates and by *selective increases in vertical dimension* which are used to support the TMJ and reduce direct stress to the joints by increasing the vertical dimension between the jaws by an occlusal onlay appliance. This appliance is usually maintained full time for 6 months (not 3 years). As the symptoms decrease, the vertical level between the jaws is reduced by occlusal grinding of the appliance weekly. In a short period of time this appliance can be maintained in position without violating the normal space between the jaws, thus triggering clenching which intrudes the teeth into the sockets.

CONCLUSIONS

Minimum opening anterior appliances that disocclude the posterior teeth are used to treat TMJ dysfunction pain of nontraumatic origin (Fig. 10.35). In the treatment of TMJ dysfunction pain of traumatic origin, posterior support appliances are used to cover the teeth of one arch and support and separate the joints that have intracapsular edema (Fig. 10.34). These appliances are reduced in vertical dimension (by occlusal grinding weekly) as symptoms decrease, so as not to cause intrusion of the teeth.

Definitive Treatment

Occlusal adjustment is designed to bring about a "centralization" of the condyles in

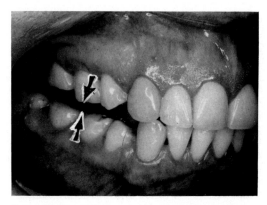

Figure 10.37. With the appliance out of the mouth and the remaining anterior teeth in contact, the degree of intrusion of the posterior teeth into the sockets is apparent. (Adapted from Weinberg LA: Treatment prostheses in TMJ dysfunction-pain syndrome. *J Prosthet Dent* 39:654, 1978.)

the fossae and/or to eliminate the locking effect of a malocclusion that displaces the condyles into a dysfunctional position (displaced from the central position). When the disc is displaced or dislocated anteriorly, special procedures are required which vary from unlocking the occlusion and permitting self-reduction, to mandibular repositioning (utilizing the teeth) to recapture the disc-condyle relationship, to surgery which reattaches the anterior dislocated disc.

CONDYLAR DISPLACEMENT

The condyles can be displaced anteriorly, posteriorly, and superiorly. The closing muscles of the mandible are extremely powerful; therefore, the normal tonus acts as a muscular strap keeping the condyle superiorly against the disc and fossa. This is not a ligamentous attachment, since research with general anesthesia and succinylcholine (muscle relaxant) resulted in the condyles literally dropping out of the fossae 7–8 mm which is 2–3 times the normal joint thickness. When the teeth are together, they dominate the condylar position in the fossae to produce anterior or posterior displacement. If there is a lack of occlusal support on one side, however, the condyle on that side can be displaced superiorly, as was originally described by Gerber (4). The treatment for each is briefly described in nondental terms.

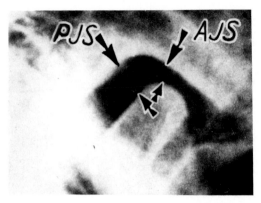

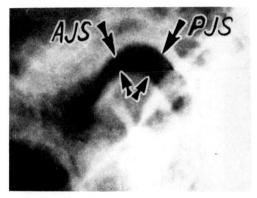

Figures 10.38 and 10.39. The occlusion can deviate the jaw to an acquired position by sliding anteriorly. The posterior joint spaces *(PJS)* are wider than the anterior joint spaces *(AJS)*, illustrating bilateral anterior condylar displacement. (Adapted from Weinberg LA: The etiology, diagnosis, and treatment of TMJ dysfunction-pain syndrome. Parts I–IV. *J Prosthet Dent* 42:654, 1979; 43:58, 1980; 43:186, 1980.)

Figure 10.39.

Anterior Condylar Displacement

Interfering cusps of the teeth prevent the jaw from closing into the relaxed "hinge" or central position. This deviates the jaw to an acquired position by sliding anteriorly with or without a lateral compo-

nent (Figs. 10.38 and 10.39). Various techniques are used to deprogram the musculature from closing into the habitual place in order to find, mark (with articulating paper that leaves a colored mark on the offending surface), and correct the deflection. The deflective cusp is ground down with diamond stones, and the process is repeated over and over until the relaxed hinge or central closure produces simultaneous contact of all the teeth, thus eliminating the deflective contacts and the slide into the habitual bite (3). The condyles are centered in the fossae (Figs. 10.40 and 10.41). This process takes considerable skill and experience, but invariably the patient will say he or she feels more comfortable. The neuromuscular complex receives less noxious stimuli, and the muscle spasm pain decreases and most of the time is eliminated. Often, the deflective contacts trig-

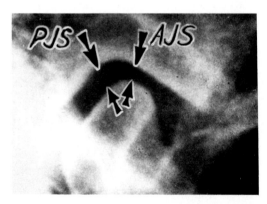

Figures 10.40 and 10.41. The occlusion is corrected by eliminating the deflective contacts and the slide into the habitual bite. The condyles are centered in the fossa (the posterior joint space (PJS) is equal to the anterior joint space (AJS) on both sides). (Adapted from Weinberg LA: The etiology, diagnosis, and treatment of TMJ dysfunction-pain syndrome. Parts I–IV. *J Prosthet Dent* 42:654, 1979; 43:58, 1980; 43:186, 1980.)

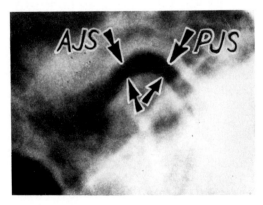

Figure 10.41.

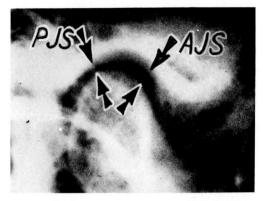

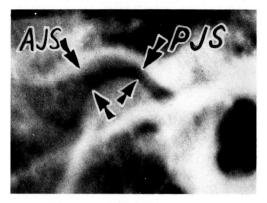

Figures 10.42 and 10.43.   Bilateral posterior condylar displacement is shown, as the posterior joint space (*PJS*) is narrower than the anterior joint space (*AJS*) on both sides. (Adapted from Weinberg LA: The etiology, diagnosis, and treatment of TMJ dysfunction-pain syndrome. Parts I–IV. *J Prosthet Dent* 42:654, 1979; 43:58, 1980; 43:186, 1980.)

Figure 10.43.

ger clenching and hypermuscular activity. The combination of palliative and causative treatment (occlusion) effectively eliminates symptoms.

Posterior Condylar Displacement

Posterior condylar displacement (Figs. 10.42 and 10.43) results in a dysfunctional joint, in that the disc is no longer in the proper relationship with the condyle. The radiograph when used in combination with the findings of joint noise is sufficient evidence for the diagnosis. If there is reciprocal clicking (on immediate opening and closing), the disc derangement is self-reducing. The absence of joint noise when considered in combination with restricted opening on the affected side may indicate anterior disc *dislocation* which may require surgery if conservative treatment is not effective in eliminating symptoms. In this case, soft tissue imaging (arthrography, CT, MRI) is required to confirm the diagnosis. One third of the population have posterior condylar displacement without pain symptoms, which means they are functioning "off the disc" (posterior to the disc when the teeth occlude). There is evidence that the retrodiscal tissue undergoes adaptive changes to accommodate to this new function (BC Moffett, personal communication). The occlusal treatment is designed to

unlock the bite and provide freedom of movement anteriorly so the condyles are not locked into a posterior displacement whenever the teeth occlude (18). Most often this treatment eliminates symptoms, allowing the patient to exist "off the disc" without mandibular repositioning.

Occasionally, a posterior condylar displacement (Figs. 10.42 and 10.43) does not respond to conservative treatment which requires anterior condylar repositioning. The occlusion is adjusted to provide anterior freedom during the conservative aspect of treatment (described previously). The mandible is repositioned anteriorly with the aid of a plastic appliance that covers the occlusal surfaces of the upper posterior teeth, which is constructed on an articulator that is adjusted for the desired anterior correction of the condyles. The patient will wear this appliance 24 hours/day for 3 months before a gold onlay is constructed (on the same model for accuracy) (Fig. 10.44). TMJ radiographs are obtained of the planned anterior condylar repositioning with the temporary plastic appliance which is then confirmed with the final gold onlay in position (Figs. 10.45–10.47). This procedure recaptures the disc and recreates a more functional relationship between the disc and the condylar head, utilizing the occlusion to maintain the corrective position.

Disc Surgery.   Occasionally, a posterior displaced condyle will initiate anterior disc displacement which can later fold on itself anterior to the condyle and become dislocated (Fig. 10.8) (not able to be recap-

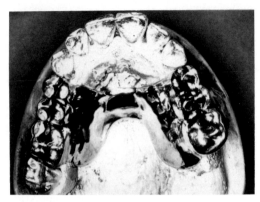

Figure 10.44. A gold onlay is constructed to reposition the condyles anteriorly.

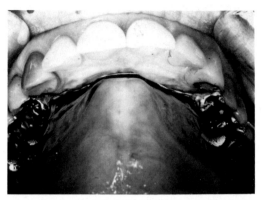

Figure 10.45. Gold onlay in position. (Adapted from Weinberg LA: The etiology, diagnosis, and treatment of TMJ dysfunction-pain syndrome. Parts I–IV. *J Prosthet Dent* 42:654, 1979; 43:58, 1980; 43:186, 1980.)

tured by itself or by manipulation). There is no clicking, but motion is limited on that side so that the mandible on opening is deflected toward the affected side. Conservative treatment for posterior condylar displacement, including condylar repositioning, should be attempted before surgery is contemplated. In this instance, after soft tissue imaging has confirmed the diagnosis, joint surgery can be attempted.

The procedure as developed by Farrar and McCarty (17, 45) consists of returning the folded disc back into the fossa and suturing its posterior portion to the retrodiscal tissue. Usually, a small portion of this tissue is removed and the posterior portion

of the condyle is "shaved" to provide space posterior to the condylar head in the fossa. This procedure is not a cure-all and is usually attempted in only 5% of patients with TMJ dysfunction (45) when all else fails.

Superior Condylar Displacement

In approximately 5% of patients with TMJ dysfunction, one condyle is superiorly displaced due to lack of posterior support on one side (Fig. 10.48), while the other side has normal joint space (4) (Fig. 10.49). Pain develops from pressure on the periphery of the disc. The planned inferior condylar repositioning is accomplished on an articulator, and a plastic onlay is temporarily positioned on the affected side. After a 3-month successful therapeutic trial, the

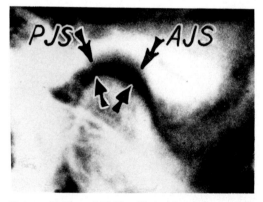

Figures 10.46 and 10.47. Bilateral anterior condylar repositioning is confirmed radiographically when the anterior (*AJS*) and posterior (*PJS*) joint spaces are equal on both sides. (Adapted from Weinberg LA: The etiology, diagnosis, and treatment of TMJ dysfunction-pain syndrome. Parts I–IV. *J Prosthet Dent* 42:654, 1979; 43:58, 1980; 43:186, 1980.)

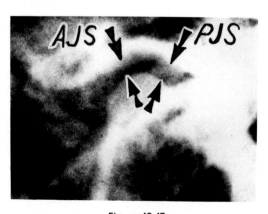

Figure 10.47.

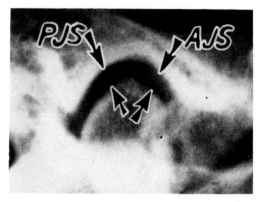

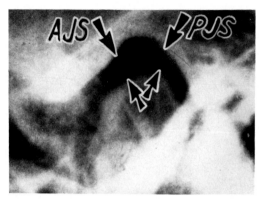

Figures 10.48 and 10.49. One condyle is superiorly displaced on one side (Fig. 10.48), while on the other side (Fig. 10.49) a normal joint space is seen. (Adapted from Weinberg LA: The etiology, diagnosis, and treatment of TMJ dysfunction-pain syndrome. Parts I–IV. *J Prosthet Dent* 42:654, 1979; 43:58, 1980; 43:186, 1980.)

Figure 10.49.

onlay is cast in gold and cemented over the teeth. Figures 10.50 and 10.51 are before and after radiographs, respectively, of the successful treatment of superior condylar displacement. Postoperative TMJ radiographs (Figs. 10.52 and 10.53) confirm inferior condylar repositioning (5). After a year of symptom-free function, the gold onlay can be replaced with individual porcelain crowns; every other tooth is completed and cemented before the alternate crowns are begun, however, in order to guarantee that the therapeutic position is maintained.

HIGH-STRESS PATIENTS

Sometimes (10%), patients with acute TMJ dysfunction have no condylar displacement and/or malocclusion. Most often these patients are suspected of having a high stress level that either directly (through physiology) or indirectly (behavioral clenching) causes TMJ dysfunction pain. The data base on condylar displacement indicates a 90% incidence of TMJ dysfunction. Therefore, when TMJ dysfunction exists without condylar displacement, stress is most often the cause, and the prognosis is guarded. Stress clenching most often is the main etiological agent. Intraoral appliances of any design usually result in *more* clenching and worsening of symptoms. Ju-

dicious occlusal adjustment to eliminate pressure areas, tripping, or trauma in nonfunctional movements can be of help. Tranquilizers and psychotherapy are most effective in these patients, since the etiology is stress related rather than occlusal in nature. Adjunctive therapy, such as chiropractic, physiotherapy, biofeedback, and close attention to diet and allergy, also is of benefit. Whiplash injury with this type of patient is very difficult to treat.

Whiplash Injury-TMJ Patient

The whiplash-TMJ patient requires a team effort because of the nature of the scope of the injury and the special de-

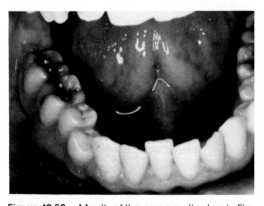

Figure 10.50. Mouth of the same patient as in Figure 10.48 before treatment. (Adapted from Weinberg LA: The etiology, diagnosis, and treatment of TMJ dysfunction-pain syndrome. Parts I–IV. *J Prosthet Dent* 42:654, 1979; 43:58, 1980; 43:186, 1980.)

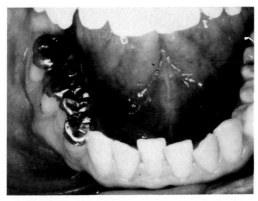

Figure 10.51. The final restoration in the mouth of the same patient shown in Figures 10.48 and 10.50 is in position. (Adapted from Weinberg LA: The etiology, diagnosis, and treatment of TMJ dysfunction-pain syndrome. Parts I–IV. *J Prosthet Dent* 42:654, 1979; 43:58, 1980; 43:186, 1980.)

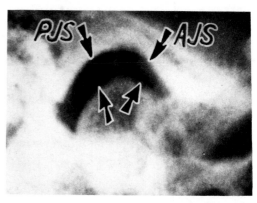

Figure 10.52. Postoperative TMJ radiograph confirms inferior condylar repositioning by the widening of the anterior (*AJS*) and posterior (*PJS*) joint spaces. Compare with the radiograph taken before operation (Fig. 10.48) of the same joint.

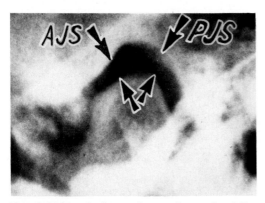

Figure 10.53. Postoperative radiograph of the opposite side in the same patient shown in Figure 10.48.

mands of the TMJ area that require some alteration of the jaw relationship to protect the joints to permit healing as well as during traction or neck brace utilization. Even if no apparent TMJ injury has been sustained and confirmed by a dental consultation, TMJ radiographs are absolutely essential to determine whether posterior condylar displacement exists. In this case, the minimum treatment is the construction of an overlay appliance (1 mm thick at the first molar) if traction or a neck brace is used. Although the onlay appliance is preventive in nature when no acute TMJ dysfunction pain is present, it would be an unnecessary risk to precipitate a complicating TMJ prob-

lem iatrogenically. It should be remembered that fully one third of the asymptomatic population has one or both condyles displaced posteriorly. It would, therefore, follow that 1 of 3 patients should have protective occlusal appliances when traction or a neck brace is utilized.

Trismus or TMJ dysfunction pain should be treated in conjunction with chiropractic, physiotherapy, and medical care because of the interrelationship of the musculature of the cervical and TMJ area. It would not be effective to attempt to treat one area without the other as well. Any postural change in the cervical area would have a direct relationship on the postural position of the mandible, while changes in muscle tone could have an adverse effect on the occlusion. Joint injury, however, should be treated with an occlusal onlay plastic appliance for up to 6 months until the patient is symptom-free, before definitive occlusal adjustment, when required, is attempted. The intracapsular inflammation and the muscle spasm pain that accompanies it prevent normal mandibular movements that preclude definitive occlusal treatment. The purpose of the onlay appliance is to protect the joints and to reduce symptoms rather than to cause mandibular repositioning. The occlusal level of the appliance is reduced by weekly grinding until holes are produced and the appliance can be discarded.

If trismus is present, a bite plate that provides posterior disocclusion to break the spasm should be constructed. A second onlay appliance is constructed right away if traction or a neck brace is used. It is important to emphasize that if either of these cervical therapeutic modalities are used *with a bite plate in position*, it will have a deleterious effect on the joints because of the posterior opening. This should be made perfectly clear to the patient.

Conclusion

The normal anatomy and biomechanics and the abnormal anatomy of the TMJ and its effect on function are discussed. This information is provided so that the relationship of the condyle, disc, muscles, and teeth to each other can be better visualized so that the effect of whiplash injury on normal and previously dysfunctional joints can be better understood. During whiplash trauma, the main TMJ injury is to the anterior portion of the joint while the head moves rapidly backward. The general signs and symptoms of TMJ dysfunction are indicated. General examination procedures are reviewed, as well as suggested factors that can help determine whether TMJ injury has also occurred. These factors are concerned with information on ear symptoms, trismus, life-style habits, dental and medical history, and psychological screening that is associated with TMJ disorders.

The clinical examination of the patient includes muscle palpation, joint noise, and occlusion. The TMJ radiographic findings are reviewed, as well as the relationship of the whiplash injury to previously existing dysfunction. The historical background and review of the conceptual development of the diagnosis and treatment of TMJ disorders are discussed in relation to current controversies in order to better acquaint the nondental specialist with the current state of the art. This should improve interdisciplinary communication. General treatment procedures for TMJ dysfunction are discussed, starting with palliative remedies and including a brief outline of definitive occlusal treatment. These include occlusal adjustment and the desired objectives of each procedure. Stress, its relation to TMJ disorders, and its effect on whiplash injury patients are also explored. Specific recommendations are made for the patient with acute and chronic TMJ dysfunction to prevent iatrogenic injury during traction or cervical collar therapy.

References

1. Weinberg LA: A radiographic investigation into temporomandibular joint function. *J Prosthet Dent* 33:672, 1975.
2. Lundeen HC: Centric relation records: the effect of muscle action. *J Prosthet Dent* 31:244, 1974.
3. Weinberg LA: Anterior condylar displacement: its diagnosis and treatment. *J Prosthet Dent* 34:195, 1975.
4. Gerber V: Kiefergelenk und Zahnolljusion. *Dtsch Zahnaerztl* 26:119, 1971.
5. Weinberg LA: Superior condylar displacement, its diagnosis and treatment. *J Prosthet Dent* 34:59, 1975.
6. Grasso J, Sharry J: The duplicability of arrow-point tracing in dentulous subjects. *J Prosthet Dent* 20:106, 1968.
7. Kabcenell JL: Effect of clinical procedures on mandibular position. *J Prosthet Dent* 14:266, 1964.
8. Kantor M, Silverman S, Garfinkel L: Centric relation recording techniques: a comparative investigation. *J Prosthet Dent* 28:593, 1972.
9. Strohaver RA: A comparison of articulator mountings made with centric relation and myocentric position records. *J Prosthet Dent* 28:379, 1972.
10. McMillen L: Border movements of the human mandible. *J Prosthet Dent* 27:524, 1972.
11. Boucher LJ, Jacoby J: Posterior border movements of the human mandible.*J Prosthet Dent* 11:836, 1961.
12. Posselt U: Studies in the mobility of the human mandible. *Acta Odontol Scand* 10 (Suppl 10):3, 1952.
13. Mahan PE, Wilkinson TM, Gibbs CH, Mauderli A, Brannon LS: Superior and inferior bellies of the lateral pterygoid muscle TMJ activity at basic jaw position. *J Prosthet Dent* 50:710, 1983.
14. Agerberg G, Carlsson GE, Hasseler O: Vascularization of the temporomandibular disk, a microangiographic study of human autopsy material. *Sartyrk Odontol Tidskr* 77:5, 1969.
15. Weinberg LA: The role of condylar position in TMJ dysfunction pain syndrome. *J Prosthet Dent* 41:636, 1979.
16. Mikhail M, Rosen H: The validity of temporomandibular joint radiographs using the head positioner. *J Prosthet Dent* 42:441, 1979.
17. Farrar W: Differentiation of temporomandibular joint dysfunction to simplify treatment. *J Prosthet Dent* 28:629, 1972.
18. Weinberg LA: Posterior bilateral condylar displacement: its diagnosis and treatment. *J Prosthet Dent* 36:426, 1976.
19. Wilkes CH: Structural and functional alterations of the temporomandibular joint. *Northwest Dent* 57:287, 1978.
20. Moffett BC, Johnson LC, McCabe JB, Askew HC: Articular remodeling in the adult human temporomandibular joint. *Am J Anat* 115:119, 1964.
21. Thilander B: Innervation of the temporomandibular joint capsule in man. *Trans R Sch Stockh Umea* 7:1–69, 1961.
22. Hilton J: In Jacobson WHA (ed): *Rest and Pain*, ed 2. New York, William Wood & Co, 1879, p 96.
23. Weinberg LA, Lager L: Clinical report on the etiology and diagnosis of TMJ dysfunction-pain syndrome. *J Prosthet Dent* 44:642, 1980.
24. Weinberg LA: The etiology, diagnosis, and treatment of TMJ dysfunction-pain syndrome. Part II: Differential diagnosis. *J Prosthet Dent* 43:186, 1980.
25. Laskin DM: Etiology of the pain dysfunction syndrome. *J Am Dent Assoc* 79:147, 1969.

26. Christensen V: Facial pain and internal pressure of masseter muscle in experimental bruxism in man. *Arch Oral Biol* 16:1021, 1971.

27. Weinberg LA: Technique for temporomandibular joint radiographs. *J Prosthet Dent* 28:284, 1972.

28. Weinberg LA: An evaluation of duplicability of temporomandibular joint radiographs. *J Prosthet Dent* 24:512, 1970.

29. Weinberg LA: Practical evaluation of the lateral temporomandibular joint radiograph. *J Prosthet Dent* 51:676, 1984.

30. Mongini F: The importance of radiography in the diagnosis of TMJ dysfunctions. *J Prosthet Dent* 45:186, 1981.

31. Omnell KA, Lysell L: In Krogh-Poulsen W, Carlsen O (eds): *Rontgendiagnostik in Bidfunktion Bettfysiologo II.* Copenhagen, Munksgaard, 1974.

32. Costen JP: Syndrome of ear and sinus symptoms dependent upon disturbed function of the temporomandibular joint. *Ann Otolaryngol* 43:55, 1934.

33. Block LS: Diagnosis and treatment of disturbances of the temporomandibular joint, especially in relation to vertical dimension. *J Am Dent Assoc* 34:253, 1947.

34. Sicher H: Structural and functional basis for disorders of the temporomandibular articulation. *J Oral Surg* 13:275, 1955.

35. Schwartz L, Cobin HP: Symptoms associated with temporomandibular joint. *Oral Surg* 10:339, 1957.

36. Bakal D: Headache: a biopsychological perspective. *Psychol Bull* 82:369, 1957.

37. Helkimo M, Carlsson B, Hedegard B, Helkimo E, Lewin T: Function and dysfunction of the masticatory system in Lapps in Northern Finland. *Sven Tandlak Tidskr* 65:95, 1972.

38. Weinberg LA: Temporomandibular joint function and its effect on centric relation. *J Prosthet Dent* 30:176, 1973.

39. Pullinger AG: Tomographic analysis of mandibular condyle position in diagnostic subgroups of temporomandibular disorders. *J Pediatr Dent* 55:723, 1986.

40. Rieder CE: The interrelationship of various temporomandibular joint examination data in an initial survey population. *J Prosthet Dent* 35:299, 1976.

41. Hannam AG: Recent advances in the study of muscle activity in mandibular function and dysfunction. Paper given at American Academy of Craniomandibular Disorders, May 20, 1981.

42. Ramfjord SP, Ash MM: *Occlusion.* Philadelphia, WB Saunders, 1966.

43. Kovaleski WC, DeBoever J: Influence of occlusal splints on jaw position and musculature in patients with temporomandibular joint dysfunction. *J Prosthet Dent* 33:321, 1975.

44. Ramfjord S, Blankenship J: Increased occlusal vertical dimension in adult monkeys. *J Prosthet Dent* 45:74, 1981.

45. McCarty WL, Farrar WB: Surgery for internal derangements of the temporomandibular joint. *J Prosthet Dent* 42:191, 1979.

11

Prognosis in Cervical Acceleration/ Deceleration Injuries

STEPHEN M. FOREMAN, DC, DABCO

Along with the industrial revolution and the subsequent production of the automobile in quantity have come hundreds of thousands of new opportunities for the occurrence of spinal injury. By the 1940's the automobile had become an intricate part of life in the United States, and the victims of acceleration/deceleration injuries began presenting themselves for treatment.

Physicians quickly discovered the typical complex symptomatic picture, consisting usually of cervical stiffness, headache, and a lack of objective evidence. The patient's condition was quickly attributed to "psychological overlay" because of the symptomatic picture of unexplained pain, anxiety, and emotional lability (1).

Such early observers as Gay and Abbott (2) noted a variety of conditions that arose from the "trivial accident." Among the conditions noted were, in varying degrees, cervical radiculitis, cerebral concussion, protruded intervertebral discs, psychoneurotic reactions, and low back pain.

In some of the early studies, investigators attempted to evaluate the affect of successful litigation on the patient's recovery. In 1956, Gotten (3) reviewed the cases of 100 patients and came to the conclusion that "the injury was being used as a convenient lever for personal gain." This opinion was endorsed for a number of years and allowed physicians to dismiss as malingerers and frauds those patients who suffered chronic pain.

Continued observations found that some patients healed and recovered as expected, while others did not. The contention that the majority of the symptoms were either consciously or subconsciously related to monetary gain became suspect. One such observer studied the situation and found it "difficult to understand why patients became neurotic only if their head is thrown backward" (4). (The point is well taken.) In a later study (5), this same investigator found that 45% of his 266 patients continued to have pain after settlement of their lawsuit.

Within several years the consensus was that the desire for monetary gain played a small role in the patient's symptomatic picture. This opinion was small comfort, however. Physicians still understood little, and theories began to be presented in an attempt to explain the residual symptoms. Nerve root compression, muscular injury, and pain arising from ligamentous damage were obvious areas of consideration. Some reserchers believed that spinal cord injury caused by traction, ischemia, or compression was responsible for the clinical picture.

Pathological confirmation from postmortem specimens was not easily obtained because the majority of the injuries were not fatal. Researchers, therefore, turned to animal models to re-create the injury in the laboratory.

Experimental Studies

Experimental duplication of acceleration/deceleration injuries was designed to demonstrate not only the soft tissue response to trauma but also the biomechanics of the injury. Severy et al. (6) were among the first to use anthropomorphic dummies and movie cameras to document the biomechanical changes that occurred during impact. With an accelerometer they calculated the force of impact of five consecutive rear-end collisions. Results of their study revealed that the driver's head, owing to the lack of intimate contact with the seat, accelerates at a greater speed than that of his or her vehicle. In one experiment, for example, the head of the dummy accelerated to a force as high as 11.4 G. This acceleration rate, when applied to the human head, results in loads in excess of 100 lb affecting the cervical structrues. The star-

tling fact to come from this study is that these forces on the cervical spine were produced in automobiles that were traveling only 15 miles/hour! These initial studies proved that low-speed accidents are capable of producing substantial damage.

Studies involving primates, completed in the 1950's by Macnab (5) and by Wickstrom et al. (7), were designed to demonstrate the range of injuries possible following whiplash. Macnab's study exposed primates to hyperextension forces that caused various injuries of the sternocleidomastoid and longus colli muscles. Also noted were damage to the anterior longitudinal ligament, avulsion of the disc, and disruption of the cervical sympathetic chain.

In the study by Wickstrom et al., a wide variety of soft tissue injuries and a small number of skeletal lesions were demonstrated. Of particular interest was the frequent damage to the apophyseal joint that was unapparent on x-ray (7). Other factors that have a direct influence on the degree of injury sustained by the patient have been identified and are discussed in detail below.

Nonpathological Factors Influencing Injury

Injuries resulting from vehicular trauma can differ, at least in one respect, in that variations in the physical condition and anatomy of the patient can alter the course of recovery. Two nonpathological factors that influence the injury resulting from this type of trauma are age and spinal canal size.

AGE

The effects of age can influence the degree of injury sustained by a patient. Younger patients, ages 0–16 years, are susceptible to cord damage but will usually suffer very few fractures. The elasticity of the paraspinal ligaments allows some degree of extra flexibility that appears to help them avoid spinal fractures.

In patients over 60 years of age, such age-related changes as osteoporosis may make them more vulnerable to fractures. Brain et al. (8) were among the first to recognize the significance of age-related degenative changes in the discs and posterior facets. Hyperextension injuries in the patient suffering from spondylitic changes may cause an acute central cord syndrome.

CANAL SIZE

The size of the spinal canal has been studied in relation to cervical myelopathy (9, 10) and disc herniations (11–13) and has been found to be an important factor in both of these processes (14). Patients with a narrow spinal canal are at a far greater risk of suffering a complete neurological deficit than are those with a "large" spinal canal.

Canal size has been classified both anatomically and radiographically in various ways. Verbiest (15) studied spinal canal size and devised the classification of relative and absolute spinal stenosis. "Absolute spinal stenosis" refers to canals that have a midsagittal diameter of 10 mm or less. Absolute stenosis is so named because the bony canal is placing direct pressure on the spinal cord. There is no excess room, and the most trivial injury may cause enough cord swelling to result in either a partial or a complete neurological deficit. "Relative stenosis" refers to spinal canals with a midsagittal diameter of 13 mm. In the presence of relative stenosis, hyperextension injuries are able to produce sufficient spinal cord swelling to cause a neurological deficit.

The spinal cord is vulnerable to injury in the absence of a relative or an absolute stenosis as just defined. Eismont et al. (14) conducted a retrospective analysis of 98 patients and found that every patient with a canal size of 16 mm or less suffered from a complete neurological deficit after his or her vehicular accident. Patients with a spinal canal size of 19 mm at the same C4-C5 level did not suffer a neurological deficit.

Narrowing of the spinal canal can be caused by various lesions including hypertrophic posterior facets (Fig. 11.1), ossification of the posterior longitudinal ligament (Fig. 11.2A and B), pseudospondylolisthesis (Fig. 11.3), and congenital malformation. One nonosseous cause of the spinal canal narrowing results from the infolding of the yellow ligaments on the posterior aspect of the spinal canal. The overlapping

of the articular facets on hyperextension is responsible for this phenomenon (16). Patients who develop a hyperlordosis may experience pressure on the spinal cord on an ongoing basis.

Cervical Vertebral Pathology

Each patient who presents for examination has structrual variations, degenerative changes, or inflammatory processes that may affect both healing ability and the damage sustained during the accident. These underlying conditions are of obvious importance, especially since they may influence the patient's prognosis, and their possible effect on the patient's injury must be assessed.

ARTHRITIC PROCESSES

Inflammatory and noninflammatory (degenerative) processes can alter the structrual integrity of the cervical spine. Some inflammatory processes may damage the ligaments and erode portions of the vertebrae. Noninflammatory processes tend to change the architecture of the joints and cause distortion; they can affect both the biomechanics and the neurological function of the area. Among the noninflammatory processes that may affect the prognosis are osteoarthritis, degenertion of the joints of Luschka, and disc degeneration.

Noninflammatory (Degenerative) Processes

Osteoarthritis. Osteoarthritis, a noninflammatory condition affecting the synovial joints, is the most common degenerative process that affects the cervical spine (17). The enlarged facets may cause cervical radiculopathy and pain. Pain due to cervical radiculopathy is more frequent than arm and shoulder pain caused by neuritis, tumors, thoracic outlet syndrome, and all other causes combined, with the exception of referred pain due to myocardial infarction (18).

The posterior facets are small synovial joints that often undergo degeneration similar to the type seen in the distal inter-

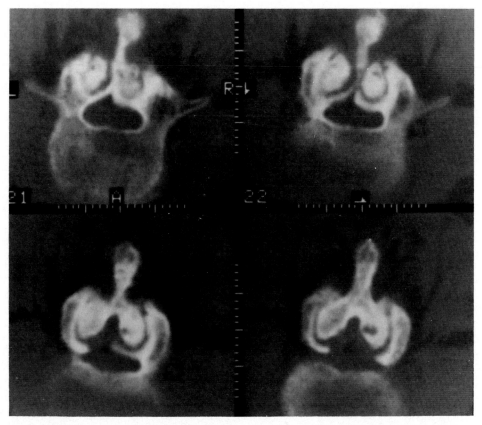

Figure 11.1.   Axial computed tomography views demonstrate the changes of degeneration in the posterior facets. Joint narrowing and spur formation are typical findings.

phalangeal joints of the hands. The degeneration causes changes such as joint space narrowing, hypertrophic spur formation, subchondral sclerosis, and joint irregularity.

Degenerative and hypertrophic changes may result in encroachment either upon the spinal canal or into the intervertebral foramen. Encroachment upon the spinal canal may narrow the canal as described previously. Encroachment into the intervertebral foramen may cause a compromise of the cervical root.

The question of clinical application arises when the articular facets are discussed. In legal cases, the physician may be required to give his or her opinion as to the probability of future degenerative changes in a patient. La Rocca (1) noted that anatomical studies revealed sprains of the zygapophyseal joints and a loss of normal juxtaposition of the articular surfaces. A better indicator of long-term posttraumatic changes

was noted by Hohl (19). In his retrospective study of 146 cervical trauma patients over a 7-year period, he found that no patient in the study had demonstrated preexisting degenerative changes on initial radiographic examination but that 39% later experienced degenerative changes. This is in contrast to the 6% in an aged-matched control group who did not experience cervical trauma (20).

Among the 39% of patients in Hohl's study who had experienced a "normal" whiplash injury without fracture or dislocation, a significant subgroup was noted. Degenerative changes were found at the time of final evaluation in more than 60% of the individuals who (a) were knocked unconscious, (b) had vertebral fixation on flexion extension films, or (c) wore a cervical support for more than 12 weeks for symptom relief.

These degenerative changes were found

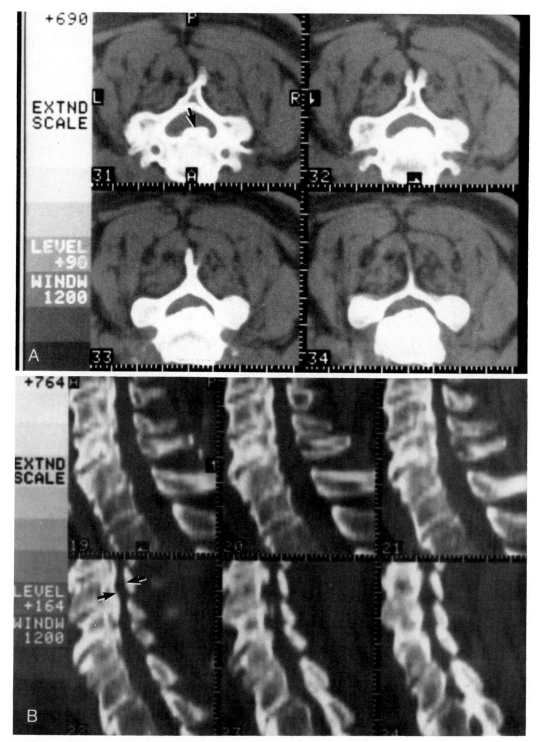

Figure 11.2   A. Axial computed tomography views of the cervical spine demonstrate ossification of the posterior longitudinal ligament (*arrow*). **B.** Sagittal views of the cervical spine show extreme narrowing of the neural canal (*arrows*).

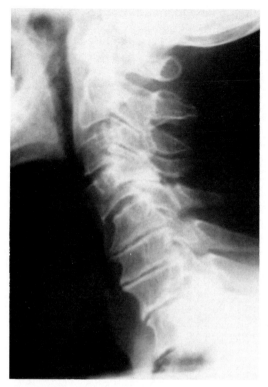

Figure 11.3 Lateral cervical spine view demonstrates degenerative changes at levels C5-T1. The resultant hypermobility at C4-C5 has caused a "degenerative spondylolisthesis."

in patients who had been normal at the time of the accident. Patients who had had preexisting degenerative changes had a poor prognosis. Norris and Watt (21) found that every patient in their study who suffered neurological loss had abnormal x-rays on initial evaluation. Forty percent of these patients had preexisting degenerative joint disease. According to the investigators, "the presence of preexisting degenerative changes, no matter how slight, appears to alter the prognosis adversely."

Degeneration of Joints of Luschka. The uncovertebral joints or the joints of Luschka are located on the posterolateral border of the vertebral bodies and, in contradistinction to the true joints, are part of the intervertebral articulation (Fig. 11.4). These joints are, as are the other articulations, prone to degenerative changes but only as part of a generalized rather than a specific process. The generalized process of joint

space narrowing, deformity, and spur formation is typically seen in the lower cervical spine.

Hypertrophic bone formation from the joints of Luschka can extend within the intervertebral foramen. The subsequent narrowing of the foramen may result in radicular symptoms because of a combination of nerve root pressure and subsequent nerve root ischemia (22). These hypertrophic changes may also intrude into the foramina transversaria and cause vertebral artery compression (23).

The clinical picture is often one of hypertrophic spurs coming from both the joints of Luschka and the posterior articular joints. This combination typically causes cervicoradiculopathy, as the intervertebral foramen, usually only 5–6 mm wide, is unable to protect the cervical nerve root when encroachment occurs.

Disc Degeneration. Disc degeneration, more accurately termed intervertebral osteochondrosis, is the third corner of the noninflammatory degenerative triad. The aging process results in dehydration of the disc, particularly the nucleus pulposus. The dehydration produces linear clefts within the discs, which can become filled with nitrogen. The nitrogen-filled clefts are visible on lateral radiographs; this process is termed the vacuum phenomenon.

The degenerative disc is a common en-

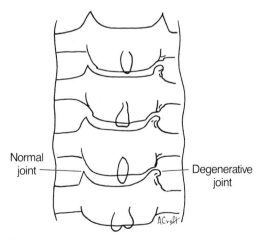

Figure 11.4. Line drawing of an anteroposterior lower cervical view depicts a normal joint of Luschka on the left and degenerative changes to the joint on the right.

tity, usually affecting men in the older age groups. The lower cervical spine is typically affected first. The diminishment in disc height is the primary consequence of degeneration. But how does this change affect the patient who has sustained a whiplash injury?

First, there is the obvious problem of disc degeneration as it relates to spinal biomechanics. Normal function of the vertebral motor unit is predicated upon the proper function of the posterior facets. A disc that is diminished in height causes dysfunction of the posterior facets. The normal elasticity of the intervertebral disc is lost, and this adds to the restriction of intersegmental movement. The added stress on the posterior facets causes typical degenerative changes, which may cause asymmetry of the intersegmental movement.

The end result of this process is a near-total loss of normal biomechanical function at the affected level. This joint fixation is a serious biomechanical lesion because the levels directly above and below have an increased susceptibility to disc herniations and spur formation (22, 24, 25) from the increased work loads imposed on them by the lack of motion of the degenerated disc. Hohl (19) recognized the importance of these preexisting fixated segments. He found that 63% of the patients who had undergone flexion and extension radiographs and had restricted motion at one intervertebral level demonstrated an increased incidence in future degenerative changes.

Disc degeneration may also cause a second significant problem both during and after the accident. Spur or osteophyte bar formation on the posterior-inferior border of the vertebral bodies may cause localized or general stenosis of the canal. The posterior osteophytes may damage the spinal cord during hyperextension.

Continued spur formation may cause a posterior bar that can cause compression of the anterior spinal artery. The compression has various effects on the spinal cord, including a lack of oxygen to the cord, stasis of intraneural blood flow (26) and, in chronic cases, necrosis of the cord.

Another change to consider is the ana-tomical alteration of the intervertebral foramen after disc degeneration. The height of the disc allows a separation of the superior and inferior articular facets that comprise the majority of the bony canal. When the disc material undergoes degeneration, the available space within the intervertebral foramen decreases (Fig. 11.5*A* and *B*).

Inflammatory Processes

Severe inflammatory processes such as ankylosing spondylitis may complicate the apparently moderate injury. If the ankylosing spondylitis has progressed to the cervical spine, several significant changes may allow fractures, dislocations, or neurological injury.

The process of ankylosing spondylitis may cause total fusion of the cervical spine.

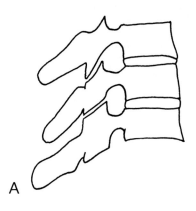

A

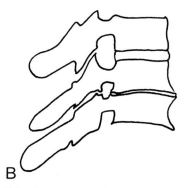

B

Figure 11.5 **A.** Line drawing depicts the role the intervertebral disc plays in intervertebral foramen size. **B.** Line drawing demonstrates reduction in the size of the intervertebral foramen after intervertebral disc degeneration.

The fusion allows a rapid onset of disuse osteoporosis, much like that which occurs in an area immobilized by casting. The osteoporosis makes the spine far more susceptible to fractures (27).

The second effect from ankylosing spondylitis is the muscle atrophy associated with vertebral immobilization. The muscles also suffer from disuse because they are rarely used to move the cervical area. The natural protective ability of the cervical musculature seems to be diminished as a result of the disease.

Rheumatoid arthritis is another inflammatory process that commonly affects the osseous and ligamentous structures of the cervical spine. The cervical area is commonly affected by rheumatoid arthritis (28),

as are the metacarpophalangeal joints (28–30). In the study by Bland et al. (28), 86% of the patients with classic rheumatoid arthritis had cervical involvement.

The rheumatoid complex has an affinity for the upper cervical area. The involvement in this area weakens the ligamentous structures, and because 85% of the motion in the cervical spine occurs in the upper cervical area, dislocation is likely to occur (31).

The damage caused by rheumatoid arthritis may include odontoid erosion (32, 33) and atlas subluxation, as is revealed by an increase in the atlantodental interval (Fig. 11.6). The atlas subluxation varies in onset, from as early as 2 weeks to as late as 13 years (34). Due to the propensity for

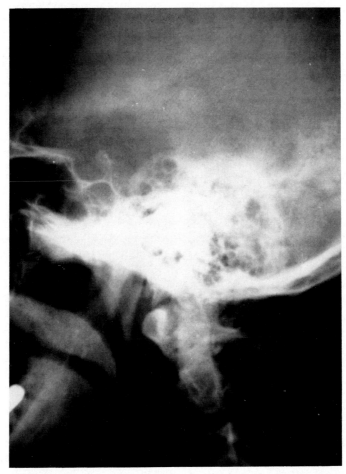

Figure 11.6. Lateral radiograph reveals an increased atlantodental interval in a patient suffering from rheumatoid arthritis.

ligament damage and subsequent subluxation, the spine of a patient with rheumatoid arthritis who has had an automobile accident should be viewed with suspicion until structural integrity is established by flexion and extension films.

BIOMECHANICAL LESIONS

Various biomechanical lesions may affect the severity of the injury. Congenital lesions such as a block vertebra may alter the motion of the cervical unit during the injury. The absence of motion may also have stressed the intervertebral disc above and below the block, resulting in an increased susceptibility to disc herniations or spur formation (23, 24).

Congenital fusion of multiple cervical levels, such as in the Klippel-Feil syndrome (Fig. 11.7), reduces the available motion of

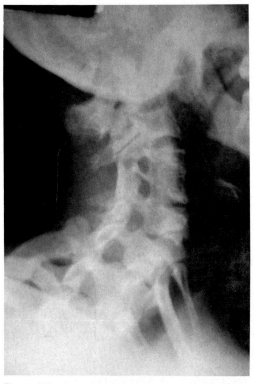

Figure 11.7. Lateral radiograph of the cervical spine allows visualization of the nonsegmentation of C1-C2 and C4-C5. Congenital fusion of both the anterior and posterior segments is noted at the C4-C5 level. This patient has Klippel-Feil syndrome.

the cervical segments and usually presents as a significant stenosis of the spinal canal (35). The fusion may take place in the anterior or posterior elements (36, 37). This change, along with the stenosis, is most commonly seen at C2-C3 (36, 37). Minor trauma may cause high-level cord symptoms or even quadriparesis (35).

Prognosis Scale

NEED FOR ACCURATE PROGNOSTIC SYSTEM IN MEDICAL-LEGAL ARENA

Most cases of cervical acceleration/deceleration syndrome today have two things in common: automobiles and attorneys. The case often involves the carrier (and attorney) for the patient's group insurance policy, the carrier (and attorney) for the medical portion of the patient's automobile insurance policy, and the carrier (and attorney) for the other person's policy. Each of these requires timely information concerning the extent of the patient's injury in order to allocate the appropriate funds.

The system is adversarial; it often requires opposing opinions regarding the patient's injury and, more importantly, the problems it may cause in the future. Unfortunately, the party with the best narrative report often "wins."

One of the biggest problems faced by the physician, the patient, and the attorney is the length of time that passes before the patient is released from treatment. The lack of an accepted system for establishing an accurate prognosis often results in prolonging the treatment period for months in an attempt to relieve symptoms that will probably never be resolved. This has allowed some practitioners to abuse the system and has caused the industry to view most whiplash injuries with suspicion.

The "abusive" case is usually only recognized at the end of the patient's treatment. The attorney is then faced with the monumental task of attempting to settle a case that is burdened with unreasonable medical charges. When physicians are unable to recognize symptoms that will not resolve due to the patient's injury, the following problems result:

1. Excessive medical charges accumulate in an attempt to relieve those symptoms that will not resolve.
2. Attorneys request large monetary settlements in an attempt to pay medical charges. Generally, there is a lack of objective data to prove the patient's injury.
3. Insurance carriers deny payment and force the claim to litigation.

The need for an accurate prognostic scale has been evident for years, and a numerical scale has been developed that allows the physician to render a prognosis on the day the injury occurs. The advantages of using such a scale include the following:

1. The physican can predict, with some accuracy, the approximate length of treatment and the probability of future problems.
2. The attorney can monitor the patient's progress, knowing in advance the approximate degree of probable improvement.
3. The insurance carrier can establish accurate settlement reserves and decrease the number of litigated cases.
4. The patient can better understand what future problems may result from the injury.

CLASSIFICATION SYSTEM OF FOREMAN AND CROFT

The exact degree of injury and the probability of future pain in patients who have suffered cervical acceleration/decleration injuries are often difficult to ascertain. It may take years for the physician to acquire the sufficient clinical experience needed to render an accurate prognosis. Foreman and Croft have developed a numerical scale with which to classify whiplash injuries objectively. The findings on physical examination provide the information needed for the patient's initial classification into a major injury category (MIC). The radiographic examination and a patient questionnaire provide the data from which are obtained the clinical modifiers to this system.

Categories

MIC 1.   MIC 1 is used for patients who present with symptoms directly relating to their injury. On physical examination, however, there are no objective findings to the patient's complaint(s).

MIC 2.   Patients who present with a decreased range of motion of the cervical spine in addition to MIC 1 symptoms are placed in MIC 2. A measurable increase in cervical diameter may also be expected. MIC 2 patients do not present with neurological signs.

MIC 3.   MIC 3 patients present with MIC 1 and MIC 2 symptoms plus objective neurological loss (either sensory or motor).

Norris and Watt (21) classified a series of 61 patients according to this system and found a significant relationship between the category and the presence of residual pain. Fifty-six percent of patients in MIC 1, 81% in MIC 2, and 90% in MIC 3 suffered residual pain. Typically, the symptoms that remained were neck pain, headache, and paresthesias.

Each patient, after the physical examination, should be classified into the appropriate MIC group. Each group is self-explanatory, and each is discussed below in relation to point values.

The work done by Norris and Watt (21) demonstrated the efficacy of this system of classification, but they did not address a multitude of individual "modifiers" that might affect the prognosis. Patients differ anatomically and in the amount of degenerative changes that may be present. Each of these factors should be considered when determining the patient's final prognosis.

Modifiers to Prognosis

A wide variety of problems can influence the patient's recovery. Some significant variations were studied and were found to be valuable in the evaluation of the patient (19, 21). Those found to be the most significant modifiers to prognosis are considered next.

Canal Size of 10–12 mm.   The narrow spinal canal has been found to be associated with a higher incidence of neurological damage (9, 10). An absolute stenosis (15) of 10 mm magnifies the effects of minor trauma and subjects the patient to neurological deficits when posttraumatic degeneration occurs.

This modifier has been given the largest value because of its potential for causing cord pressure. In combination with degenerative changes, it can produce neurological symptoms that are reversible only with surgery.

Canal Size of 13–15 mm.   Relative stenosis (15) will have many of the same effects as absolute stenosis. There is slightly more space within the canal, but the prognosis still includes the possibility of future neurological deficit.

Straight Cervical Spine.   The loss of the normal lordotic curve may be caused by either muscle spasm, ligamentous damage, or both (Fig. 11.8). The weight of the head usually rests primarily on the articular facets rather than on the vertebral bodies. The loss of the normal curve causes an uneven distribution of weight within the cervical area. The loss of the curve has been

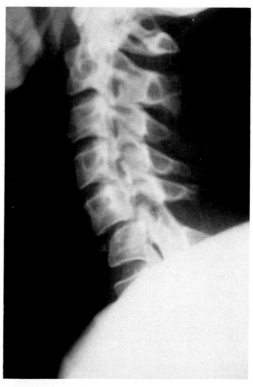

Figure 11.9.   Acute kyphosis of the cervical spine at C5-C6 is demonstrated. This change is secondary to tearing of the interspinous ligament between C5 and C6.

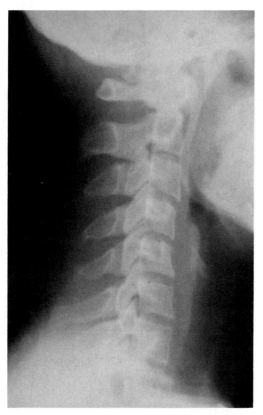

Figure 11.8.   Lateral cervical spine view demonstrates a loss of the normal cervical curve after a "whiplash" injury.

found in patients who experienced residual pain and stiffness on final examination (21).

Kyphotic Cervical Curve.   A sharp reversal or kyphotic curve is typically seen in association with posterior ligament damage (Fig. 11.9). There is a significantly higher incidence of degenerative changes in patients who have a kyphotic curve.

Care should be exercised when a kyphotic curve is being evaluated during the initial examination. Further angulation deformity can be expected if the posterior ligaments are totally disrupted. Disruption of these ligaments causes the most unstable type of cervical spine injury (25, 38, 39).

Fixated Segments.   Fixated segments, whether congenital, as in Klippel-Feil syndrome, or caused by surgical or degenerative changes (Fig. 11.10), may exacerbate the patient's injury. Chronic changes include increased spur formation at the levels above and below the fixation (25).

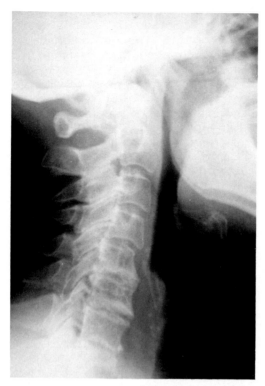

Figure 11.10. Fixation of the lower cervical spine at C5–C7 is demonstrated. Intervertebral osteochondrosis has effectively fused the area.

Hohl, in his study (19), found that those with fixated segments at one level had a poorer clinical recovery and a significantly higher incidence of degenerative changes. Sixty-three percent of those with fixations developed degenerative changes.

Preexisting Degenerative Changes. Degenerative changes, as previously discussed, may enhance the effects of the injury, due to the arthropathy of the joints and the ligamentous laxity associated with the conditions. Preexisting degenerative changes, "no matter how slight," adversely affect the prognosis (21) (Fig. 11.11).

Loss of Consciousness. A patient who strikes his or her head during the accident may lose consciousness for a brief period of time. The impact to the head is, essentially, a second, separate accident. Therefore, the structures of the cervical spine are subjected to a second trauma and have almost twice the amount of posttraumatic degeneration. Hohl (19) studied, as a subgroup, those patients who had lost con-

sciousness during the accident; he found that 64% experienced degenerative changes within the study period.

Point Values Assigned by Category

The patient who has suffered a cervical acceleration/deceleration injury should be evaluated and placed in one of the MIC groups. Each MIC group has been assigned a numerical point value.

MIC 1. MIC 1 has been assigned a value of 10 points, since there are no objective findings to verify the patient's symptoms. Some modifiers have been assigned a higher point value than that for MCI 1, but the significance of these modifiers is dependent on the initial injury.

MIC 2. MIC 2 has been assigned a value of 50 points. The loss of motion in patients in this group represents objective evidence of injury.

MIC 3. MIC 3, with its neurological deficits, has been assigned the highest point value of 90.

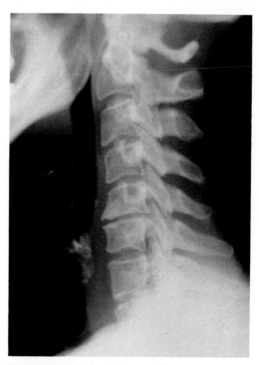

Figure 11.11. Lateral view of the cervical spine demonstrates a loss of the cervical curve and early degenerative changes at C5–C6.

Point Values Assigned by Modifier

After the physical examination and categorization of the patient, the physician should evaluate the radiographs and patient history for the presence of modifiers. Modifiers are cumulative; i.e., their value may be added together. The cumulative points from these factors are added to the points from the patient's assigned MIC group.

Modifiers	Point Value
Canal size of 10–12 mm	20
Canal Size of 13–15 mm	15
Kyphotic curve	15
Fixated segment of flexion and extension films	15
Loss of consciousness	15
Straight cervical curve	10
Preexisting degeneration	10

Interpretation

Based on his or her point total, the patient is placed in one of five categories. Although the point total determines the patient's initial prognosis, the factors outlined are subject to modification during the course of treatment.

Prognosis Group 1 (10–30 Points). Prognosis group 1 is composed of MIC 1 patients who may have one major (highpoint) or two minor (low-point) modifiers. The prognosis for patients in this group is excellent because patients have no objective findings and few modifiers. The residual problems, if any, are typically occasional, mild muscle pain and/or occipital headaches.

Prognosis Group 2 (35–70 Points). Prognosis group 2 is composed of either MIC 1 or MIC 2 patients. The MIC 1 patients in this group have more modifiers than do patients in prognosis group 1. Some modifiers may have been preexisting, but they still have a bearing on the future outcome of the case. The increased number of modifiers places the patient in a higher risk position.

The MIC 2 patients in this group may have fewer modifiers but are classified in prognosis group 2 because they sustained a higher level of injury. The prognosis for patients in this group is generally good, and future neurological deficits are unlikely. Residual symptoms, consisting of occasional to intermittent, moderate neck pain may be expected. Residual objective findings, such as restricted cervical motion, may be expected in some of the patients in this group.

Prognosis Group 3 (75-100 Points). Prognosis group 3 is primarily composed of MIC 2 patients who have several modifiers. The remainder of the group is composed of MIC 3 patients.

The prognosis for patients in this group is poor, and a number of these patients develop neurological deficits. Because the MIC 3 patients in this group have few modifiers, most of their initial neurological deficits may resolve.

Residual symptoms in this group, as well as in prognosis groups 1 and 2, include areas of numbness or, on rare occasions, muscle weakness.

Prognosis Group 4 (105–125 Points). Prognosis group 4 is composed of MIC 2 patients who have many modifiers and MIC 3 patients who have few modifiers. The probability of future or persistent neurological deficits is likely, so prognosis for patients in this group is guarded.

Neurological damage may cause symptoms such as significantly decreased grip strength, muscle atrophy, radiculitis, and myelopathy. There is a fair probability that surgical intervention will be necessary in the future.

Prognosis Group 5 (130–165 Points). Prognosis group 5 is composed of patients whose prognosis might best be termed "unstable." This is not to be confused with an unstable fracture; rather, it represents the patient's unstable clinical picture.

Patients in this group have suffered neurological deficits and have most of the modifiers in the scale. Their clinical picture is not likely to improve much, and future surgical intervention will probably be necessary. Radiculopathy and myelopathy are the primary complications.

CASE STUDIES

Example 1

ARW presented with posttraumatic changes after his car had been hit from behind a few hours previously. Physical examination revealed pain upon palpation of the anterior cervical muscles. Range of motion was restricted on extension and within normal limits in all other directions.

Radiographic examination revealed a straightening of the cervical curve. There were no other radiographic abnormalities. The patient's history was unremarkable. No periods of unconsciousness were reported.

Rating. Physical examination revealed soft tissue changes and a restriction of cervical motion. These findings place the patient in MIC 2, with 50 points.

Radiographic examination revealed the presence of one modifier—a straight cervical curve (10 points).

With a combined total of 60 points, ARW should be placed in prognosis group 2. A good prognosis is indicated.

Example 2

JBS, an elderly gentleman, was involved in an accident in which his car was struck from behind. The impact forced his car into the vehicle directly ahead of him. Physical examinations revealed cervical muscle swelling, decreased motion on flexion and extension, and weakness of the right deltoid muscle.

Radiographic examination revealed a kyphotic curve, degeneration of the disc at C4-C5, C5-C6, and C6-C7, and a spinal cord that measured 14 mm. The spinal cord measurements were the result of spondylotic changes.

Rating. Physical examination revealed a neurological deficit, placing the patient in MIC 3, with 90 points.

Radiographic examination revealed the presence of the following modifiers: preexisting degeneration (10 points), narrowed canal (15 points), and a kyphotic curve (15 points), for a total of 40 points.

With a combined total of 130 points, JBS should be placed in prognosis group 5; he presents an unstable clinical picture. His degenerative changes may continue to progress, and he could need surgical intervention at a later time.

DISCUSSION

In their clinical experience, Foreman and Croft have found the prognosis scale to be valuable in dealing with both insurance carriers and attorneys. Predictions based on the scale have been quite accurate despite the variability in healing rates and other factors not considered in the scale. (Other factors that affect a person's prognosis have been identified but were not consistent enough to be included in the scale). Foreman and Croft believe that the scale is of great value and will allow an accurate prognosis despite variations in patients and treatment responses.

Summary

1. All patients may be categorized into MIC 1, 2, or 3 according to their presenting symptomatic and radiographic picture. These groups are known to correlate with levels of residual pain.

2. Other factors, such as degenerative changes, loss of cervical curve, and loss of consciousness, have been identified as being significant modifiers to the long-term prognosis.

3. The combination of the MIC groups and the individual modifiers may be utilized to determine the long-term prognosis of the patient.

4. Proper utilization of the prognosis scale will allow the treating physician to prepare the medical documentation needed at the end of the case, while at the same time rendering proper care to the patient.

5. Use of the prognosis scale will encourage a proper workup of the case to deal with later legal concerns.

References

1. La Rocca II: Acceleration injuries of the neck. *Clin Neurosurg* 25:209–217, 1978.
2. Gay JR, Abott KH: Common whiplash injuries of the neck. *JAMA* 152:1698–1704, 1953.
3. Gotten N: Survey of one hundred cases of whiplash injury after settlement of litigation. *JAMA* 162:865–867, 1956.
4. Macnab I: Acceleration injuries of the cervical spine. *J Bone Surg* 46A:1797–1799, 1964.
5. Macnab I: The whiplash syndrome. *Orthop Clin North Am* 2:399–403, 1971.
6. Severy DM, Mathewson JH, Bechtol CO: Controlled automobile rear-ended collisions; an investigation of related engineering and medical phenomena. *Can Service Med J* 11:727–759, 1955.
7. Wickstrom JK, Martinez JL, Rodriquez R, Haines DA: Hyperextension and hyperflexion injuries to the head and neck of primates. In Gurdjian ES, Thomas LM (eds): *Neck and Backache.* Springfield, IL, Charles C Thomas, 1970.
8. Brain WR, Northfield D, Wilkinson M: The neurological manifestations of cervical spondylosis. *Brain* 75:187–225, 1952.
9. Payne EE, Spillane JD: The cervical spine—an anatomical-radiological study of 70 specimens (using a special technique) with particular reference to the problem of cervical spondylosis. *Brain* 80:571–596, 1957.
10. Wolf BS, Khilnani M, Malis L: The sagittal diameter of the cervical spinal canal and its significance in cervical spondylosis. *J Mt Sinai Hosp* 23:283–292, 1956.
11. Porter RW, Hibbert CS, Wicks M: The spinal canal in symptomatic lumbar disc lesions. *J Bone Joint Surg* 60B:485–487 1973.
12. Verbiest H: A radicular syndrome from developmental narrowing of the lumbar vertebral canal. *J Bone Joint Surg* 36B:230–338, 1954.
13. Verbiest H: Further experiences on the pathological stenosis and developmental narrowness of the bony vertebral canal. *J Bone Joint Surg* 37B:576–583, 1955.
14. Eismont FJ, Clifford S, Goldberg M, Green B: Cervical sagittal spinal canal size in spine injury. *Spine* 9:663–666, 1984.
15. Verbiest H: Neurogenic intermittent claudication in cases with absolute and relative stenosis of the lumbar vertebral canal (ASLS and RSLC) in cases with narrow lumbar intervertebral foramina and in cases with both entities. *Clin Neurosurg* 20:204–214, 1972.
16. Selecki BR, Williams HBL: Injuries to the cervical spine and cord in man. In: *Australian Medical Association Mervyn Archdale Medical Monograph No. 7.* South Wales, Australian Medical Publishing, 1970.
17. Foreman S: Radiographic differential diagnosis of common degenerative spinal disorders. *J Manipulative Physiol Ther* 8(1):23–27, 1985.
18. Ehni G: *Cervical Arthrosis.* Chicago, Year Book, 1984, p 18.
19. Hohl M: Soft-tissue injuries of the neck in automobile accidents. *J Bone Joint Surg* 56A:1675 – 1682, 1974.
20. Freidenberg ZB, Miller WT: Degenerative disc disease of the cervical spine: a comparative study of asymptomatic and symptomatic patients. *J Bone Joint Surg* 45A:1171–1178, 1963.
21. Norris SH, Watt I: The prognosis of neck injuries resulting from rear-end vehicle collisions. *J Bone Joint Surg* 65B:608–611, 1983.
22. Epstein JA, Carras R, Epstein BS, Lavine LS: The importance of removing osteophytes as part of the surgical treatment of myeloradiculopathy in cervical spondylosis. *J Neurosurg* 30:219–226, 1969.
23. Holt S, Yates PO: Cervical spondylosis and nerve root lesions. *J Bone Joint Surg* 48B:407–423, 1966.
24. Scoville WB: Cervical spondylosis treated by bilateral facetectomy and laminectomy. *J Neurosurg* 18:423–428, 1961.
25. Woesner ME, Mitts MG: The evaluation of cervical spine motion below C2; a comparison of cineroentgenographic and conventional roentgenographic methods. *Am J Roentgenol Radium Ther Nucl Med* 115:148–154, 1972.
26. Foreman S: Nerve root ischemia and pain secondary to spinal stenosis syndrome: technical and clinical considerations *J Manipulative Physiol Ther* 8(2):81–85, 1985.
27. Grisolia A, Bell R, Peltier L: Fractures and dislocations of the spine complicating ankylosing spondylitis. *J Bone Joint Surg* 49A:339–345, 1967.
28. Bland JH, Davis PH, London MG, Van Buskirk FW, Duarte CG: Rheumatoid arthritis of the cervical spine. *Arch Intern Med* 112:892–893, 1963.
29. Bland JH: *Program Interim Meeting.* Pittsburgh, America Rheumatology Association, 1972, December.
30. Bland JH, Brown EW: Seronegative and seropositive rheumatoid arthritis, clinical, radiological and biochemical differences. *Ann Intern Med* 70:88, 1964.
31. Bland JH: Rheumatoid arthritis of the cervical spine. *J Rheumatol* 1(3):319–342, 1974.
32. Sharp J, Purser DW: Spontaneous atlantoaxial dislocation in ankylosing spondylitis and rheumatoid arthritis. *Ann Rheum Dis* 20:47–77, 1961.
33. Gleason IO, Urist MR: Atlanto-axial dislocation with odontoid separation in rheumatoid disease. *Clin Orthop* 42:121–129, 1965.
34. Pratt TL: Spontaneous dislocation of the atlanto-axial articulation occurring in ankylosing spondylitis and rheumatoid arthritis. *J Faculty Radiol (Lond)* 10:40–43, 1959.
35. Epstein N, Epstein J, Zilkha A: Traumatic myelopathy in a seventeen-year old child with cervical spinal stenosis (without fracture or dislocation with a C2-C3 Klippel-Feil Fusion. *Spine* 9:344–347, 1984.
36. Baird PA, Robinson CG, Buckler WJ: Klippel-Feil syndrome, a study of mirror movement detected by electromyography. *Am J Dis Child* 113:546–551, 1967.
37. Gray SW, Romine CB, Skandalakis JE: Collective reviews, central fusion of the cervical vertebrae: *Surg Obstet Gynecol* 118:373, 1964.
38. Scher AT: Anterior cervical subluxation: an unstable position. *AJR* 133:275–280, 1979.
39. Cheshire DJE: The stability of the cervical spine following conservative treatment of fractures and dislocations. *Int J Paraplegia* 7:193–203, 1970.

Glossary

ADI Atlantodental interval, the space between the posterior aspect of the anterior arch of the atlas and the anterior surface of the odontoid process.

Anisotropy Unequal responses to external stimuli.

Antalgic Pain relieving; usually refers to the position used by a patient to relieve pain in the affected area.

AP open mouth Anteroposterior open mouth; an x-ray view.

APLC Anterior-posterior lower cervical; an x-ray view.

Arthropathy Disease of a joint.

Axonotmesis Wallerian degeneration of the transport and fibrous tubules, resulting from a severe crushing injury.

Brown-Séquard syndrome Condition caused by damage to one half of the spinal cord, resulting in ipsilateral paralysis and loss of discriminatory and joint sensation and in contralateral loss of pain and temperature sensation.

Bruxism Rhythmic or spasmodic grinding of the teeth.

Café au lait Having the color of coffee with cream.

Clonus Muscular contraction and relaxation alternating in a rapid succession.

Coupling Consistent association of one motion about an axis with another motion about another axis.

Crepitus Grating noise caused by the rubbing together of abnormal synovial surfaces.

Davis series Seven-view x-ray series of the cervical spine, including lateral, flexion, extension, APLC, AP open mouth, and oblique views.

Dementia General term used for mental deterioration.

Dermatome Area of skin supplied with afferent nerve fibers by a single posterior spinal root; also termed dermatomic area.

Diplopia Perception of two images from a single object.

DISH Diffuse idiopathic skeletal hyperostosis.

Dysmetria Disturbance of the power to control the range of movement in muscular action.

Dysphagia Difficulty in swallowing.

Eminentia Eminence, a raised area.

G Force of gravity applied to an object at rest.

Gantry Portion of the computed tomography machine in which the patient is positioned and which contains the x-ray tube.

George's line Line drawn along the posterior borders of vertebral bodies on the x-ray used to assess normal alignment.

Gliosis Condition characterized by an excess of astroglia in damaged areas of the central nervous system.

Goniometric   Measured by a goniometer, an instrument designed to measure angles, usually the arc and range of motion of joints in the spine or extremities.

Hangman's fracture   Bilateral pedicle fracture of the axis.

Horner's syndrome   Condition characterized by sinking in of the eyeball, ptosis of the upper eyelid, slight elevation of the lower lid, constriction of the pupil, narrowing of the palpebral fissure, and anhidrosis.

Hypalgesia   Diminished sensitivity to pain.

Hyperpathia   Abnormally exaggerated subjective response to painful stimuli.

Hypochondriasis   Having an abnormal anxiety about one's health.

Hysteresis   Phenomenon associated with energy loss exhibited by viscoelastic materials when they are subjected to loading and unloading cycles.

Idiopathic   Of unknown cause.

Ischemia   Deficiency of blood in a part.

Jefferson fracture   "Burst" fracture of the neural ring of the atlas.

Klippel-Feil syndrome   Condition characterized by shortness of the neck and resulting from reduction in the number of cervical vertebrae or the fusion of multiple hemivertebrae into one osseous mass; the hairline is low and the motion of neck is limited in a person with this syndrome.

Laminectomy   Surgical removal of the lamina, done to relieve the pressure on the neural contents within the canal.

Lucent cleft   Small, radiolucent shadow on the anterior corner of the lower cervical vertebrae, caused by gas accumulating around torn Sharpey's fibers.

Mediastinitis   Infection of the central cavity in the chest, which contains the heart and great vessels.

Moment   Quantity equal to the product of one of the forces and the perpendicular distance between the forces.

MPD   Myofascial pain dysfunction.

Neuropraxia   Mild form of neuronal compression; recovery usually occurs in 3–6 weeks.

Neurotmesis   Complete disruption of a nerve.

NRC   Nerve root canal.

Nystagmus   Rapid, involuntary movement of the eyeball.

OPLL   Ossification of the posterior longitudinal ligament.

Orthogonal   At right angles.

Orthosis   Orthopaedic appliance used to support or align movable parts of the body.

Os odontoideum   Lack of ossification of the dens to the body of the axis.

Ossiculum terminale   Persistence of the secondary ossification center at the cephalic end of the odontoid process.

Pancoast tumor   Neoplasm, located in the apex of the lung, that often destroys the surrounding bone and invades the brachial plexus.

Pillar view   Radiographic position that depicts the height of the articular pillars of the cervical spine.

Pitch   Motion that, when applied to the cervical spine, equates to right and left lateral flexion.

Pseudoarthrosis   False joint; usually associated with the non-union of a fracture.

Pulse sequence   Series of controlled radiofrequency signal transmissions in a magnetic resonance imaging unit.

Radiculitis   Inflammation of the root of a spinal nerve.

Radiculopathy   Disease of the nerve root.

Roll   Motion that, when applied to the cervical spine, equates to right and left lateral flexion.

Romberg's test   Test used to assess the function of the posterior column of the spinal cord.

Scintigraphy   Two-dimensional representation (map) of the γ-rays emitted by a radioisotope, revealing its varying concentration in bone.

Scotoma   Area of depressed vision within the visual field.

Sheer   Intensity of force parallel to the surface on which it acts.

Status spongiosus   Condition characterized by formation of extensive vacuoles or fluid-filled spaces within the neural structure.

Stiffness   Resistance to external loads.

Stress   Force per unit area of a structure and a measurement of the intensity of the force.

Synchondrosis   Type of cartilage joint that is usually temporary.

Syrinx   Abnormal cavity filled with fluid in the substance of the spinal cord.

T1-weighted image   Magnetic resonance image with an echo time less than 30 msec.

T2-weighted image   Magnetic resonance image with an echo time longer than 60 msec.

TE   Echo time; the point in the pulse sequence cycle when the magnetic resonance imaging unit is receiving radiofrequencies from the patient.

Tenoperiostitis   Inflammation of the periosteum of bone at the tendinous attachment.

Tension   Stress on a material, produced by the pull of forces.

Tetraplegia   Paralysis of all four extremities.

Tinnitus   Abnormal sounds within the ear.

TMJ   Temporomandibular joint.

Torque   Force that acts to produce rotation

Torsion   Stress produced in a body by turning one end along a longitudinal axis while the other end is fixed or stationary.

TR   Repetition time; the length of time the patient is exposed to radiofrequencies in a magnetic resonance imaging unit.

Trismus   Limitation of opening.

Vacuum phenomenon   Accumulation of nitrogen within a degenerated intervertebral disc, demonstrated by radiography.

Westphal's sign   Loss of the knee jerk reflex.

Yaw   Motion that, when applied to the cervical spine, equates to right and left rotation.

Index

Page numbers in *italics* denote figures; those followed by "t" denote tables.